Primary Care: An Evidence-Based Approach

Primary Care: An Evidence-Based Approach

Edited by Esther Sinclair

hayle medical

New York

Hayle Medical,
750 Third Avenue, 9th Floor,
New York, NY 10017, USA

Visit us on the World Wide Web at:
www.haylemedical.com

ISBN: 978-1-64647-105-8

Cataloging-in-Publication Data

Primary care : an evidence-based approach / edited by Esther Sinclair.
p. cm.
Includes bibliographical references and index.
ISBN: 978-1-64647-105-8
1. Primary care (Medicine). 2. Primary health care. 3. Medical care.
4. Evidence-based medicine. I. Sinclair, Esther.

RA427.9 .P75 2022

610--dc23

Table of Contents

Preface

Primary care is the day to day healthcare that is given to the patient. It involves the broad scope of healthcare that is concerned with patients of all ages, of all socioeconomic and geographic origins and patients seeking to maintain optimal health. It also involves patients with acute and chronic physical, mental and social health issues such as multiple chronic diseases. Hypertension, depression, diabetes, asthma, COPD, anxiety, etc. are some examples of common chronic illnesses usually treated in primary care. Many basic maternal and child health care services also fall under this domain such as family planning services and vaccinations. Primary care results in better health outcomes, reduced health disparities and lower spending. This book unravels the recent studies in the field of primary care. The aim of this book is to present researches that have transformed this discipline and aided its advancement. This book will serve as a reference to a broad spectrum of readers.

This book is a comprehensive compilation of works of different researchers from varied parts of the world. It includes valuable experiences of the researchers with the sole objective of providing the readers (learners) with a proper knowledge of the concerned field. This book will be beneficial in evoking inspiration and enhancing the knowledge of the interested readers.

In the end, I would like to extend my heartiest thanks to the authors who worked with great determination on their chapters. I also appreciate the publisher's support in the course of the book. I would also like to deeply acknowledge my family who stood by me as a source of inspiration during the project.

Editor

1

Microbiological point of care testing before antibiotic prescribing in primary care: considerable variations between practices

Steffen Haldrup[1,2*], Reimar W. Thomsen[1], Flemming Bro[2], Robert Skov[3], Lars Bjerrum[4] and Mette Søgaard[1*]

Abstract

Background: Point-of-care testing (POCT) in primary care may improve rational antibiotic prescribing. We examined use of POCT in Denmark, including patient- and general practitioner (GP)-related predictors.

Methods: We linked nationwide health care databases to assess POCT use (C-reactive protein (CRP), group A streptococcal (GAS) antigen swabs, bacteriological cultures, and urine test strips) per 1,000 overall GP consultations, 2004–2013. We computed odds ratios (OR) of POCT in patients prescribed antibiotics according to patient and GP age and sex, GP practice type, location, and workload.

Results: The overall use of POCT in Denmark increased by 45.8% during 2004–2013, from 147.2 per 1,000 overall consultations to 214.8. CRP tests increased by 132%, bacteriological cultures by 101.7% while GAS swabs decreased by 8.6%. POCT preceded 28% of antibiotic prescriptions in 2004 increasing to 44% in 2013. The use of POCT varied more than 5-fold among individual practices, from 54.9 to 394.7 per 1,000 consultations in 2013. POCT use varied substantially with patient age, and males were less likely to receive POCT than females (adjusted OR = 0.75, 95% CI 0.74-0.75) driven by usage of urine test strips among females (18% vs. 7%). Odds of POCT were higher among female GPs and decreased with higher GP age, with lowest usage among male GPs >60 years. GP urban/rural location and workload had little impact.

Conclusion: GPs use POCT increasingly with the highest use among young female GPs. In 2013, 44% of all antibiotic prescriptions were preceded by POCT but testing rates vary greatly across individual GPs.

Keywords: Point-of-care, Antibiotic, Infection, General practice

Background

As much as 50% of antibiotic use in human medicine may be either unnecessary or inappropriate across all health care settings [1–3]. For instance, acute bronchitis accounts for approximately 80% of lower respiratory tract infections and despite guidelines, randomized controlled trials, and meta-analyses showing little or no benefit from antibiotics [4, 5], up to 80% of patients consulting for this condition are prescribed antibiotics [6–9].

In Denmark, general practitioners (GPs) account for more than 80% of the total antibiotic use [10]. To reduce ineffective and unnecessary antibiotics the Danish National Board of Health in 2012 issued a guideline that encourages rational antibiotic prescribing (i.e., use of narrow spectrum antibiotics), and to only prescribe antibiotics when necessary based on clinical and microbiological examination [11]. Diagnostic uncertainty increases the risk of unnecessary antibiotic prescribing [6, 12], and a key to rational prescribing is to perform point-of-care testing (POCT) [13]. POCT is defined as medical diagnostic testing at or near the site of care [14], and use of POCT such as enzyme immunoassay kits (e.g., group A streptococcal (GAS) antigen), measurement of C-reactive protein (CRP), urine test strips and bacteriological cultures may reduce diagnostic uncertainty [15–17] and thereby antibiotic prescribing [17–23]. Thus, POCT may contribute to safely withholding antibiotics

* Correspondence: steffenhaldrup@au.dk; mette.soegaard@rn.dk
[1]Department of Clinical Epidemiology, Aarhus University, Olof Palmes Alle 43-45, 8200 Aarhus N, Denmark
Full list of author information is available at the end of the article

from patients who most probably would not benefit from antibiotic treatment. Nonetheless, while there is a large body of literature on prescribing patterns among GPs, few studies have examined the use of POCT in relation to antibiotic prescribing [16, 23, 24]. Studies from Sweden and Switzerland have shown that approximately 42% of patients consulting a GP for an acute respiratory tract infection receive a CRP-test [16, 25]. Older patients, those with higher education, and those with more discomfort are more likely to receive testing [16]. Another study showed that physicians were less likely to perform streptococcal tests in children with pharyngitis at the end of the week (Thursday and Friday) (adjusted relative risk 0.75, 95% confidence interval (CI) 0.66-0.87) compared with the first days of the week [26]. In line with this, a US study showed that streptococcal testing rates varied from 59% to 83% among different health plans for children with pharyngitis who were prescribed antibiotics [27]. Still, there is limited population-based information on the prevalence and time trends of use of POCT before antibiotic prescribing in primary care and about what characterizes patients and GPs who use POCT. Information on predictors of POCT may help to identify interventions to improve the efficient use of antibiotics. We therefore undertook a nationwide population-based study to examine the use of POCT in relation to antibiotic prescribing in the Danish primary health care sector in 2004–2013, and investigated patient and GP-related predictors for use of POCT.

Methods

Setting and study population

This population-based cross-sectional study was based on the entire Danish population with approximately 5,5 million residents between 2004 and 2013. The Danish healthcare system provides tax-supported health care to all residents, guaranteeing free access to hospitals, primary medical care, and partial reimbursement for prescribed medications, including most antibiotics. A unique central personal registration number, assigned to all Danish residents at birth or upon immigration, is used to record health care services in various nationwide registries, allowing unambiguous linkage among registries [28]. The current nationwide study is based on information from the Danish National Health Insurance Service Registry (DNHSR) [29], the Danish National Health Service Prescription Database (DHSPD) [30], and data provided by Danish Regions (www.regioner.dk).

POCT and antibiotic prescriptions

We obtained information on POCT and number of GP consultations through the DNHSR. Except for 2% of the population, all Danes are enlisted with a particular general practice of their choice and all services provided to this population are recorded through activity codes in the DNHSR which contains data collected from health contractors in primary care since 1990 [29]. The DNHSR include information about patients (e.g., civil registration (CRS) number, date of entering present general practice, present and previous general practice number), the general practices (including a unique practice identification number which we used to ascertain that only GPs were included, and practice type (single-handed vs. partnership)), and health services (type of consultation (ordinary, telephone, home visit, or email) and any laboratory tests performed (including CRP measurement, GAS antigen throat swabs, bacteriological cultures, urine test strips and microscopy). Each laboratory test has a unique four-digit code and is a health service for which the GP is compensated. We utilized these four digit codes, along with the six digit practice identification number, to identify all POCT performed by GPs between 2004 and 2013.

We then obtained information on all filled antibiotic prescriptions in Denmark during 2004–2013 through the DHSPD [30]. This database records the patients' personal identifier, date of dispensing, and the type and quantity of drug prescribed (according to the Anatomical Therapeutic Chemical (ATC) Classification System) each time a prescription is redeemed at any Danish pharmacy. For all antibiotic prescriptions, we ascertained whether the patients had POCT performed within the preceding 14 days of filling the antibiotic prescription.

Patient characteristics

We categorized patients according to sex, age (0–4, 5–9, 10–14, 15–19, 20–39, 40–64, 65–79, and ≥80 years), and prescribed antibiotics categorized as; tetracycline (J01AA), beta-lactamase sensitive penicillin (J01CE), penicillin with extended spectrum (J01CA), beta-lactamase resistant penicillin (J01CF), combinations of penicillin incl. beta-lactamase inhibitors (J01CR), sulphonamide and trimethoprim (J01E), macrolide, lincosamide and streptogamin (J01F), quinolone (J01MA), and other antibiotics (J01D, G, X).

GP characteristics

Through the DNHSR, we obtained data on the GP's annual number of ordinary consultations per 1,000 registered patients as proxy for GP workload (categorized in quintiles as <5675, 5675–6354, 6355–7189, >7190) [31], type of practice (single-handed versus partnership practice), and geographical location of practice (health care administrative region, city size (<5000 inhabitants or ≥5000 inhabitants). For single-handed practices we further obtained information about the GP's age (<41, 41–50, 51–60, and ≥60 years) and sex from Danish Regions. This information was not available for partnership practices because the six-digit practice identifier is applied to the practice and not the individual GP. We restricted the study to GPs with at least 500 registered patients to reduce the impact by inactive GPs on the observed variation.

Statistical analysis

We computed the annual prevalence of use of any POCT and of specific tests per 1,000 overall consultations in general practice, and estimated the prevalence proportion of antibiotic prescriptions preceded by POCT. We truncated the data at the 1st and 99th percentiles due to ambiguous rates (outliers). To compare the rates in different years and across different GPs, we standardized the rates to the age- and sex distribution of the population of Denmark as of January 1 2013 (obtained from statistics Denmark), using direct standardization. Subsequently, we used logistic regression to compute crude and adjusted odds ratios (OR) with 95% CIs for use of POCT prior to antibiotic prescribing according to patient age and sex, practice location (geographical region and city size) as well as the GP's age, sex and workload. The predictors were mutually adjusted. As the prevalence of pre-antibiotic POCT changed over time, we restricted analyses of predictors to 2013 in order to describe predictors of POCT in the most recent year. Analyses of the impact of GP age and sex were restricted to single-handed practices as this information was not available for partnership-practices. Data management and statistical analysis was conducted in SAS version 9.2/9.4 (SAS Institute, Cary, NC) and STATA 14 (Stata Corp., College Station, TX, USA).

Results

From 2004 to 2013, 27,267,874 antibiotic prescriptions were registered in the DHSPD. Of these, we excluded 5,496,924 prescriptions issued by other authorities than GPs in the primary health care, for instance doctors from the emergency service and specialists, and 1,608,012 prescriptions due to incomplete data, e.g., missing information about the issuing GP. Thus, the study included 20,162,938 antibiotic prescriptions issued by 2,021 practices to 4,434,916 patients. A total of 1,051 (52%) of the GPs worked in single-handed practices, and 970 (48%) constituted partnership practices. The usage of POCT before antibiotic prescribing amounted to 7,344,586 tests.

Use of POCT according to type of prescribed antibiotics

In 2004, 28% of the antibiotic prescriptions were preceded by POCT compared with 44% in 2013, corresponding to a 45% increase in the use of POCT prior to antibiotic prescribing (Fig. 1). The use of POCT differed substantially by type of prescribed antibiotic. For example, in 2013 the proportion of antibiotic prescriptions preceded by POCT varied from 4% for tetracycline to 44% for sulphonamide and trimethoprim prescriptions (Fig. 2).

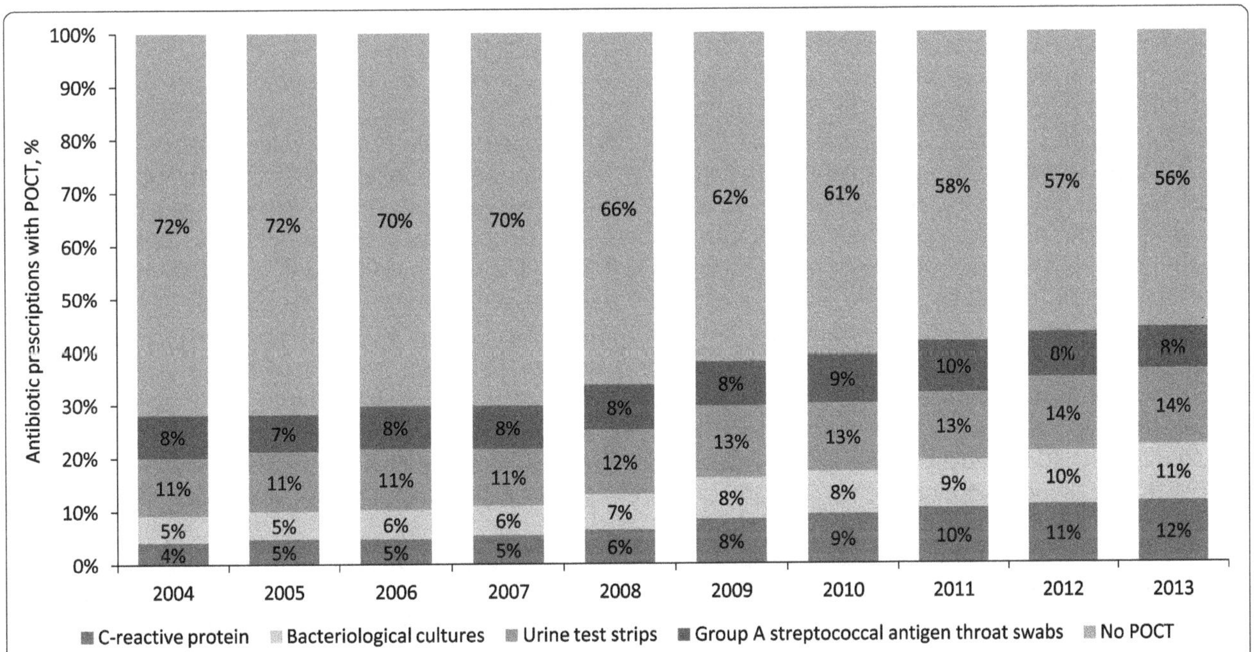

Fig. 1 Proportion of antibiotic prescriptions with and without a preceding microbiological point-of-care test (POCT) according to type of test

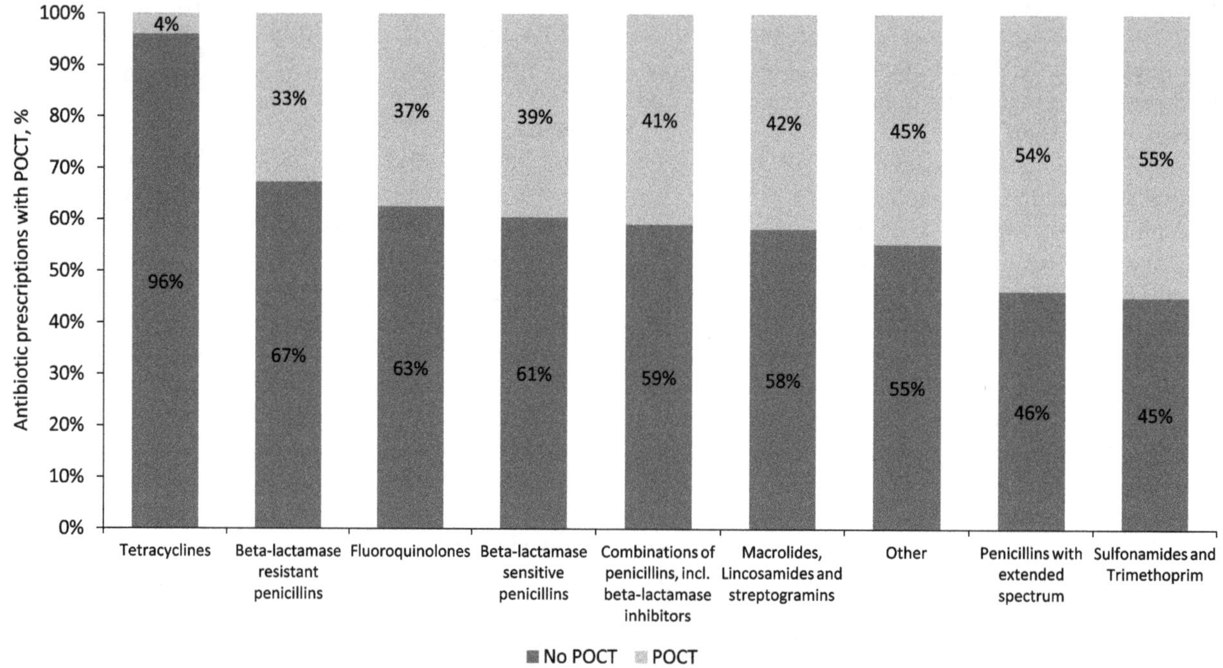

Fig. 2 Proportion of antibiotic prescriptions with and without a preceding microbiological point-of-care test (POCT) in 2013 according to type of prescribed antibiotic

Age and sex standardised rates of POCT per 1,000 overall consultations

The overall age and sex standardised prevalence rate of POCT was 147.2 per 1,000 consultations in 2004 and increased by 45.8% reaching 214.8 tests per 1,000 consultations in 2013. However, the use of individual POC tests differed markedly over time (Fig. 3). With 53.0 tests per 1,000 consultations urine test strips was by far the most frequently used test in 2004 and the usage increased by 5.5% ending at 55.9 per 1,000 consultations in 2013. Concurrently, CRP measurements increased by 132.0% (from 30.7 per 1,000 to 71.3 per 1,000) and bacteriological cultures by 101.7% (from 26.8 per 1,000 to 54.0 per 1,000). In 2013, CRP was the most frequently used test before antibiotic prescribing. In comparison, the use of GAS antigen swabs decreased by 8.6%, from 36.8 per 1,000 consultations in 2004 to 33.6 in 2013.

Rates of POCT use among the 2045 GPs varied by approximately a 5-fold, from 54.9 to 394.7 per 1,000 consultations in 2013 (median = 203, interquartile range (IQR) = 167–241) and even more for the individual tests; bacteriological cultures varied by more than 30-fold from 4.1 to 123.8 per 1,000 consultations (median = 48, IQR =32-67); urine test strips by almost a 12-fold from 11.6 to 121.3 per 1,000 (median =51, IQR =43-64); GAS antigen tests by more than 38-fold from 2.5 to 94.8 (median = 31, IQR = 24–42) and CRP measurement from 0.00 to 183.2 per 1,000 consultations (median = 63, IQR = 42–89).

Predictors of POCT use according to patient and GP characteristics

Table 1 shows patient- and GP-related predictors of POCT prior to antibiotic prescribing in 2013. The proportion of patients with POCT varied from 33% in children aged 0–4 years to 59% in teenagers aged 15–19 years, equivalent to an adjusted OR of 2.14 (95% CI 2.10-2.17). The usage of the specific tests varied greatly by age, for example 31% of children aged 5–9 years were tested for GAS antigen prior to antibiotic prescribing compared with only 1% of patients aged 65–79 years, whereas the use of urine test strips increased with age. Use of bacteriological cultures and CRP measurement also varied with age but less pronounced. Compared with women, men were less likely to receive a POCT (adjusted OR = 0.75, 95% CI 0.74-0.75). This difference was primarily driven by higher usage of urine test strips among females (18% in females vs. 7% in males), while the use of other tests differed little by sex.

Use of POCT varied across health care regions. Compared with patients living in the Capital Region of Denmark, patients in the North Denmark Region were more likely to receive POCT (adjusted OR = 1.19, 95% CI 1.18-1.20), particularly due to a higher use of urine test strips (16% vs. 12%) and CPR measurements (15% vs. 10%). Patients in the Central Denmark Region

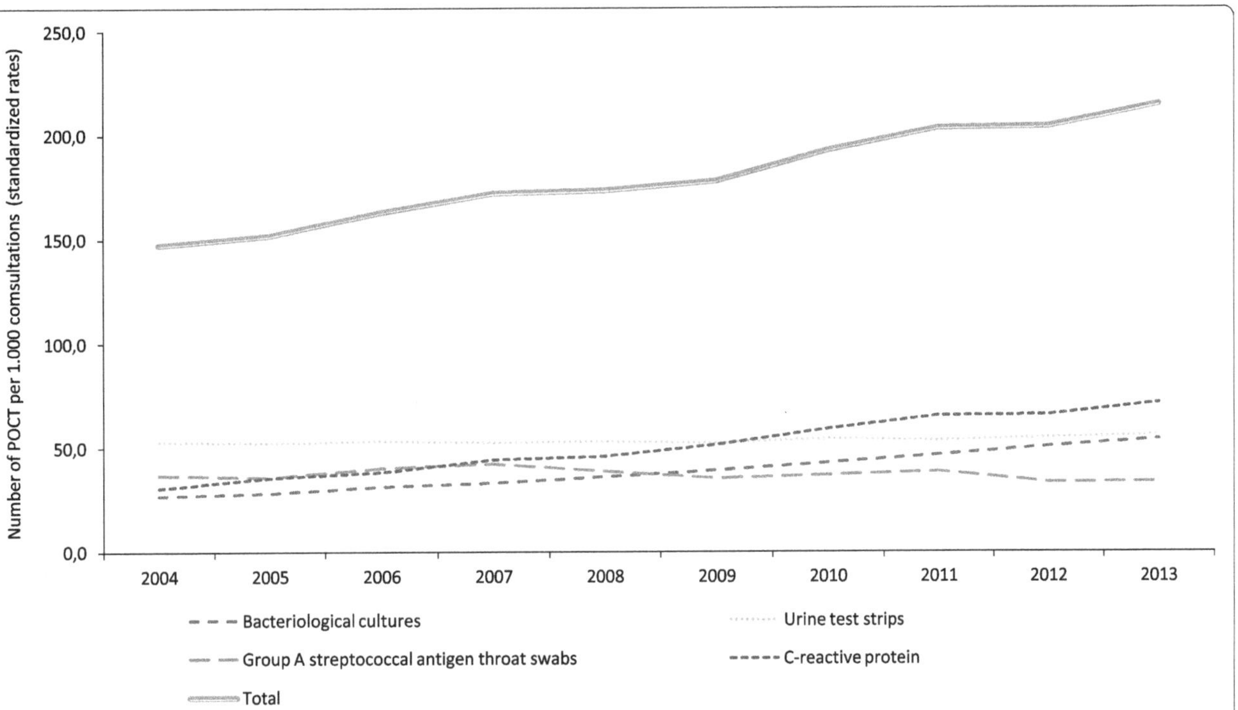

Fig. 3 Age- and sex standardized rates of microbiological point-of-care testing in individuals prescribed antibiotics and overall volume of prescribed antibiotics in general practice, 2004–2013

(adjusted OR = 0.81, 95% CI 0.80–0.82) and Region Zealand (adjusted OR = 0.91–0.92) were less likely to be tested compared with patients in the Capital Region. In contrast, there was no important rural–urban gradient, i.e., use of POCT varied little by the size of the city where the practice was located (Table 1).

Analyses restricted to GPs working in single-handed practices showed that compared with young female GPs (<41 years), female GPs aged 42–50 years were more likely to use POCT (adjusted OR = 1.06, 95% CI 1.02–1.11) while female GPs aged older than 60 years were less likely (adjusted OR = 0.84, 95% CI 0.80–0.86). Male GPs used less POCT compared with female GPs with the odds of POCT decreasing with increasing age (Table 1). The lowest use of POCT (except for use of urine test strips) was observed for male GPs older than 60 years versus female GPs < 41 years (adjusted OR = 0.61, 95% CI 0.59-0.64). In particular, a larger proportion of female GPs – except those older than 60 years – compared with male GPs used urine test strips prior to prescribing. Compared with GP age and sex, workload appeared to have little impact on odds of POCT and choice of specific tests (Table 1).

Discussion

This nationwide population-based cross-sectional study covering a 10 year period and including more than 20 million antibiotic prescriptions issued by more than 2,000 Danish practices demonstrated an increasing use of POCT before antibiotic prescribing in Denmark from 2004–2013. In 2013, GPs carried out POCT before 44% of all antibiotic prescriptions. The pattern of POCT shifted over time towards relatively higher rates of CRP measurement in 2013. Nonetheless, there was wide variability in testing rates across GPs with a more than 5 fold inter-practice variation in the overall use of POCT and considerably more for the individual tests. Odds of POCT before antibiotic prescribing varied by patient age and sex, and young female GPs were more likely to test than older male GPs, whereas workload appeared to have little influence.

Our study has strengths and weaknesses. We included the entire Danish population through the use of nationwide registries and the study was conducted in a setting in which the National Health Service provides unfettered access to health care and partial reimbursement for prescribed medications, thus largely eliminating referral and diagnostic biases. The DNHSR holds detailed data on the practices and the GPs and track changes during the study period. The registry is used for reimbursement for the GPs from the national health insurance and is considered to provide almost complete information. We do not have estimates of the validity of the activities, but it is generally considered to be high [29]. Notwithstanding, we were unable to distinguish GP consultations during ordinary working hours and out-of-hours GP service,

Table 1 Patient- and GP-related predictors of use of point-of-care (POC) testing prior to antibiotic prescribing in Denmark, 2013

Characteristic	Number of antibiotic prescriptions	Proportions of POC testing					OR for POC testing	
		POC test overall	Bacteriological cultures	Urinary test trips	Streptococcal antigen throat test	C-reactive protein	Crude OR (95% CI)	Adjusted[a] OR (95% CI)
Patient-related predictors								
Patient age, years								
0–4	129,184	33%	5%	2%	19%	7%	1.00 (reference)	1.00 (reference)
5–9	78,301	50%	8%	6%	31%	4%	1.99 (1.96–2.03)	1.98–(1.94–2.02)
10–14	45,288	47%	10%	6%	26%	6%	1.81 (1.77–1.85)	1.80 (1.77–1.84)
15–19	91,909	52%	15%	15%	15%	7%	2.23 (2.19–2.26)	2.14(2.10–2.17)
20–39	411,473	49%	14%	12%	12%	10%	1.95 (1.92-1.97)	1.85 (1.83–1.88)
40–64	620,369	42%	9%	13%	5%	15%	1.44 (1.42-1.46)	1.41(1.39-1.43)
65–79	420,459	46%	11%	19%	1%	15%	1.75 (1.72-1.77)	1.73 (1.70-1.75)
≥ 80 years	272,590	41%	11%	22%	0%	8%	1.38 (1.36-1.40)	1.33 (1.31-1.35)
Patient sex								
Female	1,320,004	47%	11%	18%	7%	11%	1.00 (reference)	1.00 (reference)
Male	749,569	39%	10%	7%	9%	13%	0.73 (0.73-0.73)	0.75 (0.74-0.75)
Geographical region of practice location								
Capital Region	597,406	45%	12%	12%	10%	10%	1.00 (reference)	1.00 (reference)
Central Denmark	428,874	40%	11%	13%	6%	11%	0.84 (0.83-0.85)	0.81 (0.80-0.82)
North Denmark Region	222,702	49%	11%	16%	7%	15%	1.19 (1.18-1.20)	1.19 (1.18-1.20)
Region Zealand	318,353	43%	8%	17%	7%	10%	0.93 (0.92-0.93)	0.91 (0.91-0.92)
Region of Southern Denmark	502,238	46%	10%	15%	8%	13%	1.07 (1.06-1.07)	1.04 (1.03-1.05)
City size								
< 5,000 inhabitants	1,820,020	44%	11%	14%	8%	11%	1.00 (reference)	1.00 (reference)
≥ 5,000 inhabitants	249,553	44%	9%	15%	7%	13%	1.02 (1.01-1.03)	1.01 (1.01-1.01)
GP-related predictors								
GP age and sex (for single-handed practices)[b]								
< 41, female	11,833	47%	12%	14%	10%	12%	1.00 (reference)	1.00 (reference)
41-50, female	51,698	49%	13%	15%	10%	12%	1.07 (1.01-1.10)	1.06 (1.02-1.11)
51-60, female	70,474	47%	13%	14%	9%	11%	0.99 (0.97-1.05)	1.01 (0.95-1.03)
> 60, female	56,098	43%	11%	12%	10%	10%	0.83 (0.81-0.88)	0.84 (0.80-0.86)
< 41, male	14,833	44%	12%	10%	9%	13%	0.88 (0.83-0.91)	0.87 (0.84-0.92)

Table 1 Patient- and GP-related predictors of use of point-of-care (POC) testing prior to antibiotic prescribing in Denmark, 2013 *(Continued)*

41-50, male	46,325	42%	9%	13%	9%	11%	0.81 (0.77-0.84)	0.80 (0.78-0.85)
51-60, male	130,236	41%	9%	13%	7%	12%	0.79 (0.74-0.80)	0.77 (0.76-0.82)
> 60, male	239,348	35%	7%	13%	6%	9%	0.62 (0.59-0.64)	0.61 (0.59-0.64)
Workload[c] in quartiles								
< 5675	475,569	44%	12%	13%	9%	11%	1.00 (reference)	1.00 (reference)
5675-6354	514,270	45%	11%	14%	8%	12%	1.02 (1.02-1.04)	1.03 (1.01-1.02)
6355-7189	535,857	44%	10%	14%	8%	12%	1.01 (0.99-1.00)	1.00 (1.00-1.02)
> 7190	543,877	43%	9%	15%	7%	12%	0.99 (0.95-0.96)	0.96 (0.98-1.00)

[a]Adjusted for patient age and sex, geographical region, city size, GP age, sex and workload (except when stratified by this variable)
[b]Excluding 1,051 (52%) GPs working in partnership-practices due to lack of data on age and sex for this practice type
[c]Defined as annual number of ordinary consultations per 1,000 registered patients

which is a main limitation of our study since these entities may differ substantially in the propensity for POCT. Moreover, we lacked data on GP age and sex working in partnership-practices. In Denmark, antibiotics are available on prescription only and a very small proportion is dispensed in hospitals. Since 2004, nationwide prescription data for antibiotic drugs have been assessable through the DHSPD. However, this registry only covers reimbursed medications and we likely underestimated the volume of tetracycline and quinolones since they were not reimbursed in 2013. According to national statistics the volume of tetracycline prescribed in the primary health care sector in 2013 amounted to 2.0 DDD per 1,000 inhabitants per day while the volume of quinolones was only 0.5 DDD per 1,000 inhabitants per day [32]. Another limitation of our study is that we do not know the indications for POCT nor the result. We used a 14-day time window to assess the use of POCT prior to antibiotic prescribing, and, in theory, the test could be unrelated to the actual antibiotic prescription. Nonetheless, we consider these events to be part of the same infectious episode. Moreover, as we only examined use of POCT in patients prescribed antibiotics, we cannot estimate to which extent use of POCT lead to non-prescribing decisions. Finally, we did not have data on practice staffing which may also influence POCT usage.

Limiting both over and under use of antibiotics in primary care is vital in reducing antibiotic resistance without exposing patients to unnecessary risks. Some of the high use of antibiotics in primary care may relate to diagnostic uncertainty [6]. GPs may be under pressure from patients who believe they need antibiotics [33]. With a negative test result at hand it may be easier for the GP to refuse prescribing an unnecessary antibiotic [15, 34, 35]. Thus, use of POCT to rule out a possible bacterial infection may reduce diagnostic uncertainty and increase confidence and acceptance of non-prescription decisions [36]. In a Dutch RCT Cals et al. [18] found that GPs assigned to CRP testing prescribed fewer antibiotics compared with those who did not use the test (31% vs. 53%). In line with this, other studies have shown that use of POCT is associated with reduced antibiotic prescribing [18, 22, 37–39] Importantly, a recent Cochrane review concluded that this reduction in antibiotic use in patients exposed to POCT is not associated with differences in recovery or duration of illness [38].

In Denmark, GPs have in-house lab facilities and potentially have a financial incentive to carry out POCT, because they are reimbursed by the National Health Service for the use of these tests. Qualitative studies have shown that GPs and patients generally report good acceptability of POCT [35, 40, 41] and economic analyses show that POCT is cost-effective [42, 43]. Increased use of CRP measurements and bacteriological cultures were the main drivers of the increased POCT, whereas urine test remained stable and GAS antigen swabs decreased. Compared with CRP measurements, bacteriological cultures requires overnight incubation and therefore cannot support "real-time" decisions. In this respect, the increase in bacteriological cultures may appear as a surprise. On the other hand, the increase could reflect cultures taken following a positive CRP test in order achieve a diagnosis and antimicrobial susceptibility. We also observed wide variability in the use of POCT across Denmark's health care regions and in particular by GP age and sex. Potential explanations for the observed differences include a preference for female GPs by young female patients and families with children. It is also likely that older GPs feel more confident with their clinical judgement, than younger GPs. Qualitative research suggest that some GPs have concerns about over reliance on test results, e.g., false positive results that may lead to unnecessary antibiotic prescriptions as well as false negatives leading to lack of necessary antibiotic treatment [35]. Interviews with 66 GPs who participated in a RCT conducted in 6 European countries revealed that the GPs felt that CRP testing was most helpful in situations of uncertainty [44]. Thus, while helpful, the GPs indicated that they would restrict the use to cases of diagnostic uncertainty because of the time taken to obtain a result [44]. They also expressed concern that POCT could lead to more consultations in future [44, 45]. In a Swedish study, 49% of all Strep-A tests were performed in patients with a diagnosis of common cold, sinusitis, acute bronchitis or pneumonia, indicating that the tests were performed in patients with a very low probability of GAS [46]. Likewise, another Swedish study reported that 42% of all patients with a diagnosis of respiratory infection were examined with a CRP test [47]. The majority of these tests (69%) were performed in patients with a diagnosis of upper respiratory infection. These findings indicate that the tests were used too liberal and often not in a population with a high probability of bacterial infection.

Conclusions

In conclusion, Danish GPs use POCT increasingly prior to antibiotic prescribing. In particular, the use of CRP measurement and bacteriological cultures increased substantially while the use of strep-A tests decreased. The proportion of patients tested and choice of test varied greatly across GPs.

Funding

This study was supported by Region Midtjyllands Praksisforskningsfond, Denmark. The sponsor did not have a role in any phase of the study conduct.

Authors' contributions

MS conceived the study idea. SHA and MS reviewed the literature. SHA and MS collected the data. SHA, RWT, and MS designed the study and directed the analyses, which were carried out by SHA. All authors participated in the interpretation of the results. SHA and MS organized the writing and wrote the initial drafts. All authors critically revised the manuscript for intellectual content and approved the final version.

Competing interests

The authors declare that they have no competing interests.

Consent for publication

Not applicable.

Author details

[1]Department of Clinical Epidemiology, Aarhus University, Olof Palmes Alle 43-45, 8200 Aarhus N, Denmark. [2]Department of General Practice, Institute of Public Health, Aarhus University, Aarhus, Denmark. [3]Antimicrobial Resistance Reference Laboratory and Surveillance Unit, Department of Microbiology and Infection Control, Statens Serum Institut, Copenhagen, Denmark. [4]Section and Research Unit of General Practice, Department of Public Health, Copenhagen University, Copenhagen, Denmark.

References

1. Dellit TH, Owens RC, McGowan JE, Gerding DN, Weinstein RA, Burke JP, et al. Infectious Diseases Society of America and the Society for Healthcare Epidemiology of America guidelines for developing an institutional program to enhance antimicrobial stewardship. Clin Infect Dis. 2007;44:159–77.
2. Hughes JM. Preserving the lifesaving power of antimicrobial agents. JAMA. 2011;305:1027–8.
3. Fleming-Dutra KE, Hersh AL, Shapiro DJ, Bartoces M, Enns EA, File TM, et al. Prevalence of Inappropriate Antibiotic Prescriptions Among US Ambulatory Care Visits, 2010–2011. JAMA. 2016;315:1864–73.
4. Woodhead M, Blasi F, Ewig S, Huchon G, Ieven M, Leven M, et al. Guidelines for the management of adult lower respiratory tract infections. Eur Respir J. 2005;26:1138–80.
5. Smucny J, Fahey T, Becker L, Glazier R. Antibiotics for acute bronchitis. Cochrane database Syst Rev. 2004;4:CD000245.
6. Whaley LE, Businger AC, Dempsey PP, Linder JA. Visit complexity, diagnostic uncertainty, and antibiotic prescribing for acute cough in primary care: a retrospective study. BMC Fam Pract. 2013;14:120.
7. Grover ML, Mookadam M, Rutkowski RH, Cullan AM, Hill DE, Patchett DC, et al. Acute respiratory tract infection: a practice examines its antibiotic prescribing habits. J Fam Pract. 2012;61:330–5.
8. Steinman MA, Landefeld CS, Gonzales R. Predictors of broad-spectrum antibiotic prescribing for acute respiratory tract infections in adult primary care. JAMA. 2003;289:719–25.
9. Grijalva CG, Nuorti JP, Griffin MR. Antibiotic prescription rates for acute respiratory tract infections in US ambulatory settings. JAMA. 2009;302:758–66.
10. Aabenhus R, Siersma V, Hansen MP, Bjerrum L. Antibiotic prescribing in Danish general practice 2004–13. J Antimicrob Chemother. 2016;71:2286–94.
11. Sundhedsstyrelsen. Vejledning om ordination af antibiotika. 2012. https://sundhedsstyrelsen.dk/~/media/34F841A604D94FD596168CAC4F2D8A3D.ashx. Accessed 15 Aug 2016.
12. McIsaac WJ, Butler CC. Does clinical error contribute to unnecessary antibiotic use? Med Decis Mak. 2000;20:33–8.
13. Jensen US, Bjerrum L. Notable increase in the consumption of antibiotics in general practice. Ugeskr Laeger. 2011;173:2853–6.
14. Kost GJ. Principles and practice of point-of-care testing. 1st ed. Philadelphia: Lippincott Williams & Wilkins; 2002.
15. van Vugt SF, Broekhuizen BDL, Lammens C, Zuithoff NPA, de Jong PA, Coenen S, et al. Use of serum C reactive protein and procalcitonin concentrations in addition to symptoms and signs to predict pneumonia in patients presenting to primary care with acute cough: diagnostic study. BMJ. 2013;346:f2450.
16. Briel M, Young J, Tschudi P, Hersberger KE, Hugenschmidt C, Langewitz W, et al. Prevalence and influence of diagnostic tests for acute respiratory tract infections in primary care. Swiss Med Wkly. 2006;136:248–53.
17. Jakobsen KA, Melbye H, Kelly MJ, Ceynowa C, Mölstad S, Hood K, et al. Influence of CRP testing and clinical findings on antibiotic prescribing in adults presenting with acute cough in primary care. Scand J Prim Health Care. 2010;28:229–36.
18. Cals JWL, Butler CC, Hopstaken RM, Hood K, Dinant G-J. Effect of point of care testing for C reactive protein and training in communication skills on antibiotic use in lower respiratory tract infections: cluster randomised trial. BMJ. 2009;338:b1374.
19. Takemura Y, Ebisawa K, Kakoi H, Saitoh H, Kure H, Ishida H, et al. Antibiotic selection patterns in acutely febrile new outpatients with or without immediate testing for C reactive protein and leucocyte count. J Clin Pathol. 2005;58:729–33.
20. Bjerrum L, Gahrn-Hansen B, Munck AP. C-reactive protein measurement in general practice may lead to lower antibiotic prescribing for sinusitis. Br J Gen Pract. 2004;54:659–62.
21. Casey JR, Marsocci SM, Murphy ML, Francis AB, Pichichero ME. White blood cell count can aid judicious antibiotic prescribing in acute upper respiratory infections in children. Clin Pediatr. 2003;42:113–9.
22. Llor C, Bjerrum L, Arranz J, García G, Cots JM, González López-Valcárcel B, et al. C-reactive protein testing in patients with acute rhinosinusitis leads to a reduction in antibiotic use. Fam Pract. 2012;29:653–8.
23. André M, Odenholt I, Schwan A, Axelsson I, Eriksson M, Hoffman M, et al. Upper respiratory tract infections in general practice: diagnosis, antibiotic prescribing, duration of symptoms and use of diagnostic tests. Scand J Infect Dis. 2002;34:880–6.
24. Sørensen HT, Steffensen FH, Schønheyder HC, Grøn P, Sabroe S. Use of microbiological diagnostics and antibiotics in Danish general practice. Int J Technol Assess Health Care. 1996;12:745–51.
25. André M, Vernby A, Odenholt I, Lundborg CS, Axelsson I, Eriksson M, et al. Diagnosis-prescribing surveys in 2000, 2002 and 2005 in Swedish general practice: consultations, diagnosis, diagnostics and treatment choices. Scand J Infect Dis. 2008;40:648–54.
26. Benin AL, Vitkauskas G, Thornquist E, Shiffman RN, Concato J, Krumholz HM, et al. Improving diagnostic testing and reducing overuse of antibiotics for children with pharyngitis: a useful role for the electronic medical record. Pediatr Infect Dis J. 2003;22:1043–7.
27. Mangione-Smith R, Elliott MN, Wong L, McDonald L, Roski J. Measuring the quality of care for group A streptococcal pharyngitis in 5 US health plans. Arch Pediatr Adolesc Med. 2005;159:491–7.
28. Pedersen CB. The Danish Civil Registration System. Scand J Public Health. 2011;39:22–5.
29. Andersen JS, Olivarius NDF, Krasnik A. The Danish National Health Service Register. Scand J Public Health. 2011;39:34–7.
30. Johannesdottir SA, Horváth-Puhó E, Ehrenstein V, Schmidt M, Pedersen L, Sørensen HT. Existing data sources for clinical epidemiology: The Danish National database of reimbursed prescriptions. Clin Epidemiol. 2012;4:303–13.
31. Gjelstad S, Straand J, Dalen I, Fetveit A, Strøm H, Lindbæk M. Do general practitioners' consultation rates influence their prescribing patterns of antibiotics for acute respiratory tract infections? J Antimicrob Chemother. 2011;66:2425–33.
32. The Danish Health Data Authority. Medstat.dk. http://www.medstat.dk/.
33. Butler CC, Rollnick S, Pill R, Maggs-Rapport F, Stott N. Understanding the culture of prescribing: qualitative study of general practitioners' and patients' perceptions of antibiotics for sore throats. BMJ. 1998;317:637–42.
34. Kolmos HJ, Little P. Should general practitioners perform diagnostic tests on patients before prescribing antibiotics? BMJ. 1999;318:799–802.
35. Butler CC, Simpson S, Wood F. General practitioners' perceptions of introducing near-patient testing for common infections into routine primary care: a qualitative study. Scand J Prim Health Care. 2008;26:17–21.
36. Stanton N, Francis NA, Butler CC. Reducing uncertainty in managing respiratory tract infections in primary care. Br J Gen Pract. 2010;60:e466–75.
37. Little P, Stuart B, Francis N, Douglas E, Tonkin-Crine S, Anthierens S, et al. Effects of internet-based training on antibiotic prescribing rates for acute respiratory-tract infections: a multinational, cluster, randomised, factorial, controlled trial. Lancet. 2013;382:1175–82.
38. Aabenhus R, Jensen J-US, Jørgensen KJ, Hróbjartsson A, Bjerrum L. Biomarkers as point-of-care tests to guide prescription of antibiotics in

patients with acute respiratory infections in primary care. Cochrane Database Syst Rev. 2014;11:CD010130.
39. Andreeva E, Melbye H. Usefulness of C-reactive protein testing in acute cough/respiratory tract infection: an open cluster-randomized clinical trial with C-reactive protein testing in the intervention group. BMC Fam Pract. 2014;15:80.
40. Cals JWL, Chappin FHF, Hopstaken RM, van Leeuwen ME, Hood K, Butler CC, et al. C-reactive protein point-of-care testing for lower respiratory tract infections: a qualitative evaluation of experiences by GPs. Fam Pract. 2010; 27:212–8.
41. Cooke J, Butler C, Hopstaken R, Dryden MS, McNulty C, Hurding S, et al. Narrative review of primary care point-of-care testing (POCT) and antibacterial use in respiratory tract infection (RTI). BMJ Open Respir Res. 2015;2:e000086.
42. Hunter R. Cost-Effectiveness of Point-of-Care C-Reactive protein tests for respiratory tract infection in primary care in England. Adv Ther. 2015;32:69–85.
43. Oppong R, Jit M, Smith RD, Butler CC, Melbye H, Mölstad S, et al. Cost-effectiveness of point-of-care C-reactive protein testing to inform antibiotic prescribing decisions. Br J Gen Pract. 2013;63:465–71.
44. Anthierens S, Tonkin-Crine S, Cals JW, Coenen S, Yardley L, Brookes-Howell L, et al. Clinicians??? Views and Experiences of Interventions to Enhance the Quality of Antibiotic Prescribing for Acute Respiratory Tract Infections. J Gen Intern Med. 2014;408–16.
45. Yardley L, Douglas E, Anthierens S, Tonkin-Crine S, O'Reilly G, Stuart B, et al. Evaluation of a web-based intervention to reduce antibiotic prescribing for LRTI in six European countries: quantitative process analysis of the GRACE/INTRO randomised controlled trial. Implement Sci. 2013;8:134.
46. Engström S, Mölstad S, Lindström K, Nilsson G, Borgquist L. Excessive use of rapid tests in respiratory tract infections in Swedish primary health care. Scand J Infect Dis. 2004;36:213–8.
47. André M, Schwan A, Odenholt I. Swedish Study Group on Antibiotic Use. The use of CRP tests in patients with respiratory tract infections in primary care in Sweden can be questioned. Scand J Infect Dis. 2004;36:192–7.

2

Managing diagnostic uncertainty in primary care

Rahul Alam[1], Sudeh Cheraghi-Sohi[1*], Maria Panagioti[1], Aneez Esmail[1], Stephen Campbell[1,2] and Efharis Panagopoulou[3]

Abstract

Background: Diagnostic uncertainty is one of the largest contributory factors to the occurrence of diagnostic errors across most specialties in medicine and arguably uncertainty is greatest in primary care due to the undifferentiated symptoms primary care physicians are often presented with. Physicians can respond to diagnostic uncertainty in various ways through the interplay of a series of cognitive, emotional and ethical reactions. The consequences of such uncertainty however can impact negatively upon the primary care practitioner, their patients and the wider healthcare system. Understanding the nature of the existing empirical literature in relation to managing diagnostic uncertainty in primary medical care is a logical and necessary first step in order to understand what solutions are already available and/or to aid the development of any training or feedback aimed at better managing this uncertainty. This review is the first to characterize the existing empirical literature on managing diagnostic uncertainty in primary care.

Methods: Sixteen databases were systematically searched from inception to present with no restrictions. Hand searches of relevant websites and reference lists of included studies were also conducted. Two authors conducted abstract/article screening and data extraction. PRISMA guidelines were adhered to.

Results: Ten studies met the inclusion criteria. A narrative and conceptual synthesis was undertaken under the premises of critical reviews. Results suggest that studies have focused on internal factors (traits, skills and strategies) associated with managing diagnostic uncertainty with only one external intervention identified. Cognitive factors ranged from the influences of epistemological viewpoints to practical approaches such as greater knowledge of the patient, utilizing resources to hand and using appropriate safety netting techniques. Emotional aspects of uncertainty management included clinicians embracing uncertainty and working with provisional diagnoses. Ethical aspects of uncertainty management centered on communicating diagnostic uncertainties with patients. Personality traits and characteristics influenced each of the three domains.

Conclusions: There is little empirical evidence on how uncertainty is managed in general practice. However we highlight how the extant literature can be conceptualised into cognitive, emotional and ethical aspects of uncertainty which may help clinicians be more aware of their own biases as well as provide a platform for future research.

Keywords: Diagnosis, Uncertainty, Primary medical care, Burnout, Training

* Correspondence: Sudeh.Cheraghi-Sohi@manchester.ac.uk
[1]NIHR Greater Manchester Primary Care Patient Safety Translational Research Centre (Greater Manchester PSTRC), The University of Manchester, Williamson Building, Oxford Road, Manchester M13 9PL, UK
Full list of author information is available at the end of the article

Background

Diagnostic uncertainty is one of the largest contributory factors to the occurrence of diagnostic errors across most specialties in medicine [1]. It is also the most common source of clinical uncertainty in primary care, as the breadth and complexity of diagnoses possible in general practice makes diagnostic uncertainty a routine inevitability [2–4]. Although diagnostic uncertainty is primarily a function of knowledge acquisition, processing and recall [4], physicians can respond to diagnostic uncertainty in various ways through the interplay of a series of cognitive, emotional and ethical reactions [5–7].

Cognitive reactions are related to difficulties in perception and interpretation of the available facts [8] and often include the use of several heuristics and biases such as unconscious "rules of thumb" or intuitive diagnostic reasoning based on stereotypes related to gender, age or occupation [9, 10].

Emotional reactions include both short and long-term stress and/or anxiety which can develop under particular uncertain or ambiguous situations and contexts [11]. They include the cultural and/or societal context in which clinical uncertainty take place (where certainty is expected and demanded by patients) alongside the affective reactions clinicians experience when their technical, personal, or conceptual resources are unable to meet the demand for certainty [4].

Ethical reactions relate to the nature of discourse between the physician and patient in relation to uncertainty and encompass elements of shared decision-making [12, 13]. Informed and shared decision-making necessitates patient understanding of their illness, options for treatment and prognosis [14]. Despite this, physicians are often hesitant to disclose uncertainty to their patients [15] leaving clinicians in an ethical dilemma.

At a dyadic level, a physician's ability to deal with uncertainty at a cognitive, emotional and ethical level influences the eventual diagnostic decision and therefore can impact on the patient and their outcomes [4]. At a wider system level, uncertainty has been shown to effect admission rates [16] and health care costs [17]. A recent study for example, has shown that General Practitioners (GPs) or family physicians respond to uncertainty by increased hospital referrals and ordering more diagnostic tests [18]. Doctors with a high intolerance of uncertainty also have higher costs of investigation and treatment [19]. Conversely, GPs who cope well with uncertainty are more likely to support shared decision-making [20]. Finally, by attempting to achieve certainty via a 'correct diagnosis', premature closure is likely to occur in the decision-making process thereby allowing hidden assumptions and unconscious biases to have more weight than they should, with increased potential for diagnostic error [21].

In summary, diagnostic uncertainty has implications for the primary care practitioner, their patients and the wider healthcare system. Understanding the nature of the existing empirical literature in relation to managing diagnostic uncertainty in primary medical care would be a logical and necessary first step in order to understand what solutions are already available and/or to aid the development of any training or feedback aimed at better managing this uncertainty.

The purpose of this systematic critical review therefore was to synthesize the strategies, skills or traits associated with or used by clinicians working in general medical practice to manage diagnostic uncertainty at any or all of the three domains of uncertainty (cognitive, emotional and/or ethical). Additionally, the review aimed to identify any existing training programs that aim to support clinicians to manage diagnostic uncertainty in order to inform the development of any future programs.

Methods

This systematic critical review was conducted and reported in accordance with the Preferred Reporting Items for Systematic Reviews and Meta-Analyses (PRISMA) [22] and registered with PROSPERO in October 2015 (available online at: http://www.crd.york.ac.uk/PROSPERO/display_record.asp?ID=CRD42015027555).

Eligibility criteria

Given that our focus was on primary medical care, any empirical studies reporting on how trainee or experienced GPs deal and manage with diagnostic uncertainty either wholly or partly in primary medical care were eligible. We also included studies where diagnostic uncertainty was included within broader clinical uncertainty assessments. Eligible study designs included randomised controlled trials, interrupted time series analysis, cohort studies, case control studies, cross-sectional studies, before and after studies, qualitative studies as well as pragmatic observational studies and studies such as process evaluations.

Exclusion criteria

Studies involving solely secondary care contexts and student participants were excluded given the potentially limited generalizability to qualified clinicians in primary care as were studies exploring patient uncertainty. Programs on uncertainty that utilized alternative forms of minimizing diagnostic uncertainty such as the use of laboratory tests [23], utilising differential diagnosis (DDx) tools [24] and studies utilizing top-down approaches such as the use of guidelines on aspects of diagnostic uncertainty were also excluded.

Information sources and searches

A combination of medical subject heading (MeSH) terms and free text words describing clinical uncertainty and tolerance were used. The following databases were searched from inception to July 2015: Ovid MEDLINE(R), Embase, CINAHL, Cochrane Database of Systematic Reviews, Cochrane Central Register of Controlled Trials, Cochrane Methodology Register, ACP Journal Club, Database of Abstracts of Reviews of Effects, Health Technology Assessment, National Health Service (NHS) Economic Evaluation Database, AMED (Allied and Complementary Medicine), CAB Abstracts, Global Health, Health and Psychosocial Instruments, Health Management Information Consortium and PsycINFO (see Additional file 1).

In addition to the articles identified by the search, we undertook hand-searches of the websites of the National Patient Safety Agency (NPSA), Patient.co.uk and Gutfeelings.eu. The reference lists of included articles were also screened for eligible papers and a Scopus search of potentially relevant articles were conducted using key words. The search was not restricted by date, language or country of publication.

Study selection

Two reviewers (RA and EP) independently screened the titles and abstracts against the eligibility criteria for inclusion. The reviewers then agreed on the papers for inclusion and full-text articles were retrieved and reviewed. Any disagreements were resolved in meetings and through discussion with the wider team until consensus was reached. High inter-rater reliability was achieved: Cohen's [25] unweighted κ coefficient = 0.74 and 0.95 for title/abstract and full-text screening, respectively.

Data extraction

A standardized data extraction form was developed and piloted. Studies meeting the inclusion criteria were then double-extracted by the review team. Data were extracted and cross-checked by the reviewers using the Microsoft Excel data extraction form and any disagreements were resolved by discussion.

Data were extracted on the participants including their grade, clinical background, specialty and setting. We then extracted data on the specific types of diagnostic uncertainty targeted by the study (cognitive, emotional, or ethical), the tools/frameworks used to assess uncertainty and any resources utilized to manage diagnostic uncertainty (internal: i.e. skills, strategies, or individual traits, or external: i.e. interventions or training programs).

Critical appraisal

The Critical Appraisal Skills Programme (CASP) checklist for qualitative research was used to assess the quality of the included qualitative studies [26]. The quantitative cross-sectional studies were critically appraised using the modified Newcastle Ottawa scale for cross sectional studies [27]. These two instruments are very well-known, easily accessible online and clearly define the meaning behind each individual criterion listed. We did not exclude studies from the synthesis based on the critical appraisal ratings.

Data synthesis

As the main focus of this review was to explore which types of skills or strategies physicians use to manage diagnostic uncertainty under its three domains, a narrative synthesis was conducted drawing on the critical review synthesis methodology described by Grant and colleagues [28]. The main advantage of the critical review methodology is that it allows a conceptual synthesis to be undertaken which is particularly suited for the purposes of this study. Following the guidelines of a critical review, the studies were conceptually grouped into the cognitive, emotional and ethical domains of uncertainty which are widely described in the empirical and theoretical literature of uncertainty as outlined in the introduction. Within the main presentation groupings (the three domains of uncertainty), we also presented the findings according to the type of evidence (qualitative or quantitative data). The small number and the moderate quality of the included studies suggest that further groupings of the studies were very unlikely to make any firm contribution, and therefore were avoided.

Results

Overview

We identified 10 studies meeting the inclusion criteria and the PRISMA flowchart demonstrates the study screening and selection process (please see Fig. 1).

Descriptive characteristics of included studies and critical appraisal

Tables 1 and 2 show the characteristics of the included studies highlighting the traits, strategies and skills influencing and impacting on managing uncertainty. Six studies were quantitative cross-sectional surveys (Table 1) [4, 6, 10, 29–31], three were qualitative process evaluations [32–34] and one was a qualitative study [13] (Table 2). All three domains of diagnostic uncertainty were equally represented in the identified literature, with eight studies per domain. Some studies were categorized across more than one domain.

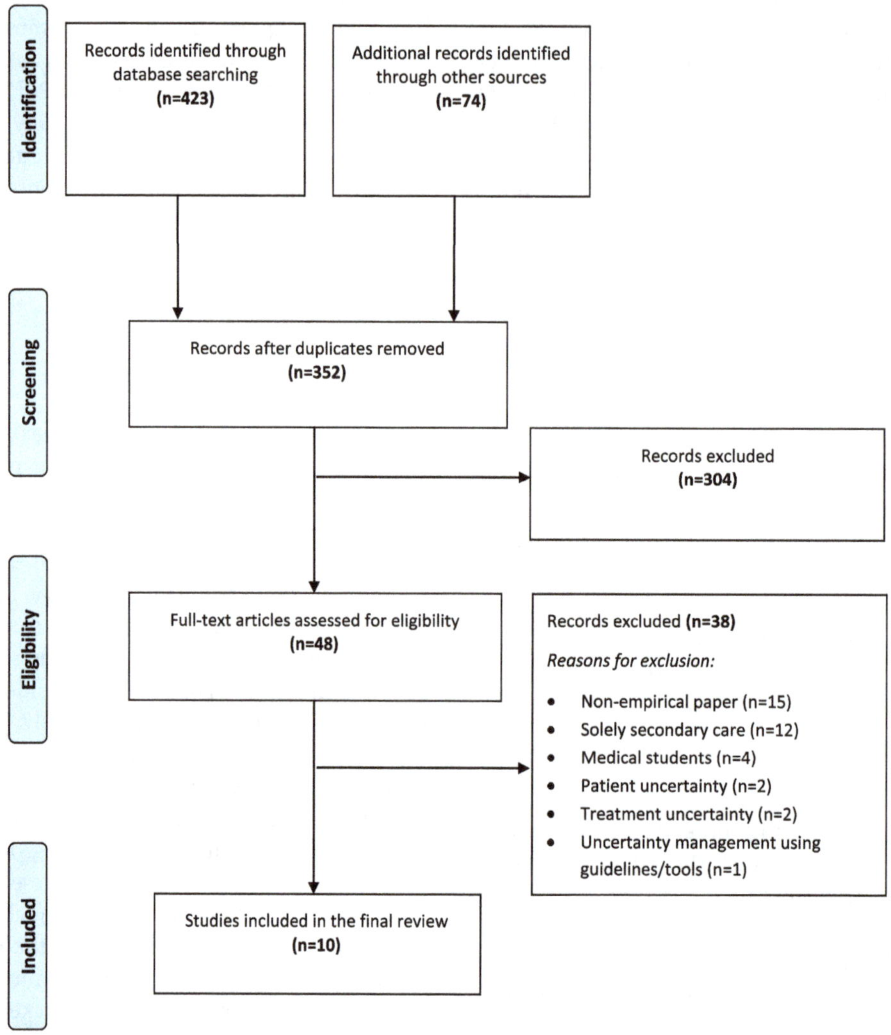

Fig. 1 PRISMA flow diagram

All 6 cross-sectional studies were low to moderate quality meeting 3 to 5 of the 7 criteria listed in the modified Newcastle Ottawa scale for cross-sectional studies (please see Additional file 2: Table S1). The qualitative study with high critical appraisal ratings (8 of the 10 criteria) identified issues across all three domains of diagnostic uncertainty which were consistent with the pattern of findings identified by the remaining qualitative and cross-sectional studies. The quality of the qualitative research was generally low to moderate. Three studies (the process evaluations) met 5 criteria while one qualitative study met 8 of the 10 criteria listed in the CASP checklist for qualitative research (please see Additional file 3: Table S2).

The majority of studies [4, 6, 10, 13, 29–33] investigated internal resources or traits/attributes for managing diagnostic uncertainty which included individual traits such as gender, experience, ethnicity, as well as the use of specific strategies used by clinicians such as skills, reasoning styles, rules of thumb and sharing the dilemma with a colleague whilst the only external resource identified related to a specific intervention in the form of an adapted Practice-based learning training program [34].

The level of detail provided in relation to how diagnostic uncertainty was managed ranged from limited preset responses in surveys to in-depth qualitative descriptions. Despite the heterogeneity with regards to their study designs and aims, the studies nonetheless provide some empirical evidence on the types of diagnostic uncertainty currently studied in the literature (emotional, ethical and cognitive) and the impact of specific characteristics on how diagnostic uncertainty manifests and on how diagnostic uncertainty is managed.

Cognitive aspects of managing uncertainty

Eight studies reported on various cognitive aspects of managing uncertainty [4, 10, 13, 29, 31–34].

Table 1 Traits, strategies and skills influencing and impacting on managing uncertainty: Quantitative cross-sectional studies

Author Year Country	Study type	Specialty or condition/ clinician grade or experience	Setting/ recruitment/ Sample size (n) and response rate (RR %)	Uncertainty assessment	Uncertainty Resource	Uncertainty type Cognitive (C) Emotional (E) Ethical (ETH)	Results
Cooke 2013 Australia [30]	Cross-sectional survey	General practice / Registrar	Survey participants recruited from advertisements and through training events; (n = 128) (RR: 90%)	Intolerance of uncertainty scale –12 (IUS-12) Physicians reactions to uncertainty Scale –8 (PRUS)	Resilience	General intolerance of uncertainty Anxiety due to uncertainty (E) Reluctance to disclose uncertainty to patients (Eth)	Lower resilience was associated with lower tolerance of uncertainty.
Evans 2009 USA [4]	Cross sectional survey	Pediatrics, family medicine and internal medicine/ Board certified and resident physicians in primary care with a mixture of experience levels	Primary care / Survey participants recruited from an academic medical centre (n = 78) (RR: 76%)	Physicians Belief Scale –32 (PBS), Physician reactions to uncertainty Scale – 8 (PRUS)	Cognitive beliefs	Conceptual uncertainty – difficulties applying abstract criteria to concrete situations (C) Stress reactions to uncertainty (E)	Physicians adopting a biopsychosocial epistemology model were associated with less stress reactions to uncertainty while a biomedical model was associated with more stress reactions to uncertainty. Clinician gender, specialty area and experience were correlated with stress reactions to uncertainty.
Nevalainen 2014 Finland [29]	Questionnaire-based survey (self-assessment)	Primary Care/Recently qualified GPs (<5 years, mean age 31.2 years) and experienced GPs (>5 years, mean age 48.4 years)	Convenience sample of GPs recruited via email. N = 165/244 (RR: 68%)	Custom made questionnaire	Experience	Access to information sources (C) Tolerance of uncertainty (E)	Experienced GPs better tolerate uncertainty (53.8% (95% CI; 42.2–65.0) in medical decision-making than their younger colleagues (25.9% (95% CI; 17.0–36.5) ($p < 0.001$).
Portnoy, 2011 USA [6]	Cross-sectional survey-representative sample	Mixed –Family practice, internists, pediatrics, obstetrics and gynecology / Mixed ¯3.9 years practicing (SD ± 7.5)	Primary care; n = 1500 total; (GPs n = 515 34.3%) (RR: 48%)	Ambiguity aversion (AA) in medicine scale.	Factors influencing physicians' attitudes towards the communication and management of scientific uncertainty in clinical practice	Physicians' attitudes about communicating and managing uncertainty and their perceptions of negative reactions to uncertainty by their patients (Eth)	Physician demographics (including medical specialty, ethnicity and gender) predicted attitudes towards communicating and managing scientific uncertainty. Physicians' perceptions of their patients' responses to ambiguity also influenced decisions to share ambiguity where physicians who thought more of their patients would have negative reactions to ambiguous information were more likely to decide what's best for the patient (p = 0.013) and to withhold an intervention that had uncertainty associated with it (p = <0.001).
Schneider 2010 Germany [10]	Survey – questionnaire (development consisting of focus groups)	General Practice / Overall experience as a doctor –mean years =22.7, experience as a GP, 15.4 years	University hospital conference & 23 "quality circles" (GP groups). Responders n = 93 (conference) & n = 232 (quality circles) (Overall RR: 68%)	Developing the Dealing with uncertainty questionnaire (DUQ); GP diagnostic action scale and GP diagnostic reasoning scale.	Cognitive heuristics	Dealing with diagnostic uncertainty and heuristics in diagnostic thinking (C) Tolerance of uncertainty (E)	The use of test of time, knowledge of family situation and occupational situation as a simple heuristic. Emotional intolerance against uncertainty correlates with an increase in diagnostic activity. Emotional responses to uncertainty might influence gender-specific reactions to uncertainty in different ways.

Table 1 Traits, strategies and skills influencing and impacting on managing uncertainty: Quantitative cross-sectional studies *(Continued)*

Schneider 2014 Germany [31]	Mixed methods study (focus groups and cross sectional survey)	Primary care, generic conditions/ clinical experience 23.9 years (SD ± 23.9 years)	Development - 10 experienced GPs and survey - n = 228 (RR: 97%)	Communicating and dealing with uncertainty questionnaire (CoDU), Physician reaction to Uncertainty (PRU), and Big Five Inventory (BFI-K)	Personality traits of GPs in relation to decision making concerning uncertainty management	Diagnostic action (C) Intuition (E) Extended social anamnesis (Eth) Anxiety due to uncertainty (E) Communicating uncertainty (Eth)	GPs scoring high in neuroticism demonstrated more anxiety due to uncertainty and higher reluctance to communicate with patients. Extraversion, conscientiousness and openness correlated negatively with anxiety due to uncertainty and positively with patient communication.

RR **Response rate, *SP* Standardized patients *NA* not applicable, *NS* not stated, *C* Cognitive, *E* emotional, *Eth* ethical**

Table 2 Traits, strategies and skills influencing and impacting on managing uncertainty: Qualitative studies

Author Year Country	Study type	Specialty or condition/ clinician grade or experience	Setting/ recruitment/ Sample size (n)	Uncertainty assessment	Uncertainty Resource	Uncertainty type Cognitive (C) Emotional (E) Ethical (ETH)	Results
Griffiths 2005 UK [13]	Qualitative study	Hormone replacement therapy, bone densitometry and breast screening/Practice nurses, general practitioners, consultants, specialist registrars, specialist nurse, radiographer	7 general practices, 3 secondary care clinics (n = 25)	Constant comparative analysis of audio recorded transcripts	Strategies health professionals use	Utilizing safety netting techniques (C) Communicating uncertainty to patients (Eth) Accepting uncertainty (E)	Three key strategies were identified: 1) Focus on certainty for now and this test; 2) providing a coherent account of the medical evidence for the risks and benefits (blurring the uncertainty); and 3) acknowledging inherent uncertainty of medical evidence and negotiating a provisional decision.
Hewson 1996 USA [32]	Process evaluation	Primary and secondary care/a range of clinical experiences (1st year residents to faculty physicians)	Primary and secondary care. 10 tapes of 9 physicians interacting with 4 standardized patient cases in phase one. 19 faculty physicians rating the strategies in phase two.	Clinicians reasoning and strategic medical management was rated using the "Medical checklist, Clinical Reasoning Skills Rating Scale, Interpersonal Skills Rating Scale & Strategic Medical Management Checklist".	Identification and frequency of strategies used by clinicians when faced with uncertainty	Behaviour patterns when clinicians are faced with diagnostic uncertainty (C) Patient communication and involvement with uncertainty (Eth).	Nine important strategies were identified: 1) defining the context of diagnosis and explaining symptoms; 2) eliminating alternative diagnoses; 3) describing the prognosis; 4) negotiating problems; 5) negotiating the plan of action; 6) keeping diagnostic options open; 7) cautious not to miss potential diagnoses; 8) appropriate time limited safety netting and 9) appropriate contingency planning.
Seaburn 2005 USA [33]	Observational study with 2 unannounced SP visits (thematic analysis)	Family practice / internists and family physicians	Community based primary care in a metropolitan area (n = 23); n = 46 interviews (the application of 7 codes from thematic analyses led to potentially >46 types of responses).	NA	NA	Greater knowledge about patient's life circumstances (C) Physician responses to ambiguous symptom presentations by patients (Eth)	Primary care physicians respond to ambiguity by either ignoring the ambiguity and becoming more directive (UC) or, less often, by acknowledging the ambiguity and attempting to explore symptoms and patient concerns in more detail (HP).
Sommers 2007 USA [34]	Intervention evaluation-thematic and frequency analysis	Primary care physicians/NS	Primary care (n = 14 practice sites, 98 clinicians with 118 patient cases)	Practice-based learning in small groups	Intervention "Practice Inquiry"	Not knowing enough about the patient and managing clinician-patient boundaries, expectations and trust (C + Eth) Using gut feelings (E)	Of the 30 sites approached between 2002 and 2005, 14 held introductory meetings and by summer 2006, 98 clinicians from 11 sites continued to hold regular Practice Inquiry group meetings suggesting the feasibility and acceptability of the intervention to clinicians.

SP Standardized patients, *NA* not applicable, *NS* not stated, *C* Cognitive *E* emotional, *Eth* ethical

Across the qualitative studies, two studies focused on the consideration of the individual patient and their unique biological, psychological and social situations whereby greater knowledge regarding the patient was one strategy by which diagnostic uncertainty could be reduced [30, 31]. Sommers et al. [34] reported how the vast majority of the clinical dilemma cases were categorized as such due to clinician-patient relationships and often involved simply "not knowing" on various fronts. Ensuring knowledge gaps were minimized and having access to a supportive environment with colleagues to reflect and build a trusting network were some of the suggested approaches to deal with cognitive uncertainty [34]. Three studies reported the use of appropriate safety netting techniques particularly using the 'test of time [13, 32, 34]. Finally, only one study provided a form of training platform to help clinicians deal with diagnostic uncertainty [34]. From 2001 to 2006, Sommers and colleagues developed small and voluntary practice-based learning groups to help clinicians deal and learn from real life case-based clinical uncertainties which included diagnostic uncertainties [34]. From the clinical group discussions of dilemma cases, clinicians were willing to reveal knowledge gaps, cognitive biases and unrealistic expectations, with the former two being associated to diagnostic uncertainties. The study demonstrated the value and usefulness of such voluntary learning groups (particularly being with colleagues) as well as the feasibility and long term sustainability which resulted in 98 clinicians partaking across 11 sites for over a period of 5 years. However, the study did not report any effects of the intervention on the ability of the clinicians at an individual, or group level, to manage their uncertainties more effectively.

The results of four quantitative cross-sectional studies [4, 10, 29, 31] were consistent and complementary to the qualitative data. Evans and Trotter [4] found that the physician's epistemological stance (biomedical vs psychosocial model) can influence the cognitive thought processes ultimately impacting on how diagnostic uncertainty is managed. Nevalainen demonstrated how as part of their cognitive thought processes, younger GPs found electronic databases more useful than experienced GPs (100% (95% CI 95.8–100.0) vs. 93.7 (95% CI 85.8–97.9), (p = 0.018) [29]. In one study, Schneider and colleagues report how intolerance to uncertainty correlates with self-rated diagnostic activity such as the increased ordering of tests [10]. Finally, in another study, Schneider demonstrates how various personality traits from the Big Five inventory (BFI-K) are also associated with diagnostic reasoning (see Table 1) [31].

Emotional management of uncertainty

Eight of the studies also briefly alluded to different emotional precursors and responses to managing uncertainty [4, 10, 13, 29–32, 34].

Accepting diagnostic uncertainty as an inevitable part of general practice and going with a provisional decision including using intuition and gut feelings was one strategy discussed across several qualitative and cross-sectional studies [10, 13, 31, 32, 34]. Cross-sectional studies also provided additional interesting findings in relation to the emotional management of diagnostic uncertainty. Cooke [30] demonstrated that positive states in physicians such as resilience, is associated with higher levels of compassion satisfaction and personal meaning in patient care. Conversely, low resilience correlated with secondary traumatic stress, inhibitory anxiety, general intolerance to uncertainty and concerns about bad outcomes. In a similar survey administering the "anxiety due to uncertainty" and "concern about bad outcomes" scales; Evans and colleagues [4] found that a biomedical epistemology is associated with more stress reactions to diagnostic uncertainty whilst a psychosocial epistemology is associated with less stress reactions to diagnostic uncertainty. In another survey, Schneider [10] suggests that affective reactions to diagnostic uncertainty may have a consistent emotional and behavioral dimension to it. They also go on to suggest that anxiety may exert gender specific reactions to diagnostic uncertainty in different ways. Female GPs stated higher anxiety due to diagnostic uncertainty ($P < 0.01$) resulting in the use of more primary care heuristics. Male GPs with higher anxiety due to diagnostic uncertainty on the other hand used fewer primary care heuristics and increased test ordering [10]. Nevalainen and colleagues [29] report that experienced GPs tolerate diagnostic uncertainty better than their less experienced counterparts with younger GPs more frequently expressed fears of committing medical errors. They also demonstrate that experienced and less experienced GPs differ with their specific coping strategies. For example experienced GPs were more likely to apologize to the patient about a medical error while their less experienced counterparts were more likely to discuss errors with colleagues instead. Finally, in a more recent survey, Schneider and colleagues [31] demonstrated how individual personality traits from the Big 5 Inventory (neuroticism, extraversion, openness, agreeableness, conscientiousness) were positively associated with diagnostic reasoning techniques as well as communication with patients. For example, physicians scoring high in neuroticism showed more anxiety due to diagnostic uncertainty whereas extraversion, conscientiousness and openness correlated negatively with anxiety due to diagnostic uncertainty [31].

Ethical management of uncertainty

Eight studies highlighted ethical aspects of diagnostic uncertainty management [6, 13, 29–34].

Across the cross-sectional studies, Portnoy [6] demonstrated that physicians' perceptions of their patients' responses to ambiguity influenced their decisions to share that ambiguity. Physicians who thought that more of their patients would have negative reactions to ambiguous information were more likely to decide what's best for the patient (p = 0.013) and to withhold an intervention that had diagnostic uncertainty associated with it (p = <0.001). Nevalainen [29] reported a reluctance to disclose uncertainty and medical errors to patients by less experienced GPs and how experienced GPs were more likely to discuss diagnostic errors with patients [29]. Moreover, in a cross-sectional quantitative survey of Australian registrars [30], showed that intolerance of uncertainty (which included diagnostic uncertainty) and reluctance to disclose uncertainty to patients were associated with a higher degree of burnout [30]. Similarly, Schneider [31] illustrated how GPs scoring high in neuroticism had a higher reluctance to communicate their uncertainties with patients and extraversion, conscientiousness and openness correlated negatively with patient communication [31]. Moreover, Seaburn and colleagues [33] using the quantitative data collected as part of their observational study, identified two distinct responses to diagnostic uncertainty. In a small proportion of GP consultations, GPs avoided acknowledging diagnostic uncertainty or uniformly denied uncertainty (n = 13; 22%). Their responses often involved premature and multiple diagnoses, the inability to respond directly to patient questions and concerns, arriving at treatment plans with little or no shared decision-making and occasionally communicating in a way that ignored the patient's concerns. A greater proportion of GPs acknowledged uncertainty in their consultations (n = 48; 77%). They spent more time gathering information, offered support in the form of empathy and completed the examination prior to suggesting potential diagnoses and the diagnostic uncertainties associated with them [33].

The negative impact of failures on disclosing diagnostic uncertainty has also been evident in the qualitative data. Sommers [34] demonstrated how recurring relationship dilemmas between the GP and patient contributed to uncertainties (which included diagnostic uncertainties) amongst their cases. They included negotiating clinician–patient boundaries, aligning patient–clinician expectations and establishing trust with the patient. Finally, Hewson [32] and Griffiths [13] go on to provide a comprehensive account of key skills and strategies (see Table 2) necessary to help manage uncertainty but highlight the need for a more patient-centered approach to managing uncertainty which includes improved communication and attending to patient concerns and fears.

Discussion

Summary

This review has provided an overview of the existing empirical literature on managing diagnostic uncertainty in primary medical care. In total, ten studies were identified as meeting the inclusion criteria and indicate that of the existing work in this area, studies have predominantly focused on traits associated with or internal resources of primary medical care clinicians for managing diagnostic uncertainty. Due to the heterogeneity, low quality (which was 1) with respect to the hierarchy of evidence and 2) moderate in terms of their conduct); and paucity of studies in this area, it is unclear however which types of internal resources are most effective for managing diagnostic uncertainty and which domains of uncertainty are most troublesome and/or amenable to intervention. Furthermore, only one external resource/intervention was identified, a training programme, which although acceptable to clinicians reported no evidence on its effectiveness in helping clinicians to better manage their diagnostic uncertainties.

Clinicians in primary care manage and deal with diagnostic uncertainty in a wide variety of ways. As a platform for work in this area, we have categorized the exiting literature on managing diagnostic uncertainty into three domains: cognitive, emotional and ethical domains. By categorizing these elements of diagnostic uncertainty, researchers, medical educators and clinicians may be able to better conceptualize the various components of diagnostic uncertainty enabling them to have an improved awareness of their existence, their potential impact(s) and ultimately to address them. We now briefly discuss some of the issues in each of these domains.

In the ethical domain, there is a need to balance paternalism and truly shared decision-making [12]. Deciding on the level of detail to communicate, finding appropriate descriptors to explain the diagnostic decision and risk – all in the context of infinitely varying degrees of patient expectations and understanding makes the process and unenviable task. This is further exacerbated with few guidelines or tools existing to help clinicians communicate diagnostic uncertainties with their patients. Despite the difficulties, in order to involve the patient in shared decision making, it is essential to share uncertainties with patients regardless of how difficult the clinician may perceive the task to be. A transparent consultation is morally and ethically obligated, is more likely to engage with the patient and lead to better outcomes for the patient and clinician [35]. Indeed, although there are well established tools for assessing communication in health care, none of these are focused primarily on discussions around diagnosis [36].

In the emotional domain, clinicians need to have an increased self-awareness of their own emotional responses to diagnostic uncertainty [37] as well as the potential influence of their individual characteristics and personality traits which may influence how they manage and perceive uncertainty. However, the lack of formal support mechanisms to help clinicians cope with the emotional drain of dealing with diagnostic uncertainties is of particular concern. Indeed, clinicians' maladaptive responses to uncertainty contribute to work-related stress [38]. More than two decades ago, Young and Spencer [39] argued for formal structured stress and emotional support for GPs and there appears to have been little progress. It would appear that one of the primary avenues for such support in the UK presents in the form of Balint Groups [40], the purpose and aims of which closely resembles the article by Sommers [34].

In the cognitive domain, most research and practice has focused on attempting to aid the cognitive aspects of diagnosis via the development and use of decision aids [41], differential diagnostic (DDX) generator tools [24] or diagnostic guidelines [42]. It is unclear however whether such approaches have succeeded in reducing uncertainty [43]. Furthermore, even the apparent cognitive clarity of dichotomous, quantitative diagnostic tests, may do little to alleviate any diagnostic uncertainty in an environment as messy as primary care where much diagnostic information is lost, as disease prevalence is low and the accuracy of the test is poor [44].

Finally, although we have categorized the included studies into three separate domains of diagnostic uncertainty, as the studies illustrate, the domains are often related and uncertainty is experienced across all or some domains for different individuals and in different scenarios. No studies have attempted to look at this variation.

Research and policy implications

Clinicians are aware in their everyday practice of the inevitability of diagnostic uncertainties yet the culture of medicine promotes the appearance of certainty, believing it to be for the good of the science, patients and the system. However, as we have discussed, clinicians' maladaptive responses to diagnostic uncertainty have implications for clinicians themselves, their patients and the health system they work in. Therefore an essential first step must be the acknowledgment and acceptance of the inevitability of diagnostic uncertainties in an area of medicine such as primary medical care [21]. Medical students, trainees and qualified clinicians should be taught to expect diagnostic uncertainty to be part of their work and then ways of effectively managing the various aspects of that uncertainty. Specifically, teaching clinicians to recognize which domains(s) of uncertainty is affecting them at that particular time point and giving them the skills to manage that particular issue/level is paramount. Indeed, we argue that nationally and internationally, all medical curricula be embedded with specific components focusing on managing diagnostic uncertainty and uncertainty more widely, in order to allow prospective doctors to identify which of the domains they are experiencing, when and how to effectively manage those uncertainties. At present it is not particularly a focus for medical education curricula or continuing medical education (CME) [45] and this needs to change. The problem here however, as our review has demonstrated, is that the educational knowledge and training programs required to do this and the good quality research underpinning them, is lacking. Some work has been done on managing uncertainty in medicine more generally [46, 47] but it is not clear if this work is transferable to diagnostic uncertainty, and what if anything is unique about diagnostic uncertainty as opposed to other aspects of uncertainty in medicine. Although changes across CME and medical education curricula could aid both trainee and experienced GPs, it is also unclear to what extent, in which ways, and which groups, if any, would benefit from training in managing diagnostic uncertainty. Some evidence from studies included in this review suggested that physicians with low clinical experience might encounter more difficulties coping with medical errors and diagnostic uncertainty compared to experienced physicians [29]. Future studies aiming to explore the relationship between physician experience and physician outcomes such as burnout would be of clear interest here.

Finally, other possible solutions to managing diagnostic uncertainty exist. For example, the use of DDX tools for cognitive aspects of diagnostic uncertainty, there is no evidence to say whether DDX tools do in fact do this. The research in this area appears to have focused on the diagnostic accuracy of the tools [24, 48, 49] rather than the *impact* of the tools and their use on the diagnostic uncertainty experienced by the clinicians themselves. For example, does the confirmation of the appearance of a clinician's working diagnosis, in the differential list generated by a DDX tool help to reduce cognitive uncertainty? One could hypothesize that the opposite is true given that the lists can be expansive. Furthermore, even if these tools help clinicians manage diagnostic uncertainty, it is unclear whether this is a more effective approach than training clinicians in different approaches to managing the various types of diagnostic uncertainty. A clear potential initial avenue for research in this area therefore, is to assess the effectiveness of currently available solutions such as DDX tools and to develop methods, tools and/or training programs which aim to teach clinicians to effectively manage diagnostic uncertainty in each of the uncertainty domains. In summary, the scope of research in this area is vast and here we have simply made some initial suggestions of areas for exploration.

Strengths and limitations

This systematic critical review had several strengths. It constitutes the first attempt to identify and conceptualize the available literature on managing diagnostic uncertainty in general practice as well as that literature into relevant domains which provides a systematic framework for the development of comprehensive interventions directed at managing or reducing diagnostic uncertainty.

We published our study protocol a priori in PROSPERO. Abstract and full paper screening were independently conducted by two authors with a high degree of inter-rater reliability and the study eligibility criteria in terms of study designs were broad and allowed flexibility to include a wide range of studies. Conversely, the significant heterogeneity, the low-moderate critical appraisal ratings and the limited number of studies retrieved, whilst demonstrating the lack of empirical studies on the topic area were a limitation and as such the findings need to be interpreted with this in mind. Moreover, the aims and objectives of the included studies were not always directly addressing our research question but were focused on the broader area of diagnostic uncertainty that met our inclusion criteria. As such there is the potential risk of reporting bias within the primary studies. For example, a survey may not have included and/or reported on all the three levels of interest to us as it was not part of their objectives.

Conclusions

Primary medical care clinicians are routinely exposed to diagnostic uncertainty. Despite the documented influence on the individual clinicians, their patients and the healthcare systems they work in, this review has demonstrated that the empirical evidence on managing diagnostic uncertainty is extremely limited and of moderate quality. Existing attempts to deal with diagnostic uncertainty have been focused on how to reduce it, rather than training physicians in how to manage or tolerate it. However, if we accept that diagnostic uncertainty is inevitable in primary care, training physicians on how to manage uncertainty at a cognitive, emotional, and ethical domain, will safeguard the quality and cost-effectiveness of the care they will provide. The three levels of diagnostic uncertainty discussed in this review are helpful in providing a platform for the development of such training and further research in this area.

What is already known on this topic

Clinicians in primary medical care are routinely confronted with diagnostic uncertainties. Intolerance to diagnostic uncertainty is increasingly acknowledged to have negative implications for the primary care practitioner, their patients and the wider healthcare system. However no reviews to date have summarized the existing empirical literature on how diagnostic uncertainty manifests and is managed.

What this study adds

This is the first review to summarise and conceptualise the existing empirical literature on managing diagnostic uncertainty in primary medical care. Included studies were categorized into three domains (cognitive, emotional and ethical) in order to provide a conceptual basis for the development of future theory based interventions. Finally, these domains are not mutually exclusive, in fact are seemingly often related and all have the potential to impact on the primary care practitioner, their patients and the wider healthcare system if not effectively managed. We propose that these three domain form the basis for future research and what form that research should take, in learning how to manage diagnostic uncertainty in primary medical care.

Abbreviations

BFI-K: Big Five inventory; CASP: The Critical Appraisal Skills Programme checklist; CI: Confidence interval; CME: Continuing medical education; DDx: Differential diagnosis; GPs: General Practitioners; MeSH: Medical subject headings; NHS: National Health Service; NPSA: National Patient Safety Agency; PRISMA: Preferred Reporting Items for Systematic Reviews and Meta-Analyses

Acknowledgements

The authors would like to thanks Dr. Avril Danczak for taking the time to review the manuscript.

Funding

This research was funded by the National Institute for Health Research (NIHR) Greater Manchester Primary Care Patient Safety Translational Research Centre. The views expressed are those of the author(s) and not necessarily those of the NHS, the NIHR or the Department of Health, Grant number: GMPSTRC-2012-1.

Authors' contributions

AE & SC are the guarantors of this article. RA, EP, SCS, AE and SC conceived and designed the study. RA and EP were involved with data acquisition and screening. RA, SCS, MP and EP undertook data extraction and analyses and RA, MP, EP and SCS were involved with interpretation and initial drafting of the manuscript. All authors had full access to all of the data and take responsibility for the integrity of the data and the accuracy of the analysis. All authors critically revised the manuscript and provided important intellectual content. All authors read and approved the final manuscript.

Consent for publication

Not applicable.

Competing interests

All authors have completed the Unified Competing Interest form at www.icmje.org/coi_disclosure.pdf (available on request from the corresponding author) and declare that (1) RA, EP, MP, SCS, AE and SC have no support from any organizations for the submitted work; (2) RA, EP, MP, SCS, AE and SC have no relationships with any companies that might have an interest in the submitted work in the previous 3 years; (3) their spouses, partners, or children have no financial relationships that may be relevant to the submitted work; and (4) RA, EP, MP, SCS, AE and SC have no non-financial interests that may be relevant to the submitted work.

Author details

[1]NIHR Greater Manchester Primary Care Patient Safety Translational Research Centre (Greater Manchester PSTRC), The University of Manchester, Williamson Building, Oxford Road, Manchester M13 9PL, UK. [2]Centre for Research and Action in Public Health, University of Canberra, ACT 2601, Australia. [3]Medical School, Department Social Medicine, Aristotle University, Thessaloniki, Greece.

References

1. Graber ML, Kissam S, Payne VL, Meyer A, Sorensen A, Lenfestey N, Tant E, Henriksen K, LaBresh K, Singh H. Cognitive interventions to reduce diagnostic error: a narrative review. BMJ Qual Saf. 2012;21:535–57.
2. Bowman D, Spicer J. Should doctors observe a moral duty to care for themselves? In primary care ethics. Oxford: Radcliffe publishing; 2007.
3. Heath I, Sweeney K. Medical generalists: connecting the map and the territory. BMJ British Med J. 2005;331:1462–4.
4. Evans L, Trotter DR. Epistemology and uncertainty in primary care: an exploratory study. Fam Med. 2009;41:319–26.
5. Kaplan SH, Greenfield S, Gandek B, Rogers WH, Ware JE Jr. Characteristics of physicians with participatory decision-making styles. Ann Intern Med. 1996;124:497–504.
6. Portnoy DB, Han PK, Ferrer RA, Klein WM, Clauser SB. Physician' attitudes about communicating and managing scientific uncertainty differ by perceived ambiguity aversion of their patients. Health Expect. 2011;16:362–72.
7. Beresford EB. Uncertainty and the shaping of medical decisions. Hast Cent Rep. 1991;21:6–11.
8. O'Riordan M, Dahinden A, Akturk Z, Ortiz JM, Dagdeviren N, Elwyn G, Micallef A, Murtonen M, Samuelson M, Struk P, et al. Dealing with uncertainty in general practice: an essential skill for the general practitioner. Qual Prim Care. 2011;19:175–81.
9. Berner ES, Graber ML. Overconfidence as a cause of diagnostic error in medicine. Am J Med. 2008;121:S2–23.
10. Schneider A, Lowe B, Barie S, Joos S, Engeser P, Szecsenyi J. How do primary care doctors deal with uncertainty in making diagnostic decisions?: the development of the 'Dealing with uncertainty Questionnaire' (DUQ). J Eval Clin Pract. 2010;16:431–7.
11. Gerrity MS, White KP, DeVellis RF, Dittus RS. Physicians' reactions to uncertainty: refining the constructs and scales. Motiv Emot. 1995;19:175–91.
12. Than MP, Flaws DF. Communicating diagnostic uncertainties to patients: the problems of explaining unclear diagnosis and risk. Evid Based Med. 2009;14:66–7.
13. Griffiths F, Green E, Tsouroufli M. The nature of medical evidence and its inherent uncertainty for the clinical consultation: qualitative study. BMJ. 2005;330:511.
14. Politi MC, Han PKJ, Col NF. Communicating the uncertainty of harms and benefits of medical interventions. Med Decis Mak. 2007;27:681–95.
15. Braddock CH 3rd, Edwards KA, Hasenberg NM, Laidley TL, Levinson W. Informed decision making in outpatient practice: time to get back to basics. JAMA. 1999;282:2313–20.
16. Pearson SD, Goldman L, Orav EJ, Guadagnoli E, Garcia TB, Johnson PA, Lee TH. Triage decisions for emergency department patients with chest pain: do physicians' risk attitudes make the difference? J Gen Intern Med. 1995;10:557–64.
17. Fiscella K, Franks P, Gold MR, Clancy CM. Inequality in quality: addressing socioeconomic, racial, and ethnic disparities in health care. JAMA. 2000; 283:2579–84.
18. Tsiga E, Panagopoulou E: Risking your health while saving lives? In ICPH International Conference on Physician Health: Milestones and Transitions-Maintaining the Balance. London; 2014.
19. Allison JJ, Kiefe CI, Cook EF, Gerrity MS, Orav EJ, Centor R. The association of physician attitudes about uncertainty and risk taking with resource use in a Medicare HMO. Med Decis Mak. 1998;18:320–9.
20. Rogers M, Todd C. Information exchange in oncology outpatient clinics: source, valence and uncertainty. Psychooncology. 2002;11:336–45.
21. Simpkin AL, Schwartzstein RM. Tolerating uncertainty — the next medical revolution? N Engl J Med. 2016;375:1713–5.
22. Moher D, Liberati A, Tetzlaff J, Altman DG. PRISMA Group. Preferred reporting items for systematic reviews and meta-analyses: the PRISMA statement. Ann Intern Med. 2009;151(4):264-9.
23. Zaat JO, van Eijk JT. General practitioners' uncertainty, risk preference, and use of laboratory tests. Med Care. 1992;30:846–54.
24. Riches N, Panagioti M, Alam R, Cheraghi-Sohi S, Campbell S, Esmail A, Bower P. The effectiveness of electronic differential diagnoses (DDX) generators: a systematic review and meta-analysis. PLoS One. 2016;11: e0148991. doi:10.1371/journal.pone.0148991.
25. McHugh ML. Interrater reliability: the kappa statistic. Biochemia Medica. 2012;22:276–82.
26. CASP: Critical Appraisal Skills Programme (CASP). CASP Checklists http://www.casp-uk.net/. Oxford. 2014. Last Accessed Feb 2017.
27. Wells G, Brodsky L, O'Connell D, Shea B, Henry D, Mayank S, Tugwell P. Evaluation of the Newcastle-Ottawa scale (NOS): an assessment tool for evaluating the quality of non-randomized studies. In: XI Cochrane colloquium: evidence, health care and culture. Spain: Barcelona; 2003.
28. Grant MJ, Booth A. A typology of reviews: an analysis of 14 review types and associated methodologies. Health Inf Libr J. 2009;26:91–108.
29. Nevalainen M, Kuikka L, Pitkala K. Medical errors and uncertainty in primary healthcare: a comparative study of coping strategies among young and experienced GPs. Scand J Prim Health Care. 2014;32:84–9.
30. Cooke GP, Doust JA, Steele MC. A survey of resilience, burnout, and tolerance of uncertainty in Australian general practice registrars. BMC Med Educ. 2013;13:1–6.
31. Schneider A, Wubken M, Linde K, Buhner M. Communicating and dealing with uncertainty in general practice: the association with neuroticism. PLoS One. 2014;9:7.
32. Hewson MG, Kindy PJ, Van Kirk J, Gennis VA, Day RP. Strategies for managing uncertainty and complexity. J Gen Intern Med. 1996;11:481–5.
33. Seaburn DB, Morse D, McDaniel SH, Beckman H, Silberman J, Epstein R. Physician responses to ambiguous patient symptoms. J Gen Intern Med. 2005;20:525–30.
34. Sommers LS, Morgan L, Johnson L, Yatabe K. Practice inquiry: clinical uncertainty as a focus for small-group learning and practice improvement. J Gen Intern Med. 2007;22:246–52.
35. Kennedy AG: Managing uncertainty in diagnostic practice. J Eval Clin Pract 2015; 21.
36. Singh H, Graber ML, Hofer TP. Measures to improve diagnostic safety in clinical practice. J Patient Saf. 2016; doi:10.1097/PTS.0000000000000338.
37. Guenter D, Fowler N, Lee L. Clinical uncertainty: helping our learners. Canadian Fam Phys Med de fam canadien. 2011;57:120–5.
38. Logan RL, Scott PJ. Uncertainty in clinical practice: implications for quality and costs of health care. Lancet. 1996;347:595–8.
39. Young G, Spencer J. General practitioners' views about the need for a stress support service. Fam Pract. 1996;13:517–21.
40. Fitzgerald G, Hunter MD. Organising and evaluating a Balint group for trainees in psychiatry. Psychiatr Bull. 2003;27:434–6.
41. Reisman Y. Computer-based clinical decision aids. A review of methods and assessment of systems. Med Inform (Lond). 1996;21:179–97.
42. NICE: Guidance and advice list. National institute for health and care excellence Available online at https://www.nice.org.uk/guidance/published?type=dg.
43. Armstrong N, Hilton P. Doing diagnosis: whether and how clinicians use a diagnostic tool of uncertain clinical utility. Soc Sci Med. 2014;120:208–14.
44. Shinkins B, Perera R. Diagnostic uncertainty: dichotomies are not the answer. Br J Gen Pract. 2013;63:122–3.
45. Ledford C, Seehusen D, Chessman A, Shokar N. How we teach US medical students to negotiate uncertainty in clinical care: a CERA study. Fam Med. 2015;47:31–6.
46. Danczak A, Lea A. What do you do when you don't know what to do? GP associates in training (AiT) and their experiences of uncertainty. Educ Prim Care. 2014;25:321–6.
47. Danczak A, Lea A, Murphy G. Mapping Uncertainty in Medicine. London: Royal College of General Practitioners; 2016.
48. Bond WF, Schwartz LM, Weaver KR, Levick D, Giuliano M, Graber ML. Differential diagnosis generators: an evaluation of currently available computer programs. J Gen Intern Med. 2012;27:213–9.
49. El-Kareh R, Hasan O, Schiff G. Use of health information technology to reduce diagnostic errors. BMJ Qual Saf. 2013;22:1–12.

3

Correlation between patients' reasons for encounters/health problems and population density in Japan: a systematic review of observational studies coded by the International Classification of Health Problems in Primary Care (ICHPPC) and the International Classification of Primary care (ICPC)

Makoto Kaneko[1,2*], Ryuichi Ohta[3], Naoki Nago[4], Motoharu Fukushi[4] and Masato Matsushima[2]

Abstract

Background: The Japanese health care system has yet to establish structured training for primary care physicians; therefore, physicians who received an internal medicine based training program continue to play a principal role in the primary care setting. To promote the development of a more efficient primary health care system, the assessment of its current status in regard to the spectrum of patients' reasons for encounters (RFEs) and health problems is an important step. Recognizing the proportions of patients' RFEs and health problems, which are not generally covered by an internist, can provide valuable information to promote the development of a primary care physician-centered system.

Methods: We conducted a systematic review in which we searched six databases (PubMed, the Cochrane Library, Google Scholar, Ichushi-Web, JDreamIII and CiNii) for observational studies in Japan coded by International Classification of Health Problems in Primary Care (ICHPPC) and International Classification of Primary Care (ICPC) up to March 2015. We employed population density as index of accessibility. We calculated Spearman's rank correlation coefficient to examine the correlation between the proportion of "non-internal medicine-related" RFEs and health problems in each study area in consideration of the population density.

Results: We found 17 studies with diverse designs and settings. Among these studies, "non-internal medicine-related" RFEs, which was not thought to be covered by internists, ranged from about 4% to 40%. In addition, "non-internal medicine-related" health problems ranged from about 10% to 40%. However, no significant correlation was found between population density and the proportion of "non-internal medicine-related" RFEs and health problems.
(Continued on next page)

* Correspondence: makotokaneko0314@gmail.com
[1]Musashikoganei Clinic, Japanese Health and Welfare Co-operative Federation, 1-15-9, Honcho, Koganei-shi, Tokyo 184-0004, Japan
[2]Division of Clinical Epidemiology, Jikei University School of Medicine, 3-25-8, Nishishimbashi, Minato-ku, Tokyo 105-8461, Japan
Full list of author information is available at the end of the article

(Continued from previous page)

Conclusions: This is the first systematic review on RFEs and health problems coded by ICHPPC and ICPC undertaken to reveal the diversity of health problems in Japanese primary care. These results suggest that primary care physicians in some rural areas of Japan need to be able to deal with "non-internal-medicine-related" RFEs and health problems, and that curriculum including practical non-internal medicine-related training is likely to be important.

Keywords: Primary care, Reasons for encounters (RFEs), International Classification of Primary Care (ICPC)

Background

In 2013, the Ministry of Health, Labour and Welfare highlighted the importance of the primary care physician in the rapidly aging society of Japan [1]. However, in Japan, a boundary between primary care and secondary care is ambiguous due to free-access system [2] and there are many specialist clinics (e.g., ophthalmological clinic) which deal with health problems of each discipline [3]. In addition, the Japanese health care system has yet to establish structured training for primary care physicians; therefore, physicians who received an internal medicine based training program continue to play a principal role in the primary care setting [3].

To promote the development of a more efficient primary health care system, the assessment of its current status in regard to the spectrum of patients' reasons for encounters (RFEs) and health problems is an important step [4]. However, the International Classification of Diseases 10th revision (ICD-10) does not include a classification for RFEs or the health problems of unsolved problems [5, 6], which makes it inconsistent with the primary care setting. Therefore, the International Classification of Primary Care 2nd edition (ICPC-2) is recommended for use in primary care[7]· Although several descriptive surveys utilizing ICPC-2 have been conducted in Japan [4], there has been no systematic review which target surveys using ICPC-2. For example, recognizing the proportions of patients' RFEs and health problems, which are not generally covered by an internist, can provide valuable information to promote the development of a primary care physician-centered system. In addition, Miyazaki presumed that the less accessibility patients have to a specialist clinic and/or a secondary care hospital, the more diverse their RFEs and health problems in the primary care setting [4].

This study aimed to describe the diversity of RFEs and health problems in Japanese settings of primary care. We also examined a correlation between the proportions of non-internal medicine related RFEs/health problems and population density as index of accessibility.

Methods

Study design

Systematic review.

Search strategy

In the present study, we followed the preferred reporting items for systematic reviews and meta-analyses (PRISMA) statement [8]. We searched six databases (PubMed, the Cochrane Library, Google Scholar, Ichushi-Web, JDreamIII and CiNii) for studies in Japan coded by ICHPPC and ICPC up to March 2015. The search strategy was based on the following title/abstract keywords in English and Japanese: ("ICPC" OR "ICPC-2" OR "ICHPPC" OR "International Classification of Primary Care" OR "International Classification of Primary Care-2" OR "International Classification of Health problem in Primary Care") AND ("Japan"). We also reviewed the reference lists of relevant studies to identify research that might have been missed in the database search.

Ichushi-Web is an online Japanese literature searching system provided by the non-profit Japan Medical Abstracts Society. Ichushi-Web covers about 10 million medical papers from 6000 journals in Japan, and is often used for Japanese literature searches [9].

JDreamIII (Japan Science and Technology Agency Document Retrieval System for Academic and Medical Fields) is an online Japanese literature searching system provided by the Japan Science and Technology Agency. JDreamIII covers about 60 million articles, including serial publications, reports, conference material, public documents and proceedings on science and technology [10].

CiNii is an online Japanese literature searching system provided by the National Institute of informatics. CiNii covers about 18 million articles focusing on natural and cultural science [11].

Inclusion and exclusion criteria

Literature searches and data extraction were independently conducted by two investigators (M.K. and R.O.), and any discrepancies were resolved by discussion. In the present study, databases were searched for observational studies in Japan coded by ICHPPC, ICHPPC-2, ICHPPC-2-Defined, ICPC and ICPC-2 classifications to evaluate the correlation between patients' RFEs and health problems and population density. Studies conducted in the hospital setting were excluded because the aim of the study was to clarify the spectrum of RFEs and health problems in primary care. Details of the inclusion criteria are shown in Table 1.

Table 1 Inclusion criteria

Study design	Observational study
Date of publication	Until March 31, 2015
Setting	Japan
	Clinic only (Hospital were excluded)
Methods	Coding RFEs or health problems using ICHPPC, ICHPPC-2,
	ICHPPC-2-Defined, ICPC and ICPC-2
Results	Frequency of RFEs and health problems

ICHPPC: International Classification of Health Problems in Primary Care
ICPC: International Classification of Primary Care
RFEs: reasons for encounters

The present study included the following classifications developed by the World Organization of National Colleges, Academies and Academic Associations of General Practitioners/Family Physicians (WONCA) [6]:

ICHPPC: Developed in 1975 to classify health problems in primary care. The classification was mapped to ICD-8.

ICHPPC-2: Developed in 1979 and mapped to ICD-9.

ICHPPC-2-Defined: Developed in 1983. Explanatory remarks were added with ICHPPC-2 to improve usability.

ICPC: Developed in 1987 to combine "Reasons for Encounter Classification (RFEC)" and "International Process in Primary Care (IC-Process-PC)" with the ICHPPC. The classification contained RFEs, including feelings of patients and interventions. The classification was mapped to ICD-10.

ICPC-2: Developed in 1998 and mapped to ICD-10. Explanatory remarks were added with ICPC. This classification is frequently used in primary care settings all over the world. It has been translated into 22 languages.

Studies that did not mention the frequency of RFEs and health problems, studies conducted in countries other than Japan, unpublished data, conference presentations, and conference minutes were all excluded from the present study.

Data extraction

Extracted information is shown in Table 2. In Japan, patients who have "non-internal medicine-related" RFEs tend to visit specialists as opposed to internists [3]. Therefore, a high percentage of "non-internal medicine-related" RFEs and health problems is thought to indicate the comprehensiveness of RFEs and health problems by the primary care physician. To clarify the comprehensiveness of RFEs in Japanese primary care settings, we calculated the proportions of"non-internal medicine-related RFEs" and "non-internal medicine-related health problems" among the top 20 RFEs and health problems in each study because most of included studies did not report the rank of RFEs and health problems more than the top 20.

Table 2 Data extraction

Data	Remarks
Year of publication	
Author	
Setting	The categories of setting are based on description in each included study
Study period	
Number of facilities	
Total number of patients	
Total number of encounters	
Total number of RFEs	
Total number of health problems	
Proportion of "non-internal medicine-related" RFEs in the top 20 RFEs	
Proportion of "non-internal medicine-related" health problems in the top 20 health problems	
Classification	ICHPPC/ICHPPC/ICHPPC -2-Defined
	ICPC/ICPC2
Primary outcome measures	RFEs (first visit, periodic visit) /health problems (acute, chronic)
Distinction between acute and chronic	
Quality of coding	Prospective or retrospective
	Single or multiple evaluator
	Description of coding training
Prospective or retrospective	
Number of evaluators	

RFEs: reasons for encounters
ICHPPC: International Classification of Health Problems in Primary Care
ICPC: International Classification of Primary Care

Eighteen categories of health problems in the ICHPPC: Among these categories, "I: Infective and parasitic," "II: Neoplasms," "III: Endocrine, nutritional and metabolic" "IV: Blood disease" "VI: Nervous system and sense organs," "VII: Circulatory system," "VII: Respiratory system," "IX: Digestive system," were defined as "internal medicine-related". In contrast, "V: Mental disorder," "X: Genitourinary system(including breast)," "XI: Pregnancy, childbirth and puerperium," "XII: Skin and subcutaneous tissue," "XIII: Musculoskeletal and connective tissue," "XIV: Congenital anomalies," "XV: Perinatal morbidity," "XVII: Injuries and adverse effects," were defined as "non-internal medicine-related". ("XVI: Signs, symptoms and ill-defined conditions," and "XVII: Supplementary" were excluded.)

Seventeen categories of RFEs and *health problems* in *the ICPC* (Table 3): Among these categories, "A: General and unspecified," "B: Blood. Blood-forming organs and

Table 3 Examples of ICPC

Category	Example
A: General and unspecified	A01 Pain general/A02 Chill/A03 Fever
B: Blood. Blood-forming organs and immune mechanism	B02 Lymph gland/B04 Blood symptom/B25 Fear of AIDS
D: Digestive	D01 Abdominal pain/D02 Abdominal pain epigastric/D03 Heartburn
F: Eye	F01 Eye pain/F02 Red eyes/F03 Eye discharge
H: Ear	H01 Ear pain/H02 Hearing complaint/H03 Tinnitus
K: Cardiovascular	K01 Heart pain/K02 Pressure/K03 Cardiovascular pain
L: Musculoskeletal	L01 Neck symptom/L02 Back symptom/L03 Low back symptom
N: Neurological	N01 Headache/N02 Face pain/N04 Restless legs
P: Psychological	P01 Feeling anxious/P02 Acute stress reaction/P03 Feeling depressed
R: Respiratory	R01 Pain respiratory system/R02 Shortness of breath/R03 Wheezing
S: Skin	S01 Pain of skin/S02 Pruritus/S03 Warts
T: Endocrine/Metabolic and Nutritional	T01 Excessive thirst/T02 Excessive appetite/T03 Loss of appetite
U: Urological	U01 Dysuria/U02 Urinary frequency/U04 Incontinence Urine
W: Pregnancy, Childbearing, Family planning	W01 Question of pregnancy/W02 Fear of pregnancy/W03 Antepartum bleeding
X: Female genital	X01 Genital pain female/X02 Menstrual period/X03 Intermenstrual pain
Y: Male genital	Y01 Pain penis/Y02 Pain in testis/Y03 Urethral discharge
Z: Social problems	Z01 Poverty/Z02 Food or water problem/Z03 Housing problem

ICPC: International Classification of Primary Care

immune mechanism," "D: Digestive," "K: Cardiovascular," "N: Neurological," "R: Respiratory" and "T: Endocrine/ Metabolic and Nutritional" were defined as "internal medicine-related". In contrast, "F: Eye," "H: Ear," "L: Musculoskeletal," "P: Psychological," "S: Skin," "U: Urological" "W: Pregnancy, Childbearing, Family Planning," "X: Female genital," "Y: Male genital" and "Z: Social problems" were defined as "non-internal medicine-related".

We were not able to find the definition on the distinction between "internal medicine-related" and "non-internal medicine-related" in the previous reports. Therefore, two of authors, (MM and MK), a Fellow of the Japanese Society of Internal Medicine and a Japan Primary Care Association certified family physician, discussed and defined this distinction for the study. In detail, we discussed which clinical speciality was mainly chosen by patients having the RFEs of each ICPC/ICHPPC- chapter under the situation that both internists and other specialists such as ophthalmologists were equally available. Also, we took into consideration whether an internist referred a patient to specialists.

Statistical analysis

Usual indicators of accessibility such as "Provider-to-population ratios", "Travel impedance to nearest provider" and "Average travel impedance to provider" [12] could not be evaluated from the studies conducted in the past and past census data. That was the reason why we employed population density as an index of accessibility, because population density can be used as an indicator of rurality [13]. We then calculated Spearman's rank correlation coefficient to examine the correlation between the proportion of "non-internal medicine-related" RFEs and health problems in each study area in consideration of the population density.

We calculated the population density in each study based on census data in the administrative district area from the year closest to the study period [14, 15].

Results

After searching through the titles and abstracts of 4275 publications, 17 eligible publications were identified (Fig. 1). Details about the included studies [16–32] are shown in Additional file 1: Table S1 and the characteristics of those studies are shown in Table 4.

In these studies, "non-internal medicine-related" RFEs, which was not thought to be covered by internists, varied from approximately 4% to 40%. In addition, "non-internal medicine-related" health problems varied from 10% to 40%. The proportion of "non-internal medicine-related" RFEs reached 41.4% in a study set in rural area. Moreover, the proportion of "non-internal medicine-related" health problems reached 45.4% in another study of rural setting.

The relationship between the proportion of "non-internal-medicine-related" RFEs among all RFEs and population density is shown in Fig. 2a, while that between "non-internal-medicine-related" health problems among all health problems and population density is

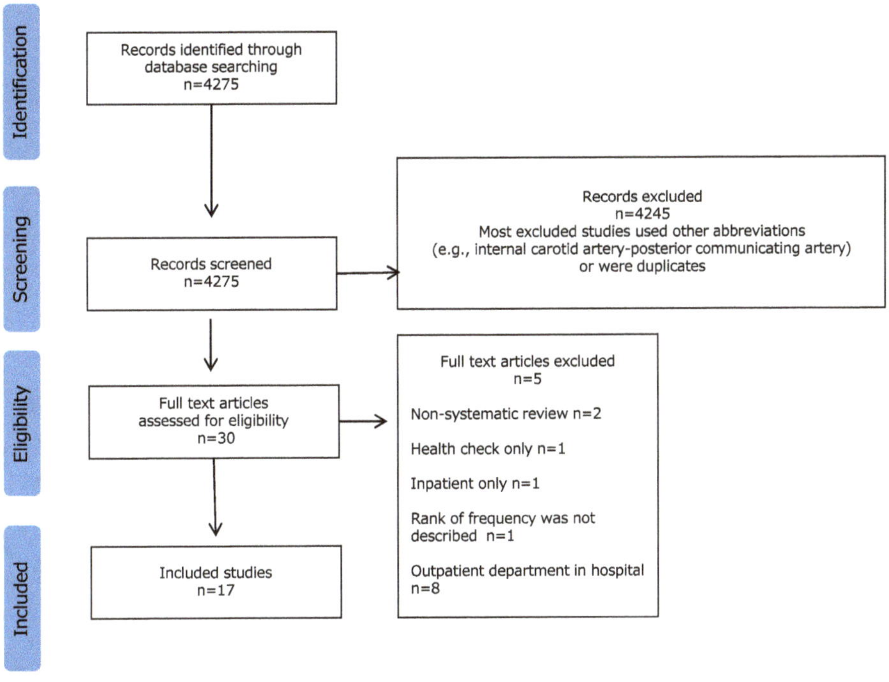

Fig. 1 Flow diagram for the selection of studies in the systematic review

shown in Fig. 2b. We used "RFEs in the first visit" for Fig. 2a and statistical analysis because most studies described only RFEs in the first visit. Five studies in which all health problems (all health problems: combination of acute and chronic health problems) had not been described were excluded from Figure2b and statistical analysis. We used Spearman's rank correlation coefficient to investigate for the presence of a dependence between RFEs/health problems and population density. In Fig. 2a, there seems to be negative correlation between proportion of non-internal medicine related RFEs and population density. However, no statistically significant correlations were found (p = 0.20): Spearman's rank correlation coefficient was −0.80 (95% Confidence Interval: −0.998 to 0.507). Also, the correlation between health problems and population density was not statistically significant (p = 0.74): Spearman's rank correlation coefficient was −0.14 (95% Confidence Interval: −0.678 to 0.729).

Discussion

The current systematic review detected 17 studies coded by ICHPPC and ICPC in Japan with diversity in both study design and settings.

In Japan, even in the primary-care setting, the proportion of "non-internal medicine-related" RFEs varies tremendously. In contrast, in other countries with an advanced primary care system, primary care physicians manage more "non-internal medicine-related" RFEs and health problems [33]. The differences between these countries and Japan in the proportion of RFEs are likely due to the Japanese free access system. In Japan, a patient can visit a specialist freely as a first encounter. A primary-care clinic located near a facility with a specialist does not need to manage "non-internal medicine-related" RFEs and health problems. For example, one of the included study [24] in urban area described the non-internal medicine related health problems were only 11.4%. However, in some studies in rural area, the percentage of "non-internal medicine-related" RFEs or health problems reached over 40% [20, 22, 25, 31]. Therefore, to refine and improve the educational system for aspiring generalists in Japan, curriculum with "non-internal medicine-related" practical training should be emphasized.

The shortage of studies in urban or suburban areas may partly explain the lack of a significant correlation between "non-internal medicine-related" RFEs/health problems and population density. For instance, most of the studies (13/17) using ICHPPC and ICPC were carried out in rural areas. In contrast, only two of the studies were conducted in an urban setting. In addition, only 2 studies described the evaluator's experience of attending ICPC-coding training program, though the quality of data collection is said to be important when using data from patient records such as ICPC [34]. Japanese primary care physicians might obtain more-precise picture by considering surveys in diverse areas and quality of methodology.

It is also important to note that far fewer Japanese studies use ICPC data for purposes such as health care

Table 4 Characteristics of included studies

	Total number (proportion %)
Eligible publications	17
Classification	
ICHPPC	1 (5.9)
ICHPPC-2-Defined	9 (52.9)
ICPC	5 (29.4)
ICPC-2	2 (11.8)
Study period	
< 1 year	4 (23.5)
1 year	10 (58.8)
> 1 year	2 (11.7)
Others: one study contained two study periods (2 years and 4 month)	1 (5.9)
Setting	
Urban clinic	1 (5.9)
Rural clinic	13 (76.5)
Comparison between	1 (76.5)
rural clinic, rural hospital and urban clinic	1 (5.9)
University hospital's affiliated primary care clinic	1 (5.9)
Number of facilities	
Single	12 (70.6)
Multiple	5 (29.4)
Study design	
Prospective	13 (76.5)
Retrospective	2 (15.4)
Prospective and retrospective	1 (5.9)
No description about study design	1 (5.9)
Number of evaluators	
1 person	11 (64.7)
≥ 2 persons	3 (17.6)
No description about number of evaluators	3 (17.6)
Quality of coding	
There are descriptions about quality of coding	2 (11.8)
There are no descriptions about quality of coding	15 (88.2)
Primary outcome measure	
Only RFEs	1 (5.9)
Only health problems	9 (52.9)
RFEs and health problems	7 (41.2)

ICHPPC: International Classification of Health Problems in Primary Care
ICPC: International Classification of Primary Care
RFEs: reasons for encounter

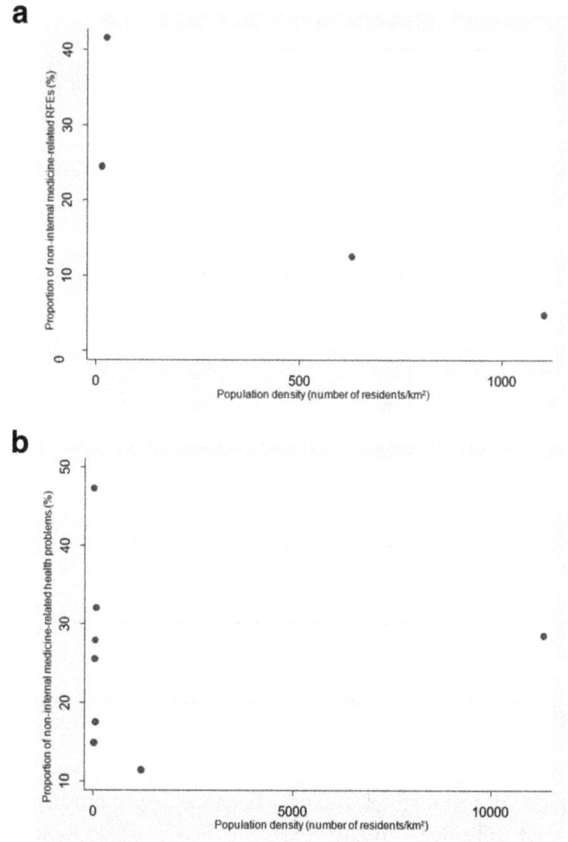

Fig. 2 **a** Proportion of "non-internal medicine-related" reasons for encounter (RFEs) among the top 20 RFEs and population density. We used "RFEs in the first visit" for the Figure because most studies described only RFEs in the first visit. **b** Proportion of "non-internal medicine-related" health problems among the top 20 health problems and population density. We included 8 studies in which all health problems (all health problems: combination of acute and chronic health problems) had been described

policy and medical education compared with other countries using ICPC data [32, 35–38]. For example, in the Netherlands, more than 300 studies have been conducted from the existing ICPC database [39].

The current study has some limitations. First, population density could only be measured retrospectively. It was not possible to consider detailed medical circumstances such as the existence of a nearby specialist clinic and/or the distance to a secondary care hospital. These factors likely had an impact on RFEs and health problems. Second, to ensure quality, only original articles published in peer-reviewed journals were included in the present systematic review. Conference presentations and unpublished articles that were excluded from this study may contain additional research conducted in urban areas or in multiple facilities. Third, unfortunately, the type of doctors (internist/primary care physicians) and the type of training were not described in the studies included by our systematic review. Fourth, the distinction between internal medicine and non-internal medicine was not judged based on actual patient behavior under the situation that the care by various specialists was easily available. The distinction was only based on the decision by the two of the authors. In addition, whether patients with non-internal medicine related RFEs/health problems choose primary care physicians or specialists, i.e. orthopedics might depend on type of training which a physician received (internist/primary care physician). If some internists in the researches included by our systematic review acquired the knowledge and skills of primary care physician by self-directed learning, however, the proportion of non-internal medicine related RFEs and health problems might be overestimated for internists in general.

Conclusions

In conclusion, the findings of review suggest that the ability to deal with "non-internal medicine-related" RFEs and health problems is required for primary care physicians in some rural areas of Japan. In addition, curriculum need to be combined with "non-internal medicine-related" practical training to foster aspiring generalists. We expect these findings to help facilitate improvements in the early stages of the educational system for generalists. More studies focusing on ICPC should be conducted in the future in order to better understand the current status of primary care in Japan.

Although the study was regionally limited, its result may suggest that a training system for primary care physicians to deal with a variety of RFEs and health problems is important even in countries not having gatekeeping function by primary care physician such as Japan.

Abbreviations

ICD: The International Classification of Diseases; ICHPPC: International Classification of Health Problems in Primary Care; ICPC: International Classification of Primary Care; WONCA: The World Organization of National Colleges, Academies and Academic Associations of General Practitioners/ Family Physicians, ; RFEs: Reasons for encounters

Acknowledgments

Not applicable.

Funding

The authors did not receive financial or other material support for the study

Consent to publish

Not applicable.

Authors' contributions

MK designed the study. MK and RO participated in the implementation, data collection, data analysis. MK took part in writing of the manuscript. MK also serves as guarantor. NN and MF supported data collection. MM analyzed the data and drafted the manuscript. All authors had full access to the data and take responsibility for the integrity of the data and accuracy of the analysis.

Author information

MK, MD., PhD
RO, MD.
NN, MD.
MF, MD.
MM, MD., PhD, MPH., Professor Division of Clinical Epidemiology

Competing interests

MM received the lecture fee and travel fee for lecture from Centre for Family Medicine Development (CFMD) of Japanese Health and Welfare Co-operative Federation. MM is an adviser of CFMD practice based research network. MM is a program director of Jikei Clinical Research Program for Primary-care. MK is a member of CFMD practice based research network. MK and RO were former trainees of Jikei Clinical Research Program for Primary-care. NN is a lecturer of Jikei Clinical Research Program for Primary-care. NN received the lecture fee and travel fee from Jikei University School of Medicine. There is no potential competing interest to be declared relevant to this work other than the above description.

Author details

[1]Musashikoganei Clinic, Japanese Health and Welfare Co-operative Federation, 1-15-9, Honcho, Koganei-shi, Tokyo 184-0004, Japan. [2]Division of Clinical Epidemiology, Jikei University School of Medicine, 3-25-8, Nishishimbashi, Minato-ku, Tokyo 105-8461, Japan. [3]Unnan City Hospital, Faculty of Community Care, 96-1, Iida, Daito-cho, Unnan city, Shimane 699-1221, Japan. [4]Musashi Kokubunji Park clinic, 2-16-34-127, Nishimoto-machi, Kokubunji-shi, Tokyo 185-0023, Japan.

References

1. Japanese Ministry of Health, Labour and Welfare. Report on the role of. specialists. [cited 2014 Jun 10] Available from: http://www.mhlw.go.jp/stf/shingi/2r985200000300ju-att/2r985200000300lb.pdf. (in Japanese).
2. Organization for Economic Co-operation and Development, OECD Reviews of Health Care Quality: Japan 2015 [cited 2017 Mar 31] Available from: http://www.oecd.org/publications/oecd-reviews-of-health-care-quality-japan-2015-9789264225817-en.htm.
3. Kusaba T. Comprehensiveness and education about common disease in outpatient care of primary care clinics. In: Yokobayashi K, editor. Recommendations: common disease in Japan generalist teachers consortium. Tokyo: Kai-shorin; 2013. p. 104–11. (in Japanese).
4. Miyazaki K. In: Yokobayashi K, editor. Common disease in adult patients. Tokyo: Kai-shorin: Recommendations: Common Disease in Japan Generalist Teachers Consortium; 2013. p. 88–97. (in Japanese).
5. Starfield B, Shi L, Macinko J. Contribution of primary care to health systems and health. Milbank Q. 2005;83:457–502.
6. Lamberts H, Wood M, Hofmans-Okkes IM. International primary care classifications: the effect of fifteen years of evolution. Fam Pract. 1992;9:330–9.
7. Soler JK, Okkes I, Wood M, Lamberts H. The coming of age of ICPC: celebrating the 21st birthday of the international classification of primary care. Fam Pract. 2008;25:312–7.
8. Moher D, Liberati A, Tetzlaff J, Altman DG. And the PRISMA group. Preferred reporting items for systematic reviews and meta-analyses: the PRISMA statement. Ann Intern Med. 2009;151(4):264–9.
9. Ichushi Web: About Ichushi Web. [cited 2014 Dec 18] Available from: http://www.jamas.or.jp/service/ichu/about.html. (in Japanese).
10. JDreamIII: About JDreamIII. [cited 2015 Jan 4]. Available from: http://jdream3.com/. (in Japanese).
11. CiNii Articles: About CiNii Articles. [cited 2015 Jan 4] Available from: http://ci.nii.ac.jp/. (in Japanese).
12. Mark F Guagliardo. Spatial accessibility of primary care: concepts, methods and challenges. International journal of health geographics. 2004; 3:3.
13. Bruce Minore, Mary Ellen Hill, Irene Pugliese and Tara Gauld. Rurality literature review. Centre for Rural and Northern Health Research, 2008. [cited 2017 Feb 23]. Available from: file:///C:/Users/makoto/Downloads/CRaNHR_NWLHIN_Rurality_FINAL_%20Feb.%2001,2008.pdf.

14. Ministry of Internal Affairs and Communications. National population census. [cited 2015 Nov 23]. Available from: http://www.stat.go.jp/data/kokusei/2015/.
15. Geospatial Information Authority of Japan. Statistical reports on the land area by prefectures and municipalities in Japan. [cited 2015 Nov 23] Available from: http://www.gsi.go.jp/KOKUJYOHO/MENCHO-title.htm. (in Japanese).
16. Miyahara S. Studies of common disease in rural districts. Japanese Journal of Primary Care. 1984;7:217–28. (in Japanese).
17. Toguchi T, Kimura H, Ueda F. Study about WHO-ICPC. Journal of Health and Welfare Statistics. 1985;32:16–23. (in Japanese).
18. Taketazu F, Ejiri T, Satoh T, Nagamatsu Y, Maezawa M. An analysis of patients of a clinic in a rural area in Japan-by using ICPHPPC-2-defined. Jichi Medical School Journal. 1995;8:157–64. (in Japanese).
19. K. Narato. What is common disease? The Japanese Journal of Family Medicine. 1988;4:339–44. (in Japanese).
20. T. Yamada. Medical aspects of elderly people in a mountain village. Japanese Journal of Primary Care. 1990;13:290–6. (in Japanese).
21. A. Ochi. Common disease in the Minami-Daito Islands. Japanese Journal of Primary Care. 1991;14:178–83. (in Japanese).
22. R. Kawamoto. Medical considerations for elderly people in rural areas. Ehime Medical Journal. 1992;11:39–45. (in Japanese).
23. Shiraishi Y, Kayaba K, Tsuruda K, Satho T, Hirata K, Kogure K, et al. Health problems treated by primary care physicians. Japanese Journal of Public Health. 1992;39:848–57. (in Japanese).
24. H. Shigemoto. Ambulatory medicine – An analysis based on the International Classification of Primary Care. Japanese Journal of Primary Care. 1994;17:148–57. (in Japanese).
25. R. Kawamoto. Health problems of elderly patients in a rural area. Japanese Journal of Geriatrics. 1994;31:38–44. (in Japanese).
26. Kunori T, Mori A. An analysis of health problems in Hokkaido prefectural clinic based on the international classification of primary care. Community Medicine. 1994;8:65–70. (in Japanese).
27. Yamada T, Mise J, Waza K, Igarashi M, Shigemot H. Application of ICPC to computer-based patient records. Japan Journal of Medical Informatics. 1997; 17:209–15. (in Japanese).
28. Waza K, Imai K, Onishi Y, Mise J, Igarashi M. A study on the reasons for encounters at the university hospital's affiliated community-oriented primary care clinic using ICPC. Japanese Journal of Primary Care. 2001;21: 182–90. (in Japanese).
29. Yamada T, Yoshimura M, Nago N, Asai Y, Koga Y, Inoue Y, et al. What is common disease and common health problem – the use of ICPC in a community-based project. Japanese Journal of Primary Care. 2000;23:80–9. (in Japanese).
30. Yamada T, Yoshimura M, Nago N, Inoue Y, Asai Y, Koga Y, et al. A study on the outcomes of health problems (the concept of "episode of care") based on clinical statistics using the international classification of primary care (ICPC). Japanese Journal of Primary Care. 2000;23:213–23.
31. Y. Morita, S. Kuroki, Alan Lefor, E. Kajii. Analysis of the reasons for visits to a clinic on an isolated island. General Medicine. 2012;13:30–6.
32. Kisa K, Kawabata H, Terashita T, Nakamura T, Maezawa M. Medical reimbursement receipt analysis to determine the relationship between disease type and patients' healthcare-seeking behavior. General Medicine. 2012;13:77–84.
33. Soler JK, Okkes I, Oskam S, van Boven K, Zivotic P, Jevtic M, et al. An international comparative family medicine study of the transition project data from the Netherlands, Malta and Serbia. Is family medicine an international discipline? Comparing diagnostic odds ratios across populations. Fam Pract. 2012;29:299–314.
34. Thiru K. Alan Hassey, and frank Sullivan. Systematic review of scope and quality of electronic patient record data in primary care BMJ. 2003; 326(7398):1070.
35. Yamamoto K, Hiraide A, Tomita N, Negoro S, Ito A, Kasahara A, et al. Experience of clinical practice during the student era at Osaka University medical school. Med Educ. 2000;31:17–21. (in Japanese).
36. Takeshima T, Kumada M, Mise J, Ishikawa Y, Yoshizawa H, Nakmura T, et al. Reasons for encounter and diagnosis of new patients at a small community hospital in Japan: an observational study. Int J Gen Med. 2014;7:259–69.
37. Tsukamoto T, Ohira Y, Noda K, Takada T, Uehara T, Ikusaka M. Investigation of diseases that cause diagnostic difficulty for Japanese general physicians. Asia Pacific Family Medicine. 2014;13:9.
38. Yamada M, Ishii K, Oda Y, Emura S, Koizumi S. The role of COOP/WONCA charts in predicting psychological distress in patients with medically unexplained symptoms and doctor-shopping behavior. General Medicine. 2006;7:9–14.
39. Transition Project Bibliography. [cited 2015 July 23] Available from: http://www.transhis.nl/language/nl/ (In Dutch).

4

Assessing and improving organizational readiness to implement substance use disorder treatment in primary care: findings from the SUMMIT study

Allison J. Ober[1*], Katherine E. Watkins[1], Sarah B. Hunter[1], Brett Ewing[1], Karen Lamp[2], Mimi Lind[2], Kirsten Becker[1], Keith Heinzerling[3], Karen C. Osilla[1], Allison L. Diamant[1,4] and Claude M. Setodji[1]

Abstract

Background: Millions of people with substance use disorders (SUDs) need, but do not receive, treatment. Delivering SUD treatment in primary care settings could increase access to treatment because most people visit their primary care doctors at least once a year, but evidence-based SUD treatments are underutilized in primary care settings. We used an organizational readiness intervention comprised of a cluster of implementation strategies to prepare a federally qualified health center to deliver SUD screening and evidence-based treatments (extended-release injectable naltrexone (XR-NTX) for alcohol use disorders, buprenorphine/naloxone (BUP/NX) for opioid use disorders and a brief motivational interviewing/cognitive behavioral –based psychotherapy for both disorders). This article reports the effects of the intervention on key implementation outcomes.

Methods: To assess changes in organizational readiness we conducted pre- and post-intervention surveys with prescribing medical providers, behavioral health providers and general clinic staff ($N = 69$). We report on changes in implementation outcomes: acceptability, perceptions of appropriateness and feasibility, and intention to adopt the evidence-based treatments. We used Wilcoxon signed rank tests to analyze pre- to post-intervention changes.

Results: After 18 months, prescribing medical providers agreed more that XR-NTX was easier to use for patients with alcohol use disorders than before the intervention, but their opinions about the effectiveness and ease of use of BUP/NX for patients with opioid use disorders did not improve. Prescribing medical providers also felt more strongly after the intervention that XR-NTX for alcohol use disorders was compatible with current practices. Opinions of general clinic staff about the appropriateness of SUD treatment in primary care improved significantly.

Conclusions: Consistent with implementation theory, we found that an organizational readiness implementation intervention enhanced perceptions in some domains of practice acceptability and appropriateness. Further research will assess whether these factors, which focus on individual staff readiness, change over time and ultimately predict adoption of SUD treatments in primary care.

Keywords: Implementation intervention, Organizational readiness, Evidence-based substance use disorder treatment, Primary care, Collaborative care, Care coordination, Medication-assisted treatment, Extended-release injectable naltrexone, Vivitrol®, Buprenorphine/naloxone, Suboxone®, Motivational interviewing

* Correspondence: ober@rand.org
[1]RAND Corporation, 1776 Main Street, Santa Monica, CA 90407, USA
Full list of author information is available at the end of the article

Background

Several evidence-based treatments for substance use disorders (SUDs)—medications in particular, but also brief therapy—are available and appropriate for delivery in primary care settings [1–7], but are underutilized [8–11]. Primary care is thought to be well-suited to provide SUD treatment because the prevalence of alcohol use disorders and use of illicit drugs is higher among primary care patients than in the general population due to comorbidity of SUDs with other illnesses that bring people into medical care [12, 13], and most individuals visit a primary care provider at least once a year [14]. Further, expanded coverage under the Patient Protection and Affordable Care Act (PPACA) has increased the number of individuals seeking medical care in primary care clinics in United States [15, 16]. Increasing identification of SUDs and availability of SUD treatment in primary care could increase access to treatment for millions of individuals who need but never receive treatment for a number of reasons, including low perceived need for treatment, lack of readiness, SUD-related stigma, or because speciality treatment centers lack the capacity to provide timely treatment [17–20]. Despite the potential benefits, few primary care providers have integrated treatment for SUDs into their practice.

Although there is little available data on barriers to the uptake of SUD treatment by primary care providers, some of the known barriers include lack of leadership buy-in for integrating SUD care into medical practices; lack of confidence among physicians in their own or their clinic's ability to treat SUDs; lack of adequate physician role models and access to decision support consultants; deficiencies in training and expertise in addiction treatment (i.e., workforce issues), Medicaid regulations that impede payment for the use of certain medications and same-day medical and mental health visits, and negative attitudes towards and biases against people with SUDs [21–26]. Other barriers common to the adoption of any new practice include perceived complexity and effectiveness of the new practice, perceived fit with and relevance to existing practices, and the feasibility of implementing the new practice [27], including inability to visualize how the new practice will fit into the existing workflow (i.e., lack of written protocols) [28–30]. Further, providers in primary care clinics face large workloads, imbalance between skills and increasing job demands, and lack of team support, all of which can lead to burnout and could impede organizational readiness for and implementation of new practices [31–33].

Organizational and behavioral change theories, such as Rogers' (1995) diffusion of innovation theory [27] and Bandura's (1977) theory of behavior change [34], posit that individuals' perceptions of the characteristics of new practices, their self-efficacy to implement the practices, and their perceptions of the capacity of their organization to implement the practices, are critical precursors of behavior change that support implementation. These precursors are often referred to in the organizational change literature as elements of "organizational readiness" [28, 29, 35–41]. Although definitions of organizational readiness vary widely, they have in common several key constructs, such as whether an organization's culture and climate are ready to make general changes (for example, organizations with stronger staff morale, less staff turnover, and openness to new practices in general typically are more likely to support implementation of new practices) [42–44], whether individual members view their organization as capable of change, or whether individual members are themselves prepared and willing to make a specific change or adopt a specific new practice [28, 43, 45]. Weiner et al. (2008) suggest that conceptualization of organizational readiness is most practical when it focuses on organization members' preparedness to implement intentional change, that is, whether individuals within an organization are psychologically and behaviorally prepared and willing to implement a specific new practice. Although some studies suggest an association between various organizational readiness constructs, including readiness of individuals as well as the culture and climate of their organizations, and adoption of new practices [46–49], no studies to date have examined the readiness of individual primary care clinic providers and other clinic staff to deliver treatment for SUDs.

To prepare a federally qualified health center (FQHC) in Los Angeles, California to deliver SUD screening and treatment to patients with opioid and alcohol use disorders (OAUDs), we employed a multi-faceted implementation intervention using a cluster of implementation strategies. FQHCs are community health clinics that receive support from the U.S. government to provide primary care and other services to medically underserved populations. We tested the intervention in a FQHC because FQHCs are responsible for delivering a large proportion of publicly funded primary care treatment in the U.S. We operationalized 'organizational readiness' as perceptions of the acceptability, appropriateness and feasibility of practices, and intentions to adopt the practices; these constructs are considered 'implementation outcomes' according to implementation researchers and theorists [27, 28, 34, 45, 50] and are based on organizational and behavioral change theory [27, 34, 50]. We focused on the treatment of OAUDs because there are FDA-approved medications to treat these disorders. Our full study design, which included an RCT phase where a collaborative care service delivery intervention was added 18 months after the start of the organizational readiness intervention, is described in the study protocol paper [51].

In this article, we describe the organizational readiness intervention and present pre- to post-intervention implementation outcomes after 18 months of the intervention and prior to the RCT. Some elements of the organizational readiness intervention, such as technical assistance and training of new staff, continued throughout the RCT. We hypothesized that the organizational readiness intervention would increase provider and staff acceptance and perceptions of appropriateness and feasibility of three evidence based SUD treatments—extended-release injectable naltrexone (XR-NTX) for alcohol use disorders, buprenorphine/naloxone (BUP/NX) for opioid use disorders, and a 6-session motivational interviewing/cognitive behavioral therapy (MI/CBT)-based psychotherapy for both disorders—and greater intention to adopt these treatments among the providers (i.e., physicians for the medications and therapists for the psychotherapy). XR-NTX is effective for people with alcohol or opioid disorders and also is feasible for delivery in primary care [52–56]; BUP/NX has been proven effective for patients with opioid use disorders and is feasible for delivery in office-based settings [1–7]; and MI/CBT-based therapies have shown efficacy in reducing substance use across settings [57–60]. For this study, prescribing medical providers were trained to deliver XR-NTX for alcohol use disorders only.

Methods

Study setting and participants

We conducted the study at a multi-site FQHC in Los Angeles, California. The FQHC's two largest adult-care sites, which serve approximately 20,000 low-income patients annually, were included in the study, and provide more than 106,000 primary care, specialty care, mental health, dental, and health education visits annually. Services include diagnosis, treatment, medications, follow-up care, and laboratory tests; prior to the study, the clinic did not provide screening or treatment for any SUDs. The sites were treated as a single site due to providers working across locations. Full-time staff working at the two clinics asked to participate in the survey consisted of 18 prescribing medical providers, 9 behavioral health providers, 42 medical assistants and 24 discharge coordinators (referred to as "general staff") in Year 1, and 18 prescribing medical providers, 9 behavioral providers, 43 medical assistants and 23 discharge coordinators in Year 2.

Organizational readiness implementation intervention

To enhance organizational readiness to provide evidence-based treatment for OAUDs, we employed multiple theory-based strategies hypothesized to increase adoption of evidence-based practices (EBP) in community organizations [28, 29, 41, 61–70]. The organizational readiness implementation intervention aimed to increase "behavioral and psychological willingness" to implement OAUD treatment in primary care among providers and staff [71].

The organizational readiness intervention consisted of six implementation strategies delivered over 18 months (see Fig. 1). The strategies fall within three key implementation process categories outlined by Powell et al. (2011): plan for change; educate at all levels; and restructure delivery systems [61].

Process category 1: Plan for change

Strategy 1: Convene a collaborative researcher-clinic implementation team [28, 64]

We convened an implementation team to engage and increase buy-in [64] from clinic leadership and staff. The core team consisted of key members of the research team (the Principal Investigator and co-Investigator, with other relevant researchers joining for some meetings to provide input on special topics) and the clinic medical director and behavioral health director. The full implementation team met bi-weekly and in-person during the first 18 months of the study and once a month during the RCT. A variety of key clinic leaders were periodically invited to attend the meeting, including the clinic Chief Operating Officer, the head of the clinic's call center (where all patient calls are received), and the nursing/medical assistant director. Core team members also conducted two briefings for the Chief Executive Officer to share updates on our implementation progress and our implementation intervention protocols—one at the organizational readiness intervention and another prior to the start of the pilot period.

Strategy 2: Assess barriers and resources and "present state" workflow [65, 66]

To assess barriers to and resources to deliver SUD treatment, we conducted focus groups with prescribing medical providers ($N = 9$) and behavioral health providers ($N = 8$), and semi-structured interviews with administrators ($N = 8$). Administrators included the Executive Director, Medical Director, Associate Medical Director, Behavioral Health Services Director, Nursing Supervisor, Case Manager Supervisor, Front Desk Supervisor, and Security Supervisor. To assess the "present state" workflow, we observed clinic procedures and interviewed multiple clinic leaders. We created detailed "present state" workflow diagrams to assess how SUD screening, assessment and treatment delivery would be incorporated (i.e., who would do what to whom, when, and where). In the interest of providing rapid feedback to the implementation team, we summarized key barriers identified in the focus groups and interviews and provided the summary to the team.

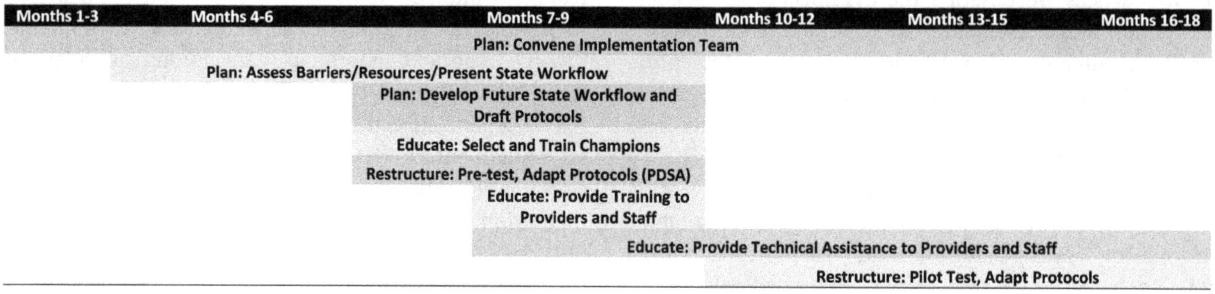

Fig. 1 Organizational readiness implementation intervention timeline

Strategy 3: Develop "future state" workflow and clinic-specific implementation protocols [28, 64]

Based on barriers identified during focus groups and interviews and on present state workflow diagrams, the research team drafted "future state" workflow and clinic-specific implementation protocols for each treatment. The implementation team then iterated until the workflow and protocols aligned with the clinic's practices and culture. The final "future state" workflow diagram and clinic-specific implementation protocols allowed staff to visualize how (when, where and by whom) the SUD treatments would be implemented [72–74].

Strategy 4: Select and train "champions" [64]

We selected and trained prescribing medical provider- and behavioral health- champions. A champion is a well-respected individual within an organization who is enthusiastic about a new practice and who can serve as a role model for adopting new practices [64]. The medical director (a primary care provider) and behavioral health director (a licensed clinical social worker), along with one additional primary care provider, became champions of the SUD treatments. An addiction medicine physician led the trainings for prescribing medical providers for both of the medications. Only physicians participated in the BUP/NX training, as nurse practitioners and physician assistants were not yet authorized to prescribe this medication. An MI/CBT-expert led the psychotherapy training. After receiving training, the two primary care providers began offering the two medications to eligible patients to identify barriers and to inform development of the clinic-specific protocols [72–74]. The behavioral health director did the same with the MI/CBT-based psychotherapy.

Process category 2: Educate at all levels

Strategy 5: Training and technical assistance [75–77]

We provided multiple trainings for prescribing medical providers, behavioral health providers, and general clinic staff on the SUD treatments. Trainings were tailored to specific staff roles within the organization and were as follows:

- All clinic providers, administrators, staff at all levels of the organization, and volunteers (approximately 100 staff members and clinic volunteers): A 30-min "all-staff" kick-off meeting that included an overview provided by the researchers of the significance of incorporating SUD treatment into primary care, a review of how clinic workflow would accommodate SUD treatment (i.e., the "future state" workflow), and a brief informative talk by a local, well-respected local psychologist who specializes in integration of SUD treatment in primary care;
- Prescribing medical providers: XR-NTX training consisting of 2.5 h of training for all prescribing medical providers (physicians, physician assistants, nurse practitioners) provided by an addiction medicine physician (7 participated in training during the first 18-months); "Provider's Clinical Support System for Medication-Assisted Treatment (PCSS-MAT)" training on BUP/NX, which required completion of a 3.75-h on-line module followed by 4.25 h of in-person training by an addiction medicine physician and receipt of the X-waiver[1] for BUP/NX prescribing (7 participated in training during the first 18-months);
- Behavioral health providers: A 1-h overview (8 participated in the first 18 months), plus 16 h of training on the MI/CBT-based brief therapy for licensed clinical social workers (LCSWs), conducted by a psychologist with expertise in MI and CBT (5 participated in the first 18 months).
- SUD care coordinators (2 care coordinators participated): 8 h of training on care coordination and motivational interviewing techniques provided by the researchers and the MI/CBT expert.
  The two care coordinators in this study were paraprofessionals who also had other responsibilities at the clinic;

- Nurse practitioners and physician assistants (3 and 2, respectively, participated in training during the first 18 months): 1 h of training on administering XR-NTX conducted by an addiction medicine physician;
- Clinic pharmacists and pharmacy technicians (4 and 3, respectively, participated): 1-h of training on medications to be provided to patients and pharmacy procedures for administering XR-NTX (BUP/NX was not provided by the clinic pharmacy), conducted by an addiction medicine physician.
- Medical assistants, call center staff, discharge coordinators: 1 h of training on SUD screening and referral procedures with two booster trainings and individual trainings for volunteers, who also conducted screenings, conducted by research staff.

We also provided ongoing technical assistance consisting of access to the addiction medicine physician and MI/CBT expert and ongoing support and monitoring of screening, referral and care coordination by research staff.

Process category 3: Restructure delivery systems

Strategy 6: Pre-test protocols using plan-do-study-act (PDSA) cycles, pilot test protocols, complete protocol adaptation

Soon after the treatment protocols were drafted, the champions began implementing the three treatments. That is, the two medical provider champions began to deliver XR-NTX and BUP/NX to eligible, interested patients and the behavioral health champion began providing the MI-based psychotherapy to eligible, interested patients. Although the designated champions initiated delivery, medication administration also involved nurse practitioners (to deliver XR-NTX injections) and pharmacy staff (to dispense and track XR-NTX). Throughout this process, the implementation team made iterative adaptations to the protocols using plan-do-study-act (PDSA) cycles [67–70], revising the protocols as feedback on implementation was received, and then repeating the cycle. PDSA cycles offer a structured approach to engaging staff in making iterative, feedback-based changes in service delivery [67, 68]. Adaptation of protocols helps ensure the fit of protocols within the organization and can lower resistance from individuals who will be affected by the change in delivery [29]. Of note, prior to the study, the clinic did not conduct screening for SUD, a sizable barrier to implementing treatment. Because the clinic needed to implement screening in order to identify patients with SUD, we included SUD screening in the future state clinic workflow and assisted in its adoption in a similar fashion as the other practices—we began with a screening protocol and tested and revised it using PDSA cycles. After all staff members were trained and protocols were developed (after 10 months of the organizational readiness intervention), we conducted an 8-month pilot study that involved screening and treating patients using draft protocols. Final protocol adaptations were made following the pilot.

Data collection procedures and measures

Procedures

For the present analysis, we used data from staff surveys conducted before the organizational readiness intervention was executed and 18-months later (and prior to the RCT) to assess changes in acceptability, perceptions of appropriateness and feasibility of, and intention to adopt SUD treatment during this period. The survey included previously developed measures, modifications of previously developed measures, as well as locally developed items. Surveys were web-based; for providers without access to clinic e-mail, we distributed paper and pencil surveys.

Measures

(1) *Acceptability*. Acceptability refers to satisfaction with the *complexity or ease of use* of a new practice and its effectiveness, or credibility [50]. To measure acceptability we adapted items from Moore and Benbasat's validated instrument [78] which measures items that parallel elements of successful diffusion of new practices [27]. Within the *acceptability* domain, we measured *ease of use* perceptions among prescribing medical providers (a two-item scale for each of the two medications) and behavioral health providers (the same two-item scale but pertaining to the MI/CBT-based psychotherapy). The two scale items were *"overall, I believe that extended-release injectable naltrexone [or other EBP] is easy to use," and "extended-release injectable naltrexone [or other EBP] is clear and understandable."* Response options ranged from 1, Extremely Disagree, to 7, Extremely Agree ($\alpha = 0.96$). We also included items from the National Center for Addiction and Substance Abuse's (CASA) National Survey of Primary Care Physicians and Patients on Substance Abuse [79]) that capture providers' opinions about the *effectiveness* of SUD EBP (one item per EBP) (response options ranged from 1, Not Effective, to 4, Very Effective), as well whether providers find it difficult to discuss SUDs with their patients (two items per EBP) (response options ranged from 1, Very Difficult, to 4, Not at all Difficult). **(2) *Appropriateness*.** Appropriateness refers to the compatibility of each EBP with current practices [50]. To measure compatibility of the EBPs with current practices we adapted an item from Moore and Benbasat for each EBP [78]. This item was *"I think buprenorphine/naloxone [or other EBP] will fit with the way I like to work."* Response options ranged from 1, Extremely Disagree, to 7, Extremely Agree. We also used locally-developed items to ask about whether providers and general staff believed SUDs could be effectively treated in primary care and the clinic itself, and also asked about fit with the clinic's mission and values (three items). Response options ranged from 1, Strongly Disagree, to 5, Strongly Agree. **(3) *Feasibility*.** Feasibility is the actual fit of an EBP within an organization [50]. We asked about feasibility using items from CASA's National Survey of Primary Care Physicians and Patients on Substance Abuse [79] that capture how prepared providers feel about identifying patients with alcohol use disorders (AUD) and opioid use disorders (OUD) (one item for AUD, one for prescription OUD, and one for street OUD/heroin) (response options ranged from 1, Not at all Prepared, to 5, Very Prepared). **(4) *Intent and/or willingness to adopt the EBP*.** To measure intention or willingness to adopt, we used the three-item "demonstrability" scale from Moore and Bensabet [78], which present statements such as "*I believe I can communicate to others the consequences of using extended-release injectable naltrexone [or other EBP].*" We also asked providers questions about whether they were willing to consider using each of the EBPs in their practice (e.g., *I would consider using buprenorphine/naloxone in my practice*). Note that for all variables that asked prescribing medical providers about medications, our pre-intervention survey items combined the two medications (XR-NTX and BUP/NX) and referred to "medication-assisted treatment (MAT) for OAUDs," as providers were not familiar with each medication. Our instructions for these items described the two medications and explained the indications of each; we use this measure as a proxy for the pre-intervention assessment of each medication. For our post-intervention measures, we asked questions about each medication separately. Post-intervention, all prescribing medical providers were asked about XR-NTX, and only physicians (not nurse practitioners or physician's assistants) were asked about BUP/NX because at the time of the survey only physicians were authorized to prescribe this medication.

Analysis

To measure changes between the two time points we conducted Wilcoxon signed rank tests. To adjust p-values for multiple tests, we used Benjamini and Hochberg false discovery rate (FDR) correction [80]. We examined responses by type of clinic staff. Due to staff turnover and post-intervention non-response, the sample size varied across variables and percentages are based on the total number of participants who responded both pre- and post-intervention. Due to the very small number of behavioral health providers who completed surveys at both time periods, we do not report on changes in behavioral health providers' perceptions.

Results

Participant characteristics

Fifteen of 18 (83%) prescribing medical providers, 8 of 9 (89%) behavioral health providers and 46 of 66 (70%) general clinic staff (medical assistants and clinic coordinators) completed the year 1 survey and 16 of 20 (80%) prescribing medical providers, 8 of 9 (89%) behavioral health providers and 46 of 66 (70%) general clinic staff completed the year 2 survey. Participating staff were mostly female (84%) and Hispanic (70%). More than half of the staff who responded (52%) had been in their current position at the clinic for more than 10 years (see Table 1).

Pre-post organizational readiness intervention results

Acceptability

As shown in Table 2, prescribing medical providers' perceptions of the acceptability of medication-assisted treatment were fairly low across most domains prior to the intervention execution, with mean scores for ease of use at 3.05 (all prescribing providers) and 2.94 (physicians only), on a 7-point scale (7 = strongly agree with statements about ease of use); mean effectiveness scores ranging from 2.33 to 2.9 on a 4-point scale (4 = very effective); and difficulty of discussing alcohol use and opioid use with patients at 3.25 and 2.67, respectively, on a 4-point scale (4 = not at all difficult).

Among all prescribing providers, ease of use of XR-NTX for alcohol use disorders changed significantly ($p < .05$) from pre- to post- intervention, with mean scores changing from 3.05 pre- to 4.77 post- intervention, with standard deviations of 1.29 and 1.23, respectively. Changes in perceptions of ease of use of BUP/NX did not change significantly, and mean scores were lower in after the intervention than XR-NTX ease of use scores. Perceptions of the effectiveness of medication for the treatment of alcohol use disorders improved, but changes were not significant after the FDR adjustment for multiple statistical tests. Perceptions of ease of use of BUP/NX and effectiveness of medication for opioid use disorders did not change significantly, but were similar to post-intervention mean scores for XR-NTX effectiveness. Prescribing medical providers' perceptions of the effectiveness of mental health counseling for either disorder was over the mid-point at both time points and did not change significantly.

Appropriateness

In the appropriateness domains, prescribing medical providers' perceptions of the compatibility of aspects of SUD treatment with primary care varied pre-intervention by the type of treatment, with the mean score for the fit of counseling for patients with alcohol and opioid use disorders at the clinic at 4.42 (the highest), the mean score for whether SUDs could be treated at this clinic at 2.83 (the lowest), on a scale from 1 to 5 (5 = strongly agree with statements about appropriateness in primary care). Among general clinic staff, pre-intervention scores were similar, with scores ranging from 2.94 (fit of providing

Table 1 Staff characteristics

	All staff			Medical providers		Behavioral health providers		Non-provider staff	
	N	Missing	Mean/%	N	Mean/%	N	Mean/%	N	Mean/%
Age	66	3	44.41	15	45.13	8	44.50	43	44.14
Female	56	13	83.58	13	86.67	5	62.50	38	86.36
Highest Education		2							
< High School/High School	9		13.43	0	0.00	1	12.50	8	18.18
Associates/Bachelor Degree	13		19.40	0	0.00	1	12.50	12	27.27
Doctoral	13		19.40	12	80.00	1	12.50	0	0.00
Masters	9		13.43	3	20.00	5	62.50	1	2.27
Other	9		13.43	0	0.00	0	0.00	9	20.45
Some College	14		20.90	0	0.00	0	0.00	14	31.82
Time at Current Position		2							
3–10 Years	19		28.36	4	26.67	3	37.50	12	27.27
< 3 Years	13		19.40	4	26.67	1	12.50	8	18.18
> 10 Years	35		52.24	7	46.67	4	50.00	24	54.55
Race/ethnicity		16							
White	12		22.64	9	75.00	1	16.67	2	5.71
Black	2		3.77	1	8.33	0	0	1	2.86
Asian	1		1.89	1	8.33	0	0	0	0
Hispanic/Latino	37		69.81	1	8.33	5	83.33	31	88.57
Other	1		1.89	0	0	0	0	1	2.86

medications to patients with OAUDs at this clinic) to 3.72 (fit of providing counseling to patients with OAUDs with clinic mission and goals), also on a 5-point scale. With regard to prescribing medical providers' perceptions of compatibility of MAT with current practices, mean scores were fairly low—3.36 among all prescribing providers and 3.13 among physicians only, on a scale from 1 to 7 (7 = strongly agree with statements about compatibility).

Prescribing medical providers agreed more post-intervention that SUDs could be treated in primary care settings (in general), with mean scores changing significantly ($p < .01$) on a scale from 1 to 5, with a 5 indicating strong agreement (M = 3.00, SD = .60 pre-intervention; M = 4.26, SD = .87 post-intervention). However, views about whether SUDs could be treated at this clinic did not change. Post-intervention, prescribing providers also thought XR-NTX was more compatible with their current practices than they did pre-intervention, with statistically significant ($p < .01$) changes in mean scores on a scale from 1 to 5, with 5 indicating a high degree of compatibility (M = 3.36, SD = 1.79 pre-intervention; M = 4.77, SD = 1.22, post-intervention); opinions of compatibility of BUP/NX with current practices, did not change significantly pre- and post-intervention. Prescribing medical providers' ratings of the fit of counseling for SUDs in primary care with the clinic's mission and goals were significantly ($p < .01$) lower post- intervention on a scale from 1 to 5, with a 5 indicating strong agreement with a statement about fit (M = 4.42, SD = .67 pre-intervention; M = 3.67, SD = .98 post-intervention).

Among general clinic staff, views about the appropriateness of SUD treatment changed significantly pre- to post-intervention ($p < .01$). Post-intervention, staff agreed more with statements suggesting that SUDs could be treated in primary care settings on a scale from 1 to 5, with 5 indicating strong agreement with the statement (M = 3.17, SD = 1.01 pre-intervention; M = 4.06, SD = .76 post-intervention), that SUDs could be effectively treated at this clinic (M = 3.17, SD.98 pre-intervention; M = 3.86, SD = .77 post-intervention), and that providing medications to patients with alcohol or opioid use disorders fit the mission and goals of the clinic (M = 2.94, SD = .97 pre-intervention; M = 3.89, SD = .76 post-intervention). General clinic staff perceptions that providing counseling to patients with alcohol and opioid use disorders fit the clinic's mission and goals was initially positive and did not change pre- to post-intervention.

Feasibility

Before the organizational readiness intervention, prescribing medical providers' mean scores on feeling prepared to identify patients with alcohol, heroin and prescription opioid use disorders were 3.0, 3.27 and 3.42, respectively, on a scale from 1 to 4 (4 = very prepared).

Table 2 Changes in organizational readiness to deliver SUD treatment in primary care

	Pre-Intervention			Post-Intervention			Difference		
	Mean	SD	Range	Mean	SD	Range	Mean	SD	*P*-value^
Acceptability									
Prescribing Medical Providers									
Ease of Use (Extremely Disagree = 1; Extremely Agree = 7)									
Ease of Use of XR-NTX (*N* = 11)†	3.05	1.29	1–4.5	4.77	1.23	3–7	1.73	1.69	0.012*
Ease of Use of BUP/NX (*N* = 9)†	2.94	1.40	1–4.5	2.50	1.09	1–4	−0.44	1.42	0.500
Effectiveness (Not Effective = 1; Very Effective = 4)									
… medical treatments for alcohol use disorders (*N* = 9)	2.33	0.71	1–3	3.22	0.44	3–4	0.89	0.78	0.031
… medical treatments for opioid use disorders (*N* = 9)	2.44	0.73	1–3	3.00	0.5	2–4	0.56	0.73	0.125
… mental health treatments for alcohol use disorders (*N* = 10)	2.90	0.74	2–4	3.20	0.42	3–4	0.30	0.67	0.193
… mental health treatments for opioid use disorders (*N* = 10)	2.90	0.74	2–4	3.10	0.57	2–4	0.20	0.63	0.343
Difficulty discussing … (Very Difficult = 1; Not at all Difficult = 4)									
… alcohol abuse with your patients (*N* = 12)	3.25	0.45	3–4	3.25	0.75	2–4	0.00	0.60	1.000
… opioid abuse with your patients (*N* = 12)	2.67	0.65	2–4	3.08	0.79	2–4	0.42	1.00	0.175
Appropriateness									
Prescribing Medical Providers									
Compatibility of SUD Treatment with Primary Care (Strongly Disagree = 1; Strongly Agree = 5)									
Substance use disorders can be effectively treated in a primary care setting (*N* = 12)	3.00	0.60	2–4	4.25	0.87	2–5	1.25	0.97	0.006*
Substance use disorders can be effectively treated at [THIS CLINIC] (*N* = 12)	2.83	0.83	1–4	3.17	0.83	2–4	0.33	0.98	0.398
Providing medications to patients with alcohol or opioid use disorders fits with [THIS CLINIC'S] mission and goals (*N* = 12)	3.17	1.19	1–5	3.17	0.83	2–4	0.00	1.21	1.000
Providing counseling to patients with alcohol or opioid use disorders fits with [THIS CLINIC'S] mission and goals (*N* = 12)	4.42	0.67	3–5	3.67	0.98	2–5	−0.75	0.62	0.002*
Compatibility with Current Practice (Extremely Disagree = 1; Extremely Agree = 7)									
Perceived Compatibility of XR-NTX with current practices (*N* = 11)†	3.36	1.79	1–7	4.77	1.33	2–7	1.41	1.14	0.004*
Perceived Compatibility of BUP/NX with current practices (*N* = 8)†	3.13	2.03	1–7	2.63	1.38	1–5	−0.50	1.34	0.375
General Clinic Staff									
Compatibility of SUD Treatment in Primary Care (Strongly Disagree = 1; Strongly Agree = 5)									
Substance use disorders can be effectively treated in a primary care setting (*N* = 35)	3.17	1.01	1–5	4.06	0.76	1–5	0.89	1.08	<.0001**
Substance use disorders can be effectively treated at [THIS CLINIC] (*N* = 35)	3.17	0.98	1–5	3.86	0.77	2–5	0.69	1.08	<.0001**
Providing medications to patients with alcohol or opioid use disorders fits with [THIS CLINIC'S] mission and goals (*N* = 35)	2.94	0.97	1–5	3.89	0.76	2–5	0.94	1.24	<.0001**
Providing counseling to patients with alcohol or opiate use disorders fits with [THIS CLINIC'S] mission and goals. (*N* = 36)	3.72	0.94	1–5	3.67	1.07	2–5	−0.06	1.43	0.817
Feasibility									
Prescribing Medical Providers									
Feel prepared to … (Not at all Prepared = 1; Very prepared = 4)									
… identify patients with alcohol use disorders (*N* = 12)	3.42	0.67	2–4	3.92	0.29	3–4	0.50	0.52	0.031
… identify patients who are using illegal opiates such as heroin (*N* = 11)	3.27	0.65	2–4	3.45	0.52	3–4	0.18	0.60	0.625
… identify patients who are misusing (*N* = 12)or abusing prescription opioids (*N* = 12)	3.00	0.60	2–4	3.33	0.65	2–4	0.33	0.49	0.125

Table 2 Changes in organizational readiness to deliver SUD treatment in primary care *(Continued)*

	Pre-Intervention			Post-Intervention			Difference		
	Mean	SD	Range	Mean	SD	Range	Mean	SD	*P*-value^
Intent/willingness to adopt ebp									
Prescribing Medical Providers									
Perceived demonstrability (Extremely Disagree = 1; Extremely Agree = 7)									
… of XR-NTX (*N* = 11)†	4.21	1.20	1.67–6.33	4.85	0.91	4–7	0.64	1.11	0.086
… of BUP/NX (*N* = 9)†	4.11	1.28	1.67–6.33	3.30	1.31	1–5.33	−0.81	1.11	0.058
Would consider using in current practice (Extremely Disagree = 1; Extremely Agree = 7)									
I would consider using XR-NTX in my practice (*N* = 11)	4.09	1.87	2–7	5.55	1.13	4–7	1.45	1.81	0.037
I would consider using BUP/NX in my practice (*N* = 10)	3.80	1.69	2–7	4.30	2.16	1–7	0.50	1.72	0.469

†Pre-intervention measures combined the two medications into one question asking about MAT for OAUD; all prescribing providers were asked about XR-NTX and only physicians were asked about BUP/NX

^The Benjamini and Hochberg false discovery rate (FDR) correction was used to assess significance given the multiple testing. *P*-values reported in this column are those prior to FDR correction

*Significance at $p < 0.05$ after FDR correction

**Significance at $p < 0.01$ after FDR correction

Post-intervention, prescribing medical providers felt more prepared than at baseline to identify patients with alcohol disorders, but these changes were not statistically significant after the FDR correction.

Intention to adopt

Pre-intervention, prescribing medical providers' scores were similar for perceived demonstrability, with mean scores of 4.21 (all prescribing providers, XR-NTX) and 4.11 (physicians, BUP/NX), on a scale from 1 to 7 (7 = strongly agree with statements of demonstrability). With respect to whether providers would consider using each medication in their practice, mean scores were 4.09 for XR-NTX and 3.80 for BUP/NX. Post-intervention, prescribing medical providers were more willing to use XR-NTX in their practice but these changes were not statistically significant after the FDR correction. Willingness to use BUP/NX did not change significantly.

Discussion

We hypothesized that a multi-component implementation intervention aimed at planning, educating providers and staff, and restructuring the care delivery system would lead to greater organizational readiness, measured by four implementation outcome domains: improved perceptions of acceptability, appropriateness, feasibility and intention or willingness to adopt evidence based treatments for OAUDs; these hypotheses were partially supported. Specifically, convening a researcher-clinic implementation team, assessing barriers, resources and workflows, creating future state workflows and protocols tested by champions and in a clinic-wide pilot, providing training and technical assistance to all providers and general clinic staff, adapting workflows and protocols to meet clinic needs, improved perceptions of the appropriateness of treating SUD in primary care among both prescribing medical providers and the general clinic staff and perceptions of the acceptability of XR-NTX among prescribing medical providers. Immediately post-intervention, prescribing medical providers showed greater changes in their perceptions of ease of use and compatibility of XR-NTX with current practice, but no changes with respect to perceptions of BUP/NX ease or compatibility. Prescribing medical providers' intention to adopt XR-NTX also increased after the organizational readiness intervention, but changes were not significant after the FDR correction. General clinic staff had significant improvements in their opinions about the appropriateness of SUD treatment in primary care on three of three measures – that SUDs can be effectively treated in primary care, that SUDs can be effectively treated at this clinic, and that providing medications for alcohol or opiate use disorders fits the clinic's mission and goals. These results suggest that the organizational readiness intervention was successful at changing at least some important implementation outcomes, which are theoretically associated with the adoption of new practices [50].

Prescribing medical providers' opinions changed significantly in a negative direction with respect to their belief that providing counseling to patients with alcohol and opioid use disorders fit with the clinic's mission and goals. This may have been because during the organizational readiness intervention period, prescribing medical providers incorrectly perceived that the question about counseling pertained to prescribing medical providers providing counseling, instead of behavioral health providers. Interestingly, opinions of general clinic staff about the fit of providing counseling for opioid and alcohol use disorders did not change significantly, but the mean score was already higher (i.e., supporting the idea that counseling was a good fit) than the mean scores of the variables that did change. Although general clinic staff will not directly "adopt" the SUD treatments, they do play an important role in screening patients and making appointments for patients seeking SUD treatment; implementation theory suggests that ultimately opinions and buy-in of staff at all levels of the organization could affect overall adoption of SUD treatment at the clinic [29].

Although our hypotheses generally were supported, the findings were somewhat nuanced. First, although prescribing medical providers and general staff opinions improved with regard to the appropriateness of providing SUD treatment in primary care in general, prescribing medical providers' opinions about the appropriateness of providing SUD treatment at their particular clinic did not change significantly. Further, and perhaps related to this, while the findings suggest that the intervention we employed may have improved prescribing medical providers' readiness in the "acceptability" and "appropriateness" domains to deliver XR-NTX to patients with alcohol use disorders, the intervention did not improve readiness in those domains for the use of BUP/NX to treat opioid disorders, despite providers having treatment protocols that were adapted for their setting and extensive training. It is possible that views about treating patients with SUDs in general and about using BUP/NX to treat patients with opioid use disorders could improve with hands-on experience treating patients. Further, although the change was not statistically significant, prescribing medical providers' opinions about the demonstrability of BUP/NX actually changed in a negative direction after the 18 months of the intervention. While we do not know the reasons for the perceived differences between XR-NTX and BUP/NX, it may be that the need to get a DEA waiver to prescribe BUP/NX, the DEA requirement that providers maintain a list of all patients being prescribed BUP/NX and participate in DEA audits, and that the clinic pharmacy does not include narcotics on the clinic formulary, influenced perceptions of BUP/NX's acceptability and appropriateness for the clinic. Further, it is also possible that opinions will change after implementation of the service delivery intervention, with champions continuing to prescribe BUP/NX and more patients with OAUDs being referred to prescribing medical providers for treatment.

Importantly, prescribing medical providers' views of the feasibility of and their intention to adopt either XR-NTX or BUP/NX did not change after we adjusted for multiple statistical tests, although there was a trend towards providers perceiving XR-NTX as more feasible and being willing to adopt this practice. The lack of statistical significance may be because of the small sample size and need to correct for multiple comparisons, or because additional interventions are needed to change these readiness outcomes.

Of note, although this study was designed to increase the clinic's capacity (i.e., infrastructure) to deliver SUD treatment, which can affect adoption of new practices [45, 81, 82], we did not objectively measure organizational capacity. However, providers' perceptions of whether the treatments are acceptable and appropriate may reflect perceptions of capacity. As noted by Weiner et al. (2008), to be motivated and willing to implement a new practice, individuals must believe that they and their organizations are capable of delivering an intervention [28]. As health care organizations attempt to integrate SUD and other EBPs, it may be important for implementation interventions to explicitly address capacity as part of improving organizational readiness. Health care organizations must also consider the feasibility of implementing the organizational readiness intervention itself, and some adaptation (for example, in meeting frequency, number of providers invited to attend training, length of training) may be needed to fit individual settings.

This study has some limitations. First, we used a pre-post design, at a single FQHC, with no control group. Therefore, our findings cannot be solely attributed to the organizational readiness intervention, as there may have been other changes in or outside of the clinic or external environment that influenced findings. Generalizability to other FQHCs and other primary care settings is limited, as organizational culture and patient populations may differ across different types of primary care practices. Future study of the effects of the intervention on organizational readiness, including measures of organizational functioning (e.g., turnover, morale), in a larger, randomized sample of primary care clinics is needed. We describe our findings using central tendency statistics (means and standard deviations) for ease of interpretation, but caution should be used in interpreting the results because of the small sample sizes. Because there are few validated measures of implementation outcomes, we included some locally developed items and items from scales that have not been validated. In addition, in our pre-intervention survey, the two medications were combined and compared with follow-up measures that asked about each medication separately. We tested a bundled intervention that comprised of several different implementation strategies designed to enhance organizational readiness, and cannot separate the effects of each strategy. Finally, because we believe that perceptions of acceptability, appropriateness and feasibility, as well as intent to adopt continue to improve as staff and providers see patients benefitting from receiving treatment for their OAUD, we do not view these outcomes as final measures of the effectiveness of the organizational readiness intervention or as final indicators of the readiness of prescribing medical providers to adopt either medication.

Conclusions

We found that an organizational readiness intervention consisting of multiple theoretically grounded implementation strategies aimed at the entire organization, improved some implementation outcomes related to integrating treatment for OAUDs in primary care, but not all. There were differences in prescribing medical providers' perceptions of XR-NTX and BUP/NX, and providers generally saw treating patients with alcohol use disorders with XR-NTX as more acceptable and appropriate than treating patients with opioid use disorders with BUP/NX immediately after 18-months of the intervention. Additional work may be needed to prepare primary care providers to treat patients with OUDs and to adopt BUP/NX. These results demonstrate the value of incorporating several implementation strategies to build support for implementation of SUD treatment in primary care settings.

Endnote

[1]In the U.S., medical providers are permitted to dispense or prescribe approved Schedule III, IV, and V narcotic medications (i.e., those that have a lower risk for abuse, like buprenorphine/naloxone) in settings other than an opioid treatment program (OTP). In order to prescribe or dispense buprenorphine, medical providers must qualify for an "X-waiver" which includes completing 8 h of required training and applying for the wavier with the drug enforcement agency (DEA) [83].

Abbreviations

AUD: Alcohol use disorder; BUP/NX: Buprenorphine/Naloxone; CASA: Center for addiction and substance abuse; CBT: Cognitive behavioral therapy; DEA: Drug enforcement agency; EBP: Evidence-based practice; FDA: Food and drug administration; FQHC: Federally Qualified Health Center; HSPC: Human subject protection committee; MI: Motivational interviewing; NIDA: National institute on drug abuse; OAUD: Opioid and alcohol use disorders; OUD: Opioid use disorder; PCSS-MAT: Provider's clinical support system for medication-assisted treatment; PDSA: Plan-Do-Study-Act; PPACA: Patient protection and affordable care act; RCT: Randomized controlled trial; SUD: Substance use disorder; SUMMIT: Substance use, motivation and medication integrated treatment; XR-NTX: Extended-release Naltrexone

Acknowledgments

We acknowledge all providers and staff at the Venice Family clinic for their contributions to and participation in the study. We thank the SUMMIT team, including Kirsten Becker and the RAND Survey Research Group, David Devries, Scot Hickey and Tiffany Hruby for their contributions to carrying out the study. We acknowledge the National Institute on Drug Abuse (NIDA) for funding the study under 1R01DA034266 and Alkermes for provision of extended-release injectable naltrexone for study patients. We also acknowledge the SUMMIT Scientific Advisory Board for their input on the study design and protocols: Frank de Gruy; Adam Gorden; Miriam Komaromy; Tom McLellan; Harold Pincus; Rick Rawson; Richard Saitz; Jurgen Unutzer.

Funding

This research was funded by National Institute on Drug Abuse (NIDA) R01DA034266 (PI: Watkins).

Authors' contributions

AJO contributed to the design and implementation of the study and drafted the manuscript; KEW contributed to the design and implementation of the study and provided substantial input on the manuscript; SBH contributed to the design of the study and provided substantial input on the manuscript; BE conducted data management and analyses; KB contributed to the design and implementation of the study and provided input on the manuscript; KL contributed to the design and implementation of the study and carried out the service delivery intervention; ML contributed to the design and implementation of the study and carried out the service delivery intervention; KH contributed to the design and implementation of the study, carried out the service delivery intervention, and provided input on the manuscript; KCO contributed to the design and implementation of the study, carried out the service delivery intervention, and provided input on the manuscript; ALD contributed to the design and implementation of the study and provided input on the manuscript; CMS contributed to the evaluation and analytic plan and provided input on the manuscript.
All authors read and approved the final manuscript.

Consent for publication

Not applicable.

Competing interests

Financial competing interests.
The authors are employees of The RAND Corporation ("RAND"), a nonprofit institution that helps improve policy and decisionmaking through research and analysis. Within the past 3 years, RAND has received funding for research projects from Alkermes plc ("Alkermes") relating to the pharmaceutical Vivitrol, which is manufactured and sold by Alkermes. Allison Ober participated in RAND research projects funded by Alkermes. Katherine Watkins participated in RAND research projects funded by Alkermes and served as Principal Investigator. To the extent that this paper suggests a benefit related to greater provider acceptance of Vivitrol, this finding may have a positive financial effect on Alkermes. Prior to submission, RAND conducted additional internal quality reviews of this article with a particular focus on the possibility of bias.
Alkermes provided Vivitrol at no charge to certain patients participating in this study. This arrangement was disclosed and approved by the National Institutes of Health project officer.
Non-financial competing interests.
Not applicable.

Author details

[1]RAND Corporation, 1776 Main Street, Santa Monica, CA 90407, USA. [2]Venice Family Clinic, 2509 Pico Boulevard, Santa Monica, CA 90405, USA. [3]UCLA Department of Family Medicine, UCLA Family Health Center, 1920 Colorado Avenue, Santa Monica, CA 90404, USA. [4]UCLA Department of Internal Medicine, Division of General Internal Medicine, 911 Broxton Avenue, Los Angeles, CA 90024, USA.

References

1. Schackman BR, et al. Cost-effectiveness of long-term outpatient buprenorphine-naloxone treatment for opioid dependence in primary care. J Gen Intern Med. 2012;27(6):669–76.
2. Myles J, Law F, Raybould T. A double-blind randomised controlled trial of buprenorphine/naloxone (suboxone) versus methadone/lofexidine for the detoxification of opiate-dependent addicts. Drug Alcohol Depend. 2000;60(Suppl 1):S156.
3. Tofighi B, et al. Outcomes among buprenorphine-naloxone primary care patients after hurricane Sandy. Addict Sci Clin Pract. 2014;9:3.
4. Mauger S, Fraser R, Gill K. Utilizing buprenorphine-naloxone to treat illicit and prescription-opioid dependence. Neuropsychiatr Dis Treat. 2014;10:587–98.
5. Drainoni ML, et al. Patient perspectives of an integrated program of medical care and substance use treatment. AIDS Patient Care STDs. 2014;28(2):71–81.
6. Doolittle B, Becker W. A case series of buprenorphine/naloxone treatment in a primary care practice. Subst Abus. 2011;32(4):262–5.

7. Balhara YP. Time to include buprenorphine-naloxone combination in the WHO model list of essential medicines. J Opioid Manag. 2014;9(4):237.
8. Aspy C, et al. Integrating screening and interventions for unhealthy behaviors into primary care practices. Am J Prev Med. 2008;35(Suppl):S373–80.
9. Bradley KA, et al. Implementation of evidence-based alcohol screening in the veterans health administration. Am J Manag Care. 2006;12(10):597–606.
10. Boldt R. Obstacles to the development and use of pharmacotherapies for addiction. J Health Care L & Policy. 2010;13:1–6.
11. Friedmann P, et al. Screening and intervention for alcohol problems: A national survey of primary care physicians and psychiatrists. J Gen Intern Med. 2000;15(2):84–91.
12. Pilowsky DJ, Wu LT. Screening for alcohol and drug use disorders among adults in primary care: a review. Subst Abuse Rehabil. 2012;3(1):25–34.
13. Cherpitel CJ, Ye Y. Trends in alcohol- and drug-related emergency department and primary care visits: data from four U.S. national surveys (1995-2010). J Stud Alcohol Drugs. 2012;73(3):454–8.
14. Blackwell D, Lucas J, Clarke T. Summary health statistics for U.S. adults: National Health Interview Survey, 2012. Vital Health Stat. 2014;10(260):1-161.
15. U.S. Department of Health and Human Services Health Resources and Services Administration. The Affordable Care Act and health centers. 2013 [cited 22 Jan 2015]; Available from: http://bphc.hrsa.gov/about/healthcenterfactsheet.pdf.
16. Glied S, Ma S. How will the affordable care act affect services? In Issue Brief, T.C. Fund, Editor. New York and Washington, D.C: The Commonwealth Fund; 2015.
17. Substance Abuse and Mental Health Services Administration, results from the 2013 national survey on drug use and health: summary of national findings, NSDUH series H-46, HHS publication no. (SMA) 14–4863. Substance Abuse and Mental Health Services Administration: Rockville, MD 2014.
18. Fortney J, et al. Factors associated with perceived stigma for alcohol use and treatment among at-risk drinkers. J Behav Health Serv Res. 2004;31(4): 418–29.
19. Luoma JB, et al. Stigma predicts treatment length in residential substance use disorder treatment. Am J Drug Alcohol Abus. 2014;40:206–12.
20. Rapp RC, et al. Treatment barriers identified by substance abusers assessed at a centralized intake unit. J Subst Abus Treat. 2006;30(3):227–35.
21. Amaral-Sabadini MB, Saitz R, Souza-Formigoni ML. Do attitudes about unhealthy alcohol and other drug (AOD) use impact primary care professionals' readiness to implement AOD-related preventive care? Drug Alcohol Rev. 2010;29(6):655–61.
22. Urada D, et al. Integration of substance use disorder services with primary care: health center surveys and qualitative interviews. Subst Abuse Treat Prev Policy. 2014;9:15.
23. Quest TL, et al. Buprenorphine therapy for opioid addiction in rural Washington: the experience of the early adopters. J Opioid Manag. 2012;8(1):29–38.
24. DeFlavio JR, et al. Analysis of barriers to adoption of buprenorphine maintenance therapy by family physicians. Rural Remote Health. 2015;15:3019.
25. Padwa H, et al. Integrating substance use disorder services with primary care: the experience in California. J Psychoactive Drugs. 2012;44(4):299–306.
26. Padwa H, et al. Barriers to serving clients with co-occurring disorders in a transformed mental health system. Psychiatr Serv. 2015;66(5):547–50.
27. Rogers E. Diffusion of innovations. 4th ed. New York: The Free Press; 1995.
28. Weiner BJ, Amick H, Lee SY. Conceptualization and measurement of organizational readiness for change: a review of the literature in health services research and other fields. Med Care Res Rev. 2008;65(4):379–436.
29. Damschroder LJ, et al. Fostering implementation of health services research findings into practice: a consolidated framework for advancing implementation science. Implement Sci. 2009;4:50.
30. Grol R, et al. Planning and studying improvement in patient care: the use of theoretical perspectives. Milbank Quarterly. 2007;85(1):93–138.
31. Shanafelt TD, et al. Potential impact of burnout on the US physician workforce. Mayo Clin Proc. 2016;91(11):1667–8.
32. Linzer M, et al. Predicting and preventing physician burnout: results from the United States and the Netherlands. Am J Med. 2001;111(2):170–5.
33. Shaw RJ, et al. Organizational factors associated with readiness to implement and translate a primary care based telemedicine behavioral program to improve blood pressure control: the HTN-IMPROVE study. Implement Sci. 2013;8:106.
34. Bandura A. Self-efficacy: towards unifying theory of behavioral change. Psychol Rev. 1977;84:191–215.
35. Amatayakul M. EHR? Assess readiness first. Healthc Financ Manage. 2005;59(5):112–3.
36. Cassidy J. System analyzes readiness for integrated delivery. Health Prog. 1994;75(3):18–20. 22
37. Hardison C. Readiness, action, and resolve for change: do health care leaders have what it takes? Qual Manag Health Care. 1998;6(2):44–51.
38. O'Connor EJ, Fiol CM. Creating readiness and involvement. Physician Exec. 2006;32(1):72–4.
39. Greenhalgh T, et al. Diffusion of innovations in service review organizations: systematic review and recommendations. Millbank Quarterly. 2004;82(4):581–629.
40. Aarons GA, Sommerfeld DH, Walrath-Greene CM. Evidence-based practice implementation: the impact of public versus private sector organization type on organizational support, provider attitudes, and adoption of evidence-based practice. Implement Sci. 2009;4:83.
41. Aarons GA, Hurlburt M, Horwitz SM. Advancing a conceptual model of evidence-based practice implementation in public service sectors. Admin Pol Ment Health. 2011;38(1):4–23.
42. Aarons GA. Mental health provider attitudes toward adoption of evidence-based practice: the evidence-based practice attitude scale (EBPAS). Ment Health Serv Res. 2004;6(2):61–74.
43. Lehman WE, Greener JM, Simpson DD. Assessing organizational readiness for change. J Subst Abus Treat. 2002;22(4):197–209.
44. Glisson C, et al. Assessing the organizational social context (OSC) of mental health services: implications for research and practice. Admin Pol Ment Health. 2008;35(1–2):98–113.
45. Scaccia JP, et al. A practical implementation science heuristic for organizational readiness: R = MC. J Community Psychol. 2015;43(4):484–501.
46. Fuller BE, et al. Organizational readiness for change and opinions toward treatment innovations. J Subst Abus Treat. 2007;33(2):183–92.
47. Gotham HJ, et al. Increasing program capability to provide treatment for co-occurring substance use and mental disorders: organizational characteristics. J Subst Abus Treat. 2009;38(2):160–9.
48. Saldana L, et al. The organizational readiness for change scale in adolescent programs: criterion validity. J Subst Abus Treat. 2007;33(2):159–69.
49. Simpson DD, Joe GW, Rowan-Szal GA. Linking the elements of change: program and client responses to innovation. J Subst Abus Treat. 2007;33(2):201–9.
50. Proctor E, et al. Outcomes for implementation research: conceptual distinctions, measurement challenges, and research agenda. Admin Pol Ment Health. 2011;38(2):65–76.
51. Ober AJ, et al. An organizational readiness intervention and randomized controlled trial to test strategies for implementing substance use disorder treatment into primary care: SUMMIT study protocol. Implement Sci. 2015;10
52. Lee JD, et al. Extended-release naltrexone plus medical management alcohol treatment in primary care: findings at 15 months. J Subst Abus Treat. 2012;43(4):458–62.
53. Garbutt JC, et al. Efficacy and tolerability of long-acting injectable naltrexone for alcohol dependence: a randomized controlled trial. JAMA. 2005;293(13):1617–25.
54. Kranzler H, Wesson D, Billot L. Drug abuse sciences: Naltrexone depot study group. Naltrexone depot for treatment of alcohol dependence: a multicenter, randomized, placebo-controlled clinical trial. Alcohol Clin Exp Res. 2004;28:1051–9.
55. Krupitsky E, et al. Injectable extended-release naltrexone (XR-NTX) for opioid dependence: long-term safety and effectiveness. Addiction. 2013;108(9): 1628–37.
56. Hartung DM, et al. Extended-release naltrexone for alcohol and opioid dependence: a meta-analysis of healthcare utilization studies. J Subst Abus Treat. 2014;47(2):113–21.
57. Miller WR, Benefield RG, Tonigan JS. Enhancing motivation for change in problem drinking: a controlled comparison of two therapist styles. J Consult Clin Psychol. 1993;61(3):455–61.
58. Miller WR, Sanchez VC. Motivation of young adults for treatment and lifestyle change. In: Howard G, editor. Issues in alcohol use and misuse by young adults. Notre Dame, IN: University of Notre Dame Press; 1994. p. 55–82.
59. Miller WR, et al. Motivational Enhancement Therapy: A clinical research guide for therapists treating individuals with alcohol abuse and dependence,

National Institute on Alcohol Abuse and Alcoholism. National Institutes of Health: Rockville; 1994.
60. Ball SA, et al. Site matters: multisite randomized trial of motivational enhancement therapy in community drug abuse clinics. J Consult Clin Psychol. 2007;75(4):556–67.
61. Powell BJ, et al. A compilation of strategies for implementing clinical innovations in health and mental health. Med Care Res Rev. 2012;69(2):123–57.
62. Leeman J, et al. What strategies are used to build practitioners' capacity to implement community-based interventions and are they effective?: a systematic review. Implement Sci. 2015;10:80.
63. Wandersman A, Chien VH, Katz J. Toward an evidence-based system for innovation support for implementing innovations with quality: tools, training, technical assistance, and quality assurance/quality improvement. Am J Community Psychol. 2012;50(3–4):445–59.
64. Fixsen DL, et al. Implementation Research: A Synthesis of the Literature. New York and Washington D.C: University of South Florida, Louis de la Parte Florida Mental Health Institute, The National Implementation Research Network (FMHI Publication #231); 2005.
65. Chinman M, et al. Intervening with practitioners to improve the quality of prevention: one-year findings from a randomized trial of assets-getting to outcomes. J Prim Prev. 2013;34(3):173–91.
66. Acosta J, et al. An intervention to improve program implementation: findings from a two-year cluster randomized trial of assets-getting to outcomes. Implement Sci. 2013;8:87.
67. Deming W. Out of the crisis, 1986, vol. 507. Cambridge, MA: Massachusetts Institute of Technology Center for Advanced Engineering Study iii; 1991.
68. Berwick DM. Developing and testing changes in delivery of care. Ann Intern Med. 1998;128(8):651–6.
69. Chinman M, Hunter S, Ebener P. Employing continuous quality improvement in community-based substance abuse programs. Int J Health Care Qual Assur. 2012;25(7):606–17.
70. Hunter SB, et al. Promoting success: a getting to outcomes guide to implementing continuous quality improvement for community service organizations. Santa Monica: RAND Corporation; 2015.
71. Weiner BJ, Lewis MA, Linnan LA. Using organization theory to understand the determinants of effective implementation of worksite health promotion programs. Health Educ Res. 2009;24(2):292–305.
72. Heinzerling KG, et al. SUMMIT: Procedures for Medication-Assisted Treatment of Alcohol or Opioid Dependence in Primary Care. Santa Monica: RAND Technical Manual R. Corporation; 2016.
73. Osilla K, et al. Brief treatment for substance use disorders: a guide for behavioral health providers. Santa Monica: R. Corporation; 2016.
74. Ober AJ, et al. SUMMIT study protocol: step-by-step procedures for providing screening, brief intervention and treatment services to primary care patients with alcohol or Opioid use disorders. Santa Monica: R. Corporation. In Press.
75. Beidas R, Kendall P. Training therapists in evidence-based practice: a critical review of studies from a systems-contextual perspective. Clin Psychol. 2010;17:1–30.
76. Hunter S, et al. Technical assistance as a prevention capacity-building tool: a demonstration using the getting to outcomes framework. Health Educ Behav. 2009;36:810–28.
77. Chinman M, et al. The getting to outcomes demonstration and evaluation: an illustration of the prevention support system. Am J Community Psychol. 2008;41:206–24. PMCID: PMC2964843
78. Moore G, Benbasat I. Development of an instrument to measure the perceptions of adopting an information technology innovation. Inf Syst Res. 1991;2(3):192–222.
79. CASA Columbia, Missed Opportunity: Survey of Primary Care Providers and Patients on Substance Abuse. New York and Washington D.C: CASA Columbia; 2000.
80. Benjamini Y, Hochberg Y. Controlling the false discovery rate - a practical and powerful approach to multiple testing. J R Stat Soc Series B-Methodological. 1995;57(1):289–300.
81. Simpson DD, Dansereau DF. Assessing organizational functioning as a step toward innovation. Sci Pract Perspect. 2007;3(2):20–8.
82. Meyer AM, Davis M, Mays GP. Defining organizational capacity for public health services and systems research. J Public Health Manag Pract. 2012;18(6):535–44.
83. Substance Abuse and Mental Health Services Administration. Buprenorphine Waiver Management. Medication-Assisted Treatment 2016 [cited 20 Dec 2016]; Available from: https://www.samhsa.gov/medication-assisted-treatment/buprenorphine-waiver-management.

5

The Mini-International Neuropsychiatric Interview is useful and well accepted as part of the clinical assessment for depression and anxiety in primary care

Agneta Pettersson[1,2*], Sonja Modin[3], Rolf Wahlström[4], Sandra af Winklerfelt Hammarberg[5] and Ingvar Krakau[6]

Abstract

Background: Psychiatric complaints are common among primary care patients, with depression and anxiety being the most frequent. Diagnosis of anxiety and depression can be difficult, potentially leading to over- as well as under-diagnosis. The diagnostic process can be facilitated by incorporating structured interviews as part of the assessment. One such instrument, the Mini-International Neuropsychiatric Interview (MINI), has been established and accepted in psychiatric care. The purpose of this study was to explore the experiences and perceptions of the paper-and-pen version of MINI version 6.0 among patients and staff in primary care centers in Sweden.

Methods: The MINI was introduced at three primary care centers and was conducted by either therapists or general practitioners. Patients presented with symptoms that could suggest depression or anxiety disorders. The duration of the interview was recorded. The experiences and perceptions of 125 patients and their interviewers were collected using a structured questionnaire. Global satisfaction was measured with a visual-analog scale (0–100). Semi-structured interviews were conducted with 24 patients and three therapists, and focus groups were held with 17 general practitioners. Qualitative content analysis was used for the interviews and focus groups. The findings across the groups were triangulated with results from the questionnaires.

Results: The median global satisfaction with the MINI was 80 for patients and 86 for interviewers. General practitioners appreciated that the MINI identified comorbidities, as one-third of the patients had at least two psychiatric diagnoses. The MINI helped general practitioners attain a more accurate diagnosis. Patients appreciated that the MINI helped them recognize and verbalize their problems and did not find it intrusive. Patients and interviewers had mixed experiences with the yes-no format of the MINI, and the risk of subjective interpretations was acknowledged. Patients, general practitioners and therapists stated that the MINI contributed to appropriate treatment. The MINI assessment lasted 26 min on average (range 12 to 60 min).

Conclusions: The paper-and-pen version of the MINI could be useful in primary care as part of the clinical assessment of patients with problems suggestive of depression or anxiety disorders. The MINI was well accepted by patients, general practitioners and therapists.

Keywords: Depression, Anxiety, Differential diagnosis, Qualitative content analysis, MINI, Acceptability

* Correspondence: agneta.pettersson@ki.se
[1]Medical Management Centre, Department of Learning, Informatics, Management and Ethics, Karolinska Institutet, Tomtebodavägen 18 A, SE-171 77 Stockholm, Sweden
[2]Swedish Agency for Health Technology Assessment and Social Assessment, SE-102 33 Stockholm, Sweden
Full list of author information is available at the end of the article

Background

Psychiatric problems are common among patients in primary care [1], with depressive and anxiety disorders being the most frequent diagnoses [1–5]. Comorbidity of depressive and anxiety disorders is also common [1, 3, 6]. A correct diagnosis of any psychiatric problem is vital to enabling optimal treatment but may be difficult to establish, e.g., owing to somatic and psychiatric comorbidities [7, 8].

A governmental health technology assessment report on instruments to support the diagnosis of mood disorders [9] inspired the present study, which initially focused on depression. A previous systematic review concluded that half of patients with depression were not recognized [10]. Furthermore, some studies on depression have shown that a substantial proportion of patients remain undiagnosed after several visits to a general practitioner (GP) [4, 11]. However, other studies have indicated that awareness of depression may result in a diagnosis even when the patient has only subthreshold symptoms [12, 13].

Attempts have been made to help GPs improve their skills in diagnosing depression, including by providing training in consultation techniques [14–17] and through the use of short questionnaires or structured interviews to complement the consultation [18–20]. However, a systematic review concluded that few of these instruments had acceptable sensitivity and specificity for depression [21]. One exception was the Mini-International Neuropsychiatric Interview (MINI) instrument, which is a structured interview; at the time of the study, the MINI 6.0, based on the DSM-IV, was available. The MINI comprises modules for 17 psychiatric diagnoses. Questions are phrased to allow only "yes" or "no" answers. Examples are provided to facilitate responses and should be read word for word. The MINI is available in both a paper-and-pen and a web-based version.

For structured interviews to have utility in practice, they must also be acceptable to patients and staff. However, no studies on primary care patients' perspectives of the MINI could be retrieved (August 2016). One study, from Brazil, found that general practitioners (GPs) who used the MINI were satisfied with the interview [22]. Two studies, from Italy and Norway, showed that the MINI was well accepted by patients and interviewers in psychiatric care [23, 24]. In Sweden, few GPs use the MINI. According to a postal survey in 2011 of 300 randomly chosen Swedish GPs (42% response rate), only five of them (4%) had used the MINI [9].

As the MINI is not limited to depression and as there is significant co-morbidity of depression and anxiety, the focus of the present study shifted toward evaluating the use of the MINI for patients with symptoms suggestive of any of these diagnoses. This expansion better mirrored the primary care patient population. The MINI has shown high accuracy for depression in psychiatric as well as in primary care [9, 22, 25]. There is less information about its accuracy for other diagnoses, but it is acceptable for panic disorder and generalized anxiety disorder in psychiatric and primary care settings [22, 25, 26]. The accuracy of the MINI for agoraphobia and social anxiety disorders has been found to be acceptable when measured in psychiatric settings [25, 26].

The purpose of the present study was to explore the experiences of and perceptions of the paper-and-pen version of the MINI among staff and patients for patients with problems suggestive of depression or anxiety disorders in Swedish primary care centers (PCCs).

Methods

This was a pragmatic mixed-methods study that did not provide any financial support to the participating PCCs. The study was designed to minimize extra administrative work by participating staff.

Setting and participants

This study was carried out in Stockholm County between February 2014 and March 2015. After establishing the study with relevant decision-makers in the county council and political leadership, PCCs were recruited through personal contacts. Seven PCCs were approached, and three agreed to participate, here called PCC1, PCC2 and PCC3. The PCCs had two introductory meetings, 1 h each, led by three of the authors (AP, IK and SW). The MINI and supportive evidence were presented during the first meeting, whereas the study protocol was addressed in the second meeting. Some characteristics of the PCCs are described in Table 1. At PCC1, the MINI was implemented as part of the study. Patients were referred to a medical social worker experienced in Cognitive Behavior Therapy who conducted the MINI interview. The interviewer received a full-day training on the use of the MINI led by one of the authors (SW). At PCC2 and PPC3, the MINI was already in routine use, and the interview was conducted by certified psychologists or by GPs themselves. The psychologists and the medical social worker are referred to as therapists in this article.

Eligible patients met at least one of the following criteria: an ongoing episode of major depression that had not responded adequately to treatment after 2 months; a new episode of a mental health problem; somatic symptoms in which depression could be a differential diagnosis; and frequent attendance at the PCC as perceived by the GP [27]. Patients had to be 18 years or older, sufficiently capable in the Swedish language to participate in the interview and lacking cognitive deficiencies. Patients who needed immediate treatment were excluded. Only patients who consented to completing a questionnaire after the MINI were included in the study. The MINI assessment was performed by three employed therapists (1 at PCC1

Table 1 Characteristics of participating primary care centers (PCC)

PCC ID	Location, listed patients (n); CNI[a]	Number parti-cipating GPs (number employed)	MINI interviewer	Procedure
1	Suburb, 18,000 patients; CNI = 1.26	9 (15)	1 medical social worker after referral from a GP	MINI results fed back to the GP for decision on further management
2	Suburb, 21,000 patients; CNI = 0.93	≥8 (14)	Psychologists after referral from a GP **or** the GPs themselves	Psychologists made a full assessment including MINI and initiated CBT if relevant **or** the GPs initiated treatment.
3	Central Stockholm, 10,000 patients; CNI = 0.72	1 (3)	The GP	The GP initiated treatment

[a]*CNI* Care Need Index [45] a measure of psychosocial burden, where higher values indicate larger problems; average CNI = 1.0; *GP* general practitioner

and 2 at PCC2) and four GPs (three at PCC2 and one at PCC3). The number of contract therapists who contributed ten questionnaires at PCC2 was not retrieved.

Data collection

The perceptions and experiences of patients and interviewers were gathered from a structured questionnaire on acceptance. To obtain a deeper understanding, the questionnaires were supplemented with semi-structured interviews or focus groups.

Questionnaires

The questionnaire addressed the emotional and mental aspects of using the MINI, with one version for the patients and another for the interviewers (Additional file 1). The questionnaires were developed and validated in Germany for a study [28] on the acceptance of another structured interview, Diagnostisches Interview bei Psychischen Störungen (DIPS for the DSM-IV-TR), and were used with the permission of the research group. The questionnaires were translated into Swedish by one of the authors (AP) and back-translated by a teacher working in Sweden whose native language was German. The accuracy of the back-translated text was verified by one of the leading researchers working with the DIPS. In short, the questionnaire comprised ten Likert-type statements scored from 0 = do not agree at all to 3 = agree fully. The respondents also estimated their global satisfaction with the MINI on a Visual Analog scale (VAS, 0 to 100). In addition to completing the questionnaire, the patients shared their reasons for visiting the PCC. The interviewers also recorded the time required for the MINI assessment, including the administration and scoring, the gender and age of the patients and the results of the assessment. The questionnaires were completed directly after the MINI assessment.

Interviews and focus group discussions

The interviews and focus group discussions were based on topic guides that included probing questions when necessary (Additional file 1). They were audio-recorded and supplemented with field notes.

Patients were interviewed individually by one of the authors (AP). A purposeful sample was recruited with the goal of obtaining an even distribution between PCCs and a wide variation in gender, age and ethnicity. All patients who completed the questionnaire were asked to participate in a face-to-face interview. Those who volunteered were contacted, and the interviews were performed concurrently. The participants could choose the time and location of the interview (home, the interviewer's office or the PCC). The interviews took an average of 25 min, and the participants were compensated with a voucher for a cinema ticket (value of 12 euro). Out of 125 patients, 49 signed up for an interview. Nine (four men) did not consent, and 16 women aged 25–60 years were not contacted. Thus, 24 persons, six men and 18 women, were interviewed; four were younger than 25 years, and five were older than 60 years. Six persons were first- or second-generation immigrants. Transcripts were not returned to the participants for verification, and feedback of results was not provided.

The first author (AP) interviewed the three therapists at their respective PCCs after study completion. All GPs at PCC1 and PCC2 were invited to a focus group discussion. Focus groups were chosen because the interactions between participants can facilitate the emergence of different aspects of interest, which is especially fruitful when there is scarce information about the phenomenon beforehand [29]. Two focus groups were held at PCC1 (4 and 5 participants), and one at PCC2 (8 participants). Three of the GPs were men, and 14 were women. Three were receiving specialist training, and seven had worked as GPs for more than 20 years. The GP at PCC3 was one of the authors and did not participate in a focus group. The focus groups were moderated by AP and IK, who ensured that all participants shared their experiences. The average duration of the group discussions was 45 min. The therapists and GPs did not receive compensation other than a light meal. Neither AP nor IK knew the GPs and therapists beforehand. Interviewees were informed that the study was part of the interviewer's thesis and was of interest to the Stockholm County Council.

Data analysis

Data from the acceptance questionnaires were managed in Excel 2013. The VAS scores regarding global satisfaction with the MINI assessment were estimated with a ruler. The scores had a right-skewed distribution; therefore; the medians and interquartile range (IQR) were calculated. For the ten items on the acceptance questionnaires, the proportion of participants who almost or fully agreed with the statement (rated 2 or 3) was calculated.

The time required for the assessments was analyzed as the mean (SD) number of minutes.

The interviews and focus group discussions were transcribed verbatim by a secretary who was external to the study, and the transcripts were validated against the recordings by AP. The analytical approach was based on qualitative content analysis [30, 31] and was inductive, as research on this phenomenon is scarce [31]. Coding was performed separately for patients, interviewers and GPs. Excerpts regarding the structure and questions of the MINI from the GPs who conducted the MINI were analyzed together with the other interviewers' statements.

The preliminary extraction, condensing, and coding of meaning units was performed by AP and verified by SM. The subcategories and categories were first defined independently by SM and AP and were then confirmed by consensus. In the next step, categories across participant groups were grouped under common main categories. The entire process was conducted iteratively, continuously considering other possibilities and involving all authors. Finally, the items from the questionnaires were mapped onto the main categories for integration of the data sets. Data were managed in Word 2013 and Excel 2013. The results were presented at a meeting with GPs at PCC1, who expressed that the findings were in line with their experiences.

Results

In total, 125 patients participated completed the questionnaire (Table 2). Of these, 22% had no MINI diagnosis, 47% had one diagnosis, and 31% fulfilled the criteria for at least two diagnoses. At PCC1, 67 patients fulfilled the inclusion criteria. Of these, five declined the MINI assessment, and another seven did not consent to the questionnaire. All patients who fulfilled the inclusion criteria at PCC3 consented to the study, but one did not complete the questionnaire. Drop-out data for the patients were not reported by PCC2. The interviewers at the three PCCs completed 115

Table 2 Characteristics of responding patients ($n = 125$), reasons for visits and MINI diagnosis

Characteristics	PCC1	PCC2	PCC3	Total
Number of patients	55	54	16	125
Number female patients	39 (72%)	45 (83%)	13 (81%)	97 (78%)
Age distribution[a]				
< 25 years	5	4	4	13 (12%)
25–60 years	41	31	12	84 (78%)
> 60 years	9	5	0	14 (13%)
Main reason to visit the PCC				
Depressive symptoms	16	18	7	41 (33%)
Anxiety	6	9	4	19 (15%)
Stress, tired, sleep problems	9	6	0	15 (12%)
Other psychiatric complaints	9	14	2	15 (20%)
Somatic complaints	12	3	2	17 (14%)
Not answered	3	4	1	8 (6%)
MINI diagnosis[b]				
Depression only	10	5	7	22 (18%)
One anxiety disorder only	11	21	0	32 (27%)
More than one anxiety disorder	3	2	0	5 (4%)
Both depression and anxiety disorder	11	3	7	21 (18%)
Depression or anxiety or both with other MINI diagnoses	6	3	2	11 (9%)
Other MINI diagnoses	1	2	9	3 (2%)
None	13	13	0	26 (22%)

[a]age reported for $n = 40$ at PCC2; [b] MINI diagnoses reported for $n = 49$ patients at PCC2

questionnaires related to the participating patient; ten questionnaires were missing from PCC2.

The experiences of patients, interviewers and referring GPs expressed in the interviews and focus groups centered around six main categories: Perceived strengths of the MINI; Perceived advantages of using the MINI for GPs; Perceived advantages of using the MINI for patients; Perceived weaknesses of the MINI; The duration of the MINI as a potential concern; and The MINI is an additional tool and a personal contact with the interviewer is important. An example coding scheme is shown in Additional file 2.

All items in the acceptance questionnaires corresponded to one of the main categories, with the exception of three items from the interviewer questionnaire. These items concerned their satisfaction with the assessment. The interviewers perceived that they felt competent and did not make any mistakes during the MINI. This issue was not discussed at all during the interviews and is not described further. Table 3 summarizes the main categories, their underlying categories and the corresponding items from the acceptance questionnaires (Table 3).

The results of the questionnaires are shown in Table 4. They largely mirrored the findings of the interviews and focus groups. The overall satisfaction with the MINI as measured in the questionnaires was high. The median satisfaction among patients ($n = 124$) was 80 (IQR 64 to 92), with a range from 0 to 100. For the interviewers ($n = 115$ assessments), the median satisfaction was 86 (IQR 75 to 95), with a range from 25 to 100. In the interviews, patients and interviewers stated that the MINI was a good test.

Perceived strengths of the MINI

Structured format and detailed questions that often capture the problem

According to the questionnaires, most patients felt that the MINI had sufficiently detailed questions for the interviewer to understand the patient (Table 4). Less than 5 % perceived that there were too many questions (Table 4). The interviewers reported that they seldom

Table 3 Summary of findings for experiences and perceptions of using the MINI

Main category	PATIENTS category	INTERVIEWERS category	REFERRING GPs category	Corresponding item in the questionnaires
Perceived strengths of the MINI	Structured format and detailed questions that often capture the problem			P4, P10, I2
	The MINI does not evoke negative emotions		MINI does not evoke emotions	P3, P5, I8
Perceived advantages of using the MINI for GPs		More accurate diagnoses facilitate the work of the GP		
			A useful standard test for deeper investigations and selected patients	
Perceived advantages of using the MINI for patients	New insight into the problem			P2, P9, I5
	The MINI is mostly meaningful			P1, P6, I10
	The MINI may lead to better treatment			
Perceived weaknesses of the MINI	It is a constraint to only answer yes and no			
	Some questions are problematic, and some common problems are not covered			
	The results of the MINI may be biased			P8, I7
The duration of the MINI as a potential concern	The duration was acceptable	The MINI most often takes a short period of time		Time recording
		It could be problematic to fit the MINI into the GP consultation scheme		
The MINI is an additional tool and a personal contact with the interviewer is important		The MINI is just one part of the diagnostic procedure and its role must be explained		P7, I6, I9
	The personal contact is important for most patients			

Categories that are similar across the participant groups, patients, interviewers (therapists or GPs) and referring GPs are placed on the same row; empty space indicates that the subject was not discussed

Table 4 Results from the acceptance questionnaires

Patient questionnaire (*P*) (*n* = 125)		Interviewer questionnaire (*I*) (*n* = 115)	
Item (no.)	Percentage agreeing fully or almost fully	Item (no.)	Percentage agreeing fully or almost fully
The procedure was helpful (P1)	68	–	
I feel unclear about the results of MINI (P2)	23		
I felt interrogated (P3)	7		
Too many questions (P4)	6		
It was exhausting (P5)	4	It was exhausting (I8)	7
I felt taken seriously (P6)	93	I was responsive to the patient (I10)	85
A positive relationship with the interviewer was established (P7)	93	A positive relationship with the patient was established (I6)	87
		The patient was cooperative (I9)	96
I did not tell everything (P8)	16	The patient did not report everything (I7)	6
I understood my problems better (P9)	33	The patient only realizes some dimensions of her problem (I5)	1
It was enough detail for the interviewer (P10)	77	Difficulties to capture all relevant information (I2)	19
–		I conducted the interview as well as I could (I1)	100
–		I felt competent (I3)	88
–		I made mistakes (I4)	1

The table shows the proportions of questionnaires from patients and interviewers where the respondents agreed fully or almost fully to the items. Items that correspond to each other in the patient and interviewer questionnaires are placed on the same row

encountered difficulties capturing all relevant information with the MINI (Table 4).

The standardized format also offered advantages. Patients appreciated that the questions were the same for everyone. One reason this consistency was appreciated was that it helped them realize that others could have the same problems and that they were not "odd or weird" (Patient 23). Interviewers agreed:

> "The MINI plays down the situation for those who have a diagnosis: Apparently, there is a paper stating that you could have obsessions, so [obsessions] seem to be reasonably frequent" (GP3, PCC2).

Patients and interviewers also stated that the questions were detailed and most often easy to understand. However, the experiences with the examples included in the MINI were mixed. Some patients appreciated them because they increased their understanding of the item, whereas the examples were not helpful for others.

Some patients felt that it was easier to respond "yes" or "no" than to have to describe their situation and symptoms in own words. Thus, the MINI could facilitate the conversation for patients who were too tired to talk, had difficulties explaining how they felt or easily lost the thread of conversation while talking:

> "...sometimes it feels as if you are only talking in circles, and you realize that you don't understand where you are. This can be tough because then you wonder, 'what was the purpose of this? Why did we talk about this?'" (Patient 23).
> Patients acknowledged that the MINI was extensive and covered many disorders. They often expressed that the MINI included their problems: "There were different questions that I liked and that were really good [...]. The questions made me feel that they were about me" (Patient 21).

The MINI does not evoke negative emotions

According to the questionnaires, few patients felt interrogated during the assessment and few found it exhausting. Similarly, the interviewers seldom felt emotionally exhausted after conducting the assessment.

These negative aspects were not raised spontaneously by the patients in the interviews. After probing, the patients mostly expressed that they were not bothered by the interview. This finding was corroborated by the interviewers, who deemed that the MINI was neither provoking nor offensive to the patients. However, the patients also expressed that it could be difficult to admit to awkward symptoms.

Perceived advantages of using the MINI for GPs

More accurate diagnoses facilitate the work of the GP

The participants acknowledged that the MINI improved the accuracy of the diagnostic procedure. Patients stated that the MINI ensured that important issues were not missed. An example of this, mentioned by the referring GPs, was that distinguishing between depression and anxiety disorders could be tricky for GPs without a special interest in psychiatry. One therapist perceived that the GPs did not probe for details and that the MINI added information by, e.g., asking specific questions about feeling weak, speaking slower than usual or being restless.

The MINI facilitated open discussion of sensitive or awkward issues. It ensured that problems such as addiction and suicide attempts were included and that symptoms suggestive of, e.g., phobias and obsessive-compulsive disorder (OCD) were communicated by the patient. The MINI could thus uncover problems that were unknown to the health care provider.

> "Sometimes the MINI confirms what you had suspected. Sometimes it doesn't, and that is when you think - what luck that I used the MINI, otherwise I wouldn't have picked up the problem" (Therapist 3).

GPs with experience conducting the MINI perceived that their assessments became more professional when they used the instrument. Instead of simply asking, "Oh, how are you?" (GP2, PCC2), they thoroughly worked through a standardized questionnaire.

A useful standard test for deeper investigation and selected patients

The GPs described various experiences and routines regarding the use of the MINI. It could be perceived as a standard test for psychiatric complaints in parallel with somatic problems:

> "The MINI has its place. I think that we (GPs) should be able to diagnose psychiatric disorders and know who should be treated in primary care and who should be referred to psychiatry. Of course, we build considerably on our own experience, for example, for those who pee frequently, we often use tests to check for diabetes. I believe that it is good to have a routine test for psychiatric problems as well" (GP2, PCC2).

The GPs chose the MINI in particular when a deeper investigation was required, for example when symptoms were not clear, or the patient had not responded to selective serotonin reuptake inhibitor (SSRI) treatments as anticipated. The MINI was also viewed as an aid for managing silent patients as well as patients with somatoform disorders.

> "The MINI is good for patients with somatoform disorders. I performed the MINI with such a patient. It was OK only because it is so standardized and not focused on just *her* psychiatric problems. I found some border psychotic problems, which I believe I never would had thought of asking myself" (GP1, PCC2).

However, some patients could be reluctant. Patients with known psychiatric problems who had been aware of their diagnosis for a long time, especially the elderly, were less motivated to participate in an extra visit to health care for the interview, as were patients with somatic complaints who did not accept that they could have a psychiatric problem.

The MINI was also useful for referrals to specialist care in psychiatry, with participants stating that the explicit information obtained from the MINI facilitated the referral. However, the belief that the MINI was not necessary for a diagnosis, that anamnesis in combination with a depression or anxiety rating scale was sufficient, was also raised. Another value to GPs was that the MINI helped rule out psychiatric diagnoses. One example was that the MINI could be a quick procedure for patients with chronic back pain. Another example was provided as follows:

> "A young girl had been at several hospitals for numbness and had gone through many examinations [...]. Then, she came to me, and my clinical instinct said depression as an underlying cause for her problems. But I referred her for the MINI, and it was negative on two occasions. So, the MINI was very good; without it, I would have prescribed an antidepressant..." (GP1, PCC1).

Perceived advantages of using the MINI for the patients

New insight into the problem

The interviewers stated that the patients obtained good insight into their problems. In the questionnaire, patients agreed to a lesser extent. One third acknowledged that they understood their problems better after the MINI, and one out of five felt unclear about the results (Table 4). However, the interviewed patients expressed that the MINI gave them better insight. Patients with a MINI diagnosis understood that they had a psychiatric problem, that there was a true cause underlying their symptoms and that they needed help. The questions helped them reflect on their wellbeing in depth and focus their attention on aspects of their problems. The MINI could also help raise issues that the patients were not aware of. One example was a patient who, during the MINI, realized that she consumed too much alcohol and described it as a "wake-up call" (Patient 1).

Additionally, the interviewers specifically mentioned the alcohol module:

> "But the largest aha-experience was with alcohol. The first question is general, so you can go on with the other questions. It is really interesting to see how people just sit there and reflect on their drinking habits – 'what relation do I have to alcohol?' I think this has been very good for many patients" (Therapist 1).

The MINI is mostly meaningful

According to the questionnaire, the MINI had been of value to the patients, and most patients agreed that they felt they had been taken seriously (Table 4). In the interviews, patients often concluded that the MINI had been meaningful for them:

> "It was great! I score it eight out of ten" (Patient 21).

Having a diagnosis was perceived as a relief and could also be the starting point for patients to read about their problems and how to address them. However, some patients felt that the interview was irrelevant and that they would have preferred spending the time talking with a psychologist instead. The interviewers mentioned that although some patients might meet the criteria for a diagnosis in the MINI, the symptoms associated with the diagnosis were not of major concern to the patient. Other mental problems such as stress bothered them more. The GPs noted that patients were willing to complete the MINI when the purpose was explained to them. Patients expressed afterwards that they were satisfied with the thorough procedure.

The MINI may lead to better treatment

Patients, interviewers and GPs expressed that the MINI could have an impact on treatment. Patients who were not satisfied with their current treatment hoped that the results of the MINI would support changing it. The GPs appreciated that the MINI could help them determine the appropriate treatment. One example of this was a patient with sleeping problems who was seeking a renewed prescription for sleeping pills. The MINI showed that the patient had severe depression. After anti-depressive treatment, the patient no longer needed the sleeping pills.

Perceived weaknesses of the MINI

It is a constraint to only answer yes and no

Both patients and interviewers often perceived that the MINI was constraining, which could result in frustration from the patient. Patients expressed that "yes" and "no" were not sufficient response options. One problem was that sometimes none of the alternatives were considered correct. Another problem was that the patients wanted to explain and report details that they themselves considered important. Some stated that the MINI lacked questions that asked for more information. Patients sometimes felt that the task was impossible and answered with their own words. The perceptions of the patients were shared by the therapists. They felt that it was necessary to complement the MINI with their own questions to obtain more detail:

> "I always use the questions (of the MINI) in a structured way, but I also ask follow-up questions such as "can you give an example?" or "OK, what do you mean by that?" Otherwise, I don't think that the MINI adds that much value" (Therapist 3).

Some questions are problematic, and some common problems are not covered

Although most questions in the MINI were not problematic, some issues did emerge. Both patients and interviewers perceived that the questions relating to pastimes and to the duration of symptoms were harder to answer than questions relating to the current situation. Some questions were seen as extreme, with patients specifically noting those on suicide and addiction. The interviewers highlighted issues with the questions about suicide ("sneaky") and compulsive behavior (the examples were not familiar to the patients). Other questions were unclear and difficult to interpret: "The questions were perhaps not laser-sharp; it [the MINI] felt like a work in progress" (Patient 4).

The therapists noted that some problems that were common in primary care were not addressed in the MINI. They would have appreciated if stress, fatigue and sleep had been included in the MINI as well. Likewise, some patients expressed that the MINI was not suitable for everybody's problems:

> "The MINI did not suit me perfectly, for example. It felt like the MINI more looked for and tried to capture bipolar problems, not the more "low-key un-gladness"- the sense of never being glad, I mean" (Patient 17).

The results of the MINI may be biased

One aspect of the MINI that was mentioned was whether the results were valid. Both interviewers and patients recognized that the results could be biased by interpretation and the extent to which the patient answered truthfully. One out of six patients reported that they had not reported everything that had bothered them, while the interviewers suspected that only one out of 17 patients had not reported everything bothering them.

In the interviews, patients noted that they had to interpret questions that they felt were imprecise. They sometimes perceived that there was no such thing as a clear cut "yes" or "no" answer, and thus they guessed, made a best estimate or responded with their own words instead. The interviewers confirmed that they often had to interpret the answer. This could take the form of a dialogue, in which patients and interviewers decided on the most correct alternative together, or patients could leave the responsibility to the interviewer to translate. The interviewers also expressed that certain words in the MINI such as "ever", "regularly" and "almost completely" were not "crystal clear" (Therapist 2).

The patients noted that the assessment could be subject to manipulation, although some described the MINI as self-correcting and not sensitive to influence. Patients emphasized that they had to be honest if they wanted to receive adequate treatment. However, some confessed that they recognized the diagnoses behind the various modules:

> "I was rather aware of how I was. I had googled a little and read about anxiety and other problems. So, I understood what the questions were aiming at, I understood that now, [this question] is about depression, now about anxiety... so it was fairly easy to see through [the intent]" (Patient 19).

The duration of the MINI as a potential concern

The recorded mean duration of the 117 MINI interviews was 26 (SD 11) minutes, ranging from 12 to 60 min. More than half of the interviews (54%) lasted 20 min or less, 29% between 21 and 30 min, and 17% between 31 and 60 min.

The duration was acceptable to the patients

The time required to perform the MINI was seldom brought up by the interviewees. Some patients, after probing, noted that the MINI was time-consuming, but as one patient stated, "... as it helped me so much, it would have been worth even more time" (Patient 11).

The MINI most often takes a short period of time according to the interviewers

The interviewers, therapists and GPs found that the MINI was most often a rapid procedure, as patients in primary care generally have a limited range of psychiatric problems. However, patients who quickly lost the thread of conversation or had cognitive difficulties could require more time.

It could be problematic to fit the MINI into the GP consultation scheme

Some GPs who conducted the MINI were wary of the time needed. Even if the assessment took only 20 min, they often had to book a separate consultation for the MINI. This could be weeks later, which was not acceptable for patients with severe problems. These GPs would have appreciated a shorter or web-based version of the MINI in order to save time. A wish to use only sections of the MINI that were perceived to be relevant to the actual patient was also expressed.

The MINI is an additional tool and a personal contact with the interviewer is important

The MINI is just one part of the diagnostic procedure and its role must be explained

Patients were not always clear about the role of the MINI in the diagnostic procedure. Some patients seemed to believe that the purpose of the MINI was to replace the clinical assessment. They stressed that, on principle, the MINI could not be sufficient for a diagnosis but must be combined with a conversation.

For the interviewers and GPs, the MINI could be more or less important for the final diagnosis. Some interviewers weighed the patient's story, the patient's behavior and the results of the MINI. If contradictory, the patient's behavior and story were more important for deciding how to manage the patient than the MINI diagnosis. Others based the final diagnosis on the MINI only but found that a short discussion after the interview could result in valuable additional information. The referring GPs found that the MINI provided useful extra information, but they emphasized that their own judgement was the most important.

Some patients found that the information and instructions for completing the MINI were not sufficient. Written instructions to read in advance or short outlines of the structure of the MINI before the interview would have been helpful. Insufficient information could have unintended consequences. Not understanding the reason for the interview could lead patients to feel uncertain about how the results would be used. Patients who did not obtain a diagnosis could perceive that the interview was irrelevant. The interviewers added that thorough instructions were vital for patients to adhere to the "yes-no" structure.

An interpersonal contact with the interviewer is important

In the questionnaires, patients as well as interviewers expressed that they had established a positive relationship during the interview. In the interviews, the importance of interpersonal contact was expressed by both patients and interviewers:

> "If I had come to the physician and felt pretty rotten and had then been interviewed by a counselor or whatever ... and that person just read from a template, then maybe, I would think, 'Please, I need help, and you are just reading from a checklist'. I could imagine that" (Patient 22).

Alternatively, a therapist noted the following:

> "Some (patients) have kind of felt that they did not have the opportunity to talk (...) So it is a question of weighing up how much [to use the] instruments... there must also be time to tell in your own words how you feel. You should not underrate personal meetings" (Therapist 1).

However, for some patients, it was viewed as an advantage that there was no need for a personal relationship with the interviewer. One perception, expressed as positive, was that no eye contact was required and that the MINI "became like armor" (Patient 3) that prevented personal boundaries from being crossed.

Discussion

This study described the experiences and perceptions of the use of a psychiatric structured interview instrument, the MINI, in primary care. The MINI was considered a useful part of the clinical assessment of selected patients with unclear psychiatric symptoms. Furthermore, the MINI helped GPs establish an accurate diagnosis as the basis for choosing treatment options. Patients were satisfied with the MINI, which helped them understand and verbalize their problems. The MINI was not emotionally disturbing for the patients. The yes-no format could be a constraint, and subjective interpretations were possible. Lack of time was a concern only when the MINI was performed by GPs.

Patients rated the MINI as a relevant procedure. Many of them expressed that they preferred to answer standardized questions, as it was difficult for them to tell their story in their own words. The MINI helped them communicate their problems. They could identify parts of themselves in the questions, which also facilitated the disclosure of shameful or embarrassing problems that they otherwise would not have shared. Although some questions might have been disturbing, very few patients found the MINI to be intrusive or problematic. Patients' perceptions of psychiatric structured interviews in primary care have not been reported previously, but our results correspond to what has been described in studies from other settings, mostly in psychiatry [23, 24, 28, 32, 33]. However, it should be noted that approximately 3% of the patients found the procedure unnecessary and would have preferred to have more time for a less structured conversation.

The referring GPs and interviewers in our study perceived that the major advantage of the MINI was that it contributed to an accurate diagnosis for patients who needed a more thorough investigation and that it helped identify comorbidities. A third of the patients presented with comorbidities, mostly depression accompanied by one or more anxiety disorders. A substantial proportion, one out of ten, had other comorbidities such as bipolar disorder, OCD, Post-Traumatic Stress Disorder, suicidal behavior or alcohol dependence, conditions that were not previously known to the GPs. These figures may, however, be an underestimate. The two therapists employed at PCC2 differed from the other interviewers regarding number and type of diagnoses. They mostly reported one diagnosis only, whereas the others were more likely to report all diagnoses indicated by the MINI. One explanation of this finding could be that the therapists at PCC2 only reported the diagnosis that was the focus of their treatment.

The GPs acknowledged that an accurate diagnosis affected the choice of treatment. One option for Swedish primary care physicians when managing patients with suspected depression or anxiety is to test whether the patient improves with selective serotonin reuptake inhibitor (SSRI) treatment. As one out of five in our study did not meet the criteria for depression or anxiety disorder, this indicates that the MINI could help decrease unnecessary treatment and shorten the duration of the search for correct management. This is in accordance with another study, which found that a proportion of patients, who had received a diagnosis of affective or anxiety disorders based on clinical parameters, were subthreshold cases, not needing medical treatment [12]. Knowledge of hidden comorbidities also affects treatment and may lead to more tailored treatment or referral to psychiatry. Psychiatric disorders that are perceived as stigmatizing to the patients are less often identified by conversations with the patient than when the conversation is supplemented with a structured interview [34].

The GPs in our study concluded that the MINI was a useful addition, especially for complicated patients, which is in line with a previously mentioned study in Brazil [22]. However, it should be underscored that the MINI, like other structured interviews, is limited to specific psychiatric diagnoses and does not cover all mental problems encountered in primary care [35]. This was also observed by patients and interviewers in our study, as some of them missed modules about stress and sadness.

We have not found any other studies that investigated GPs' experiences of using a structured interview for mental illness. However, our results are more positive than those shown in other studies on the acceptance of short, self-rating questionnaires for case-finding and severity of depression. Such tests have for example been studied as part of the introduction of the guidelines from the National Institute for Clinical Excellence (NICE) [36]. Some studies highlighted a concern that the doctor-patient relationship could be compromised, in particular that good conversations might be disturbed by introducing a document that should be followed [37–41]. This aspect was not mentioned in the present study, as GPs either had chosen to work with the MINI themselves or did not face this situation because the patients were referred to a psychologist for the MINI.

Although advantages of the MINI for patients as well as for GPs were highlighted, some other aspects should be taken into consideration. Patients and interviewers often found that the yes-no format was limiting and developed ways to communicate more information. For example, patients could refuse to answer yes or no or could talk freely and leave it to the interviewer to translate their response. Some interviewers with more experience added open-ended questions. Thus, in practice, the MINI was sometimes used as a semi-structured interview. This is acceptable according to the instructions of the MINI but requires greater skills and more in-depth training of the interviewer.

A related issue, raised by patients and interviewers, concerned the validity of the MINI. Apart from the risks of misunderstanding during the interpretation of questions and answers, patients may want the interview to have a certain outcome. Interestingly, the interviewers seldom suspected that the patients had withheld information, although a sixth of the patients reported falsely negating problems assessed in the MINI. Despite these omissions, the patients seemed to be aware that truthful answers were important for their treatment. However, regardless of the approach used to diagnose psychiatric disorders, the diagnosis is solely based on information provided by the patient and/or their relatives. During consultations, information about psychiatric problems and the interpretation of this information have been shown to be dependent on certain factors, e.g., patient's gender, marital status and quality of life [12], non-verbal communication [42] and GPs' prior knowledge of the patient's other problems and contextual factors [8]. Thus, the risk of distorted information is general and not unique to the MINI.

The time required for assessment is an important aspect of tests performed in primary care settings. In our study, the average duration of the MINI was 26 min, which is in line with the times reported in other studies [22, 26]. Time was not viewed as a major barrier to the use of the MINI. However, most interviews were performed by therapists, whose time was less restricted. Some GPs who conducted the MINI, on the other hand, perceived that the consultation time could be too short for completing the MINI. This finding is in accordance with the results of a Brazilian study [22] in which GPs used the MINI. In that study, the duration of the MINI was considered an obstacle to its use as a screening instrument but was considered acceptable for use with selected patients.

Strengths and limitations

Our study is the first to explore primary care patients' perspectives toward the use of a structured interview for mental disorders. A strength of the study was the design, which addressed the implementation of the MINI from multiple perspectives. The sample was broad, with three participating PCCs from areas with varying socioeconomic statuses, GPs who had little to substantial experience, and patients with varying characteristics with respect to gender, age, ethnicity and mental problems. Furthermore, experiences and perceptions were obtained through questionnaires that were supplemented with richer information from semi-structured interviews and focus groups. The triangulation between participant groups and data collection methods showed consistent results. The content analysis was conducted by two researchers with different backgrounds and preconceptions, which allowed for different perspectives and reflexivity [43]. It should be noted that the GP at PCC3, who was also a co-author of this publication, had no access to the primary data and did not take part in the analysis.

The study protocol stated that 10–12 patient interviews should be conducted. This was a practical consideration that was made in order to avoid obtaining an amount of information that might be difficult to grasp. As suggested by Malterud et al. [44], the sample size was reevaluated. Our preliminary analysis showed that several of the interviews resulted in a limited amount of information and that more interviews were needed to more fully capture the variations in perceptions. After another 12 interviews had been conducted, the data were broader, and the final interviews did not yield any new information.

The sampling method may have led to limitations in the transferability of the results. Owing to the lack of financial support, few PCCs felt inclined to participate, although key politicians and the primary care board deemed the project important for practice. The PCCs that participated were interested enough to invest in the study. Better management of patients with mental ill-health and thus better diagnostic procedures were important for these PCCs. The experiences and perceptions of interviewers and GPs may differ in PCCs with other values and priorities, although patient perceptions are likely more stable. Another factor that may affect transferability is that the experiences were confined to the paper-and-pen version of the MINI 6.0. Changing from the MINI 6.0 to the recently introduced MINI 7.0 would probably not influence these perceptions. However, the web version of the MINI may lead to other perceptions of the procedure from both the patients and the interviewers.

Unexpectedly, the commitment to the study differed between the sites and over time. Two PCCs had a local study coordinator who ensured that the procedures were followed. The third PCC underwent a reorganization when the study coordinator left, and the personnel had to focus on implementing new routines. This affected the data collection, which became less systematic. One of the employed therapists did not complete ten questionnaires and time recordings because of time constraints. However, there was little variability in the existing 115 questionnaires, and there is no reason to believe that the missing questionnaires would have changed the results substantially.

The credibility of the findings may be affected by time. The study was conducted during one full year, and there might be a risk that the experiences changed as a result of internal or external events, such as the reorganization of PCC2. However, the interviews and questionnaires did not indicate such a shift over time. On the other hand, during the analysis, it became apparent that some patients had changed their perspectives from the time when the questionnaire was completed to the research interview, which was conducted several weeks later. At the interview, the patients had most often been informed of their diagnosis, had started treatment, and had also had time for reflection. However, there was no clear direction to any of the changes, as patients expressed higher as well as lower acceptance at the interview.

Conclusions

The paper-and-pen version of the MINI can be useful in primary care as part of the clinical assessment of patients at risk of depression and anxiety. The MINI helped to obtain a complete picture and to identify psychiatric comorbidities, including stigmatizing disorders. Patients, GPs and therapists appreciated the MINI. It facilitated the GPs' work, provided new insight for patients and was not experienced as intrusive or exhausting.

Abbreviations

GP: General practitioner; IQR: Interquartile range; MINI: Mini-International Neuropsychiatric Interview; PCC: Primary care center; VAS: Visual Analog Scale

Acknowledgments

We thank the patients and staff at the three PCCs, as well as Tina in-Albon for approving the use of the acceptance questionnaires and their translation from German, Berit Dybäck for coordinating the study at one of the PCCs, and Måns Rosén for providing valuable comments on the manuscript.

Funding

No funding was received.

Authors' contributions

AP drafted the study protocol, coordinated the study, conducted the interviews and drafted the manuscript. AP and SM analyzed the data; IK conceived the study, recruited the study sites, co-moderated the focus group discussions, and commented on the analyses; RW and SW contributed to the design of the study and commented on the analysis. All authors contributed to the manuscript and agreed upon the final draft.

Authors' information

IK, SM, and RW are senior GPs with a doctoral degree who are experienced in research in primary care. SM and RW have extensive experience with qualitative methodology. SW is a GP with a special focus on psychiatric diagnostics who contributed to the procedures section of the protocol and initiated the study at PCC2. SW moved to PCC3 and volunteered as a study participant. AP is a doctoral student working in governmental health technology assessments and has experience in interviewing. IK and AP had previous knowledge of the MINI from participation in a systematic review on diagnostic tools for affective disorders.

Consent for publication

Participants consented that the results were to be published and that information would be presented at an aggregated level. Interviewees consented that quotations could be used but in de-identified format.

Competing interests

The authors declare that they have no competing interests.

Author details

[1]Medical Management Centre, Department of Learning, Informatics, Management and Ethics, Karolinska Institutet, Tomtebodavägen 18 A, SE-171 77 Stockholm, Sweden. [2]Swedish Agency for Health Technology Assessment and Social Assessment, SE-102 33 Stockholm, Sweden. [3]Division of Family Medicine, Department of Neurobiology, Care Sciences and Society, Karolinska Institutet, Alfred Nobels allé 23 D2, SE-141 83 Huddinge, Sweden. [4]Department of Public Health Sciences, Karolinska Institutet, Tomtebodavägen 18 A, SE-171 77 Stockholm, Sweden. [5]Department for Neurobiology, Care Sciences and Society, Karolinska Institutet, Alfred Nobels allé 23 D2, SE 141 83 Huddinge, Sweden. [6]Department of Medicine, Clinical Epidemiology Unit T2, 14, Karolinska Institutet, SE-171 77 Stockholm, Sweden.

References

1. Roca M, Gili M, Garcia-Garcia M, Salva J, Vives M, Garcia Campayo J, Comas A. Prevalence and comorbidity of common mental disorders in primary care. J Affect Disord. 2009;119:52–8.
2. King M, Nazareth I, Levy G, Walker C, Morris R, Weich S, Bellon-Saameno JA, Moreno B, Svab I, Rotar D, et al. Prevalence of common mental disorders in general practice attendees across Europe. Br J Psychiatry. 2008;192:362–7.
3. Mergl R, Seidscheck I, Allgaier AK, Moller HJ, Hegerl U, Henkel V. Depressive, anxiety, and somatoform disorders in primary care: prevalence and recognition. Depress Anxiety. 2007;24:185–95.
4. Jackson JL, Passamonti M, Kroenke K. Outcome and impact of mental disorders in primary care at 5 years. Psychosom Med. 2007;69:270–6.
5. Ansseau M, Dierick M, Buntinkx F, Cnockaert P, De Smedt J, Van Den Haute M, Vander MD. High prevalence of mental disorders in primary care. J Affect Disord. 2004;78:49–55.
6. Ghuloum S, Bener A, Abou-Saleh MT. Prevalence of mental disorders in adult population attending primary health care setting in Qatari population. JPMA. 2011;61:216–21.
7. Menear M, Dore I, Cloutier AM, Perrier L, Roberge P, Duhoux A, Houle J, Fournier L. The influence of comorbid chronic physical conditions on depression recognition in primary care: a systematic review. J Psychosom Res. 2015;78:304–13.
8. van Weel-Baumgarten EM, van den Bosch WJ, van den Hoogen HJ, Zitman FG. The validity of the diagnosis of depression in general practice: is using criteria for diagnosis as a routine the answer? Br J Gen Pract. 2000;50:284–7.
9. Statens Beredning för Medicinsk Utvärdering. Case-finding, diagnosis and follow-up of patients with affective disorders, a health technology assessment report (in Swedish). Stockholm: SBU; 2012.
10. Mitchell AJ, Vaze A, Rao S. Clinical diagnosis of depression in primary care: a meta-analysis. Lancet. 2009;374:609–19.
11. Magruder-Habib K, Zung WW, Feussner JR. Improving physicians' recognition and treatment of depression in general medical care. Results from a randomized clinical trial. Med Care. 1990;28:239–50.

12. Balestrieri M, Baldacci S, Bellomo A, Bellantuono C, Conti L, Perugi G, Nardini M, Borbotti M, Viegi G. Clinical vs. structured interview on anxiety and affective disorders by primary care physicians. Understanding diagnostic discordance. Epidemiol Psichiatr Soc. 2007;16:144–51.
13. Berardi D, Menchetti M, Cevenini N, Scaini S, Versari M, De Ronchi D. Increased recognition of depression in primary care. Comparison between primary-care physician and ICD-10 diagnosis of depression. Psychother Psychosom. 2005;74:225–30.
14. Gerrity MS, Cole SA, Dietrich AJ, Barrett JE. Improving the recognition and management of depression: is there a role for physician education? J Fam Pract. 1999;48:949–57.
15. Lin EH, Simon GE, Katzelnick DJ, Pearson SD. Does physician education on depression management improve treatment in primary care? J Gen Intern Med. 2001;16:614–9.
16. Shirazi M, Assadi SM, Sadeghi M, Zeinaloo AA, Kashani AS, Arbabi M, Alaedini F, Lonka K, Wahlstrom R. Applying a modified Prochaska's model of readiness to change for general practitioners on depressive disorders in CME programmes: validation of tool. J Eval Clin Pract. 2007;13:298–302.
17. Thompson C, Kinmonth AL, Stevens L, Peveler RC, Stevens A, Ostler KJ, Pickering RM, Baker NG, Henson A, Preece J, et al. Effects of a clinical-practice guideline and practice-based education on detection and outcome of depression in primary care: Hampshire depression project randomised controlled trial. Lancet. 2000;355:185–91.
18. Gilbody S, Sheldon T, House A. Screening and case-finding instruments for depression: a meta-analysis. CMAJ. 2008;178:997–1003.
19. Lotfi L, Flyckt L, Krakau I, Martensson B, Nilsson GH. Undetected depression in primary healthcare: occurrence, severity and co-morbidity in a two-stage procedure of opportunistic screening. Nord J Psychiatry. 2010;64:421–7.
20. Spiegel W, Tonies H, Scherer M, Katschnig H. Learning by doing: a novel approach to improving general practitioners' diagnostic skills for common mental disorders. Wien Klin Wochenschr. 2007;119:117–23.
21. Pettersson A, Bostrom KB, Gustavsson P, Ekselius L. Which instruments to support diagnosis of depression have sufficient accuracy? A systematic review. Nord J Psychiatry. 2015;69:497–508.
22. de Azevedo Marques JM, Zuardi AW. Validity and applicability of the Mini international neuropsychiatric interview administered by family medicine residents in primary health care in Brazil. Gen Hosp Psychiatry. 2008;30:303–10.
23. Mordal J, Gundersen O, Bramness JG. Norwegian version of the Mini-international neuropsychiatric interview: feasibility, acceptability and test-retest reliability in an acute psychiatric ward. Eur Psychiatry. 2010;25:172–7.
24. Pinninti NR, Madison H, Musser E, Rissmiller D. MINI international neuropsychiatric schedule: clinical utility and patient acceptance. Eur Psychiatry. 2003;18:361–4.
25. Otsubo T, Tanaka K, Koda R, Shinoda J, Sano N, Tanaka S, Aoyama H, Mimura M, Kamijima K. Reliability and validity of Japanese version of the Mini-international neuropsychiatric interview. Psychiatry Clin Neurosci. 2005;59:517–26.
26. Sheehan DV, Lecrubier Y, Sheehan KH, Amorim P, Janavs J, Weiller E, Hergueta T, Baker R, Dunbar GC. The Mini-international neuropsychiatric interview (M.I.N.I.): the development and validation of a structured diagnostic psychiatric interview for DSM-IV and ICD-10. J Clin Psychiatry. 1998;59(Suppl 20):22–33.
27. Baas KD, Wittkampf KA, van Weert HC, Lucassen P, Huyser J, van den Hoogen H, van de Lisdonk E, Bindels PE, Bockting CL, Ruhe HG, et al. Screening for depression in high-risk groups: prospective cohort study in general practice. Br J Psychiatry. 2009;194:399–403.
28. Suppiger A, In-Albon T, Hendriksen S, Hermann E, Margraf J, Schneider S. Acceptance of structured diagnostic interviews for mental disorders in clinical practice and research settings. Behav Ther. 2009;40:272–9.
29. Krueger RCM. Focus groups: a practical guide for applied research, vol. 4. Los Angeles: SAGE Publications Inc; 2009.
30. Elo S, Kyngas H. The qualitative content analysis process. J Adv Nurs. 2008;62:107–15.
31. Hsieh HF, Shannon SE. Three approaches to qualitative content analysis. Qual Health Res. 2005;15:1277–88.
32. Jonasson B, Jonasson U, Ekselius L, von Knorring L. The feasibility of a new intake routine to assess substance use disorders by means of a structured interview. Gen Hosp Psychiatry. 1997;19:36–41.
33. Sorensen MJ, Thomsen PH, Bilenberg N. Parent and child acceptability and staff evaluation of K-SADS-PL: a pilot study. Eur Child Adolesc Psychiatry. 2007;16:293–7.
34. Zimmerman M, Mattia JI. Psychiatric diagnosis in clinical practice: is comorbidity being missed? Compr Psychiatry. 1999;40:182–91.
35. Bakker IM, Terluin B, van Marwijk HW, van Mechelen W, Stalman WA. Test-retest reliability of the PRIME-MD: limitations in diagnosing mental disorders in primary care. Eur J Pub Health. 2009;19:303–7.
36. National Institute for Clinical Excellence NICE. Depression: management of depression in primary and secondary care (clinical guideline 23). London: British Psychological Society and Gaskell; 2004.
37. Leydon GM, Dowrick CF, McBride AS, Burgess HJ, Howe AC, Clarke PD, Maisey SP, Kendrick T, Team QOFDS. Questionnaire severity measures for depression: a threat to the doctor-patient relationship? Br J Gen Pract. 2011;61:117–23.
38. Mitchell C, Dwyer R, Hagan T, Mathers N. Impact of the QOF and the NICE guideline in the diagnosis and management of depression: a qualitative study. Br J Gen Pract. 2011;61:e279–89.
39. Barley EA, Murray J, Walters P, Tylee A. Managing depression in primary care: a meta-synthesis of qualitative and quantitative research from the UK to identify barriers and facilitators. BMC Fam Pract. 2011;12:47.
40. Maxwell M, Harris F, Hibberd C, Donaghy E, Pratt R, Williams C, Morrison J, Gibb J, Watson P, Burton C. A qualitative study of primary care professionals' views of case finding for depression in patients with diabetes or coronary heart disease in the UK. BMC Fam Pract. 2013;14:46.
41. Pettersson A, Bjorkelund C, Petersson EL. To score or not to score: a qualitative study on GPs views on the use of instruments for depression. Fam Pract. 2014;31:215–21.
42. Wittink MN, Barg FK, Gallo JJ. Unwritten rules of talking to doctors about depression: integrating qualitative and quantitative methods. Ann Fam Med. 2006;4:302–9.
43. Malterud K. Reflexivity and metapositions: strategies for appraisal of clinical evidence. J Eval Clin Pract. 2002;8:121–6.
44. Malterud K, Siersma VD, Guassora AD. Sample size in qualitative interview studies: guided by information power. Qual Health Res. 2015; https://doi.org/10.1177/1049732315617444.
45. Sundquist K, Malmstrom M, Johansson SE, Sundquist J. Care need index, a useful tool for the distribution of primary health care resources. J Epidemiol Community Health. 2003;5:347–52.

6

How to choose the most appropriate cognitive test to evaluate cognitive complaints in primary care

Jolien Janssen[1*], Paula S. Koekkoek[1], Eric P. Moll van Charante[3], L. Jaap Kappelle[2], Geert Jan Biessels[2] and Guy E. H. M. Rutten[1]

Abstract

Background: Despite the wealth of research devoted to the performance of individual cognitive tests for diagnosing cognitive impairment (including mild cognitive impairment and dementia), it can be difficult for general practitioners to choose the most appropriate test for a patient with cognitive complaints in daily practice. In this paper we present a diagnostic algorithm for the evaluation of cognitive complaints in primary care. The rationale behind this algorithm is that the likelihood of cognitive impairment -which can be determined after history taking and an informant interview- should determine which cognitive test is most suitable.

Methods: We distinguished three likelihoods of cognitive impairment: not likely, possible or likely. We selected cognitive tests based on pre-defined required test features for each of these three situations and a review of the literature. We incorporated the cognitive tests in a practical diagnostic algorithm.

Results: Based on the available literature, in patients with complaints but where cognitive impairment is considered to be unlikely the clock-drawing test can be used to rule out cognitive impairment. When cognitive impairment is possible the Montreal cognitive assessment can be used to rule out cognitive impairment or to make cognitive impairment more likely. When cognitive impairment is likely the Mini-Mental State Examination can be used to confirm the presence of cognitive impairment.

Conclusions: We propose a diagnostic algorithm to increase the efficiency of ruling out or diagnosing cognitive impairment in primary care. Further study is needed to validate and evaluate this stepwise diagnostic algorithm.

Keywords: Dementia, Primary care, Diagnostic tests, Aging, Alzheimer's disease/dementia

Background

In case of cognitive complaints expressed by the patient or a relative, or suspicion of cognitive impairment by the general practitioner (GP), it is important to evaluate cognitive symptoms with a reliable and efficient diagnostic procedure. Differentiating between subjective cognitive complaints and cognitive impairment, i.e. mild cognitive impairment (MCI) or early dementia, can be difficult [1]. Yet, history taking and the informant interview provide crucial information for the diagnostic procedure. The GP can complement this information with additional cognitive tests to reach more certainty about the presence or absence of cognitive impairment [2].

A wealth of research is devoted to the performance of individual cognitive tests. However, the literature gives limited consideration of and guidance on which and how cognitive tests should be used in the context of the sequential and probabilistic nature of the diagnostic procedure. Since the true value of a test is determined by the extent to which it provides information on top of the information that has already been gathered [3], the choice of the most appropriate cognitive test should be based on the estimated likelihood that the patient has cognitive impairment.

In this paper, we propose a stepwise diagnostic algorithm for the evaluation of cognitive complaints in primary care, taking into account both the GP's

* Correspondence: j.janssen-5@umcutrecht.nl
[1]Julius Centre for Health Sciences and Primary Care, University Medical Centre Utrecht, Utrecht, The Netherlands
Full list of author information is available at the end of the article

assessment of the likelihood of cognitive impairment and properties of the test.

Methods

To optimise the selection of cognitive tests we distinguished three likelihoods of objective cognitive impairment in patients with cognitive complaints, namely 1: cognitive impairment is not likely; 2: cognitive impairment is possible, but activities of daily living (ADL) appear to be preserved (i.e. MCI); and 3: cognitive impairment likely and ADL is affected (i.e. dementia).

First, the authors (including both neurologists and GPs experienced in diagnosing cognitive impairment) discussed the required test features for each of these situations. Secondly, we performed a literature search on cognitive tests used in primary care. We searched for English language articles listed on PubMed from January 2000 to January 2017. We used the search terms 'dementia' and 'cognitive' combined with 'screening', 'assessment', 'instrument', 'tool' and 'measure' combined with 'primary care'. Due to the large and heterogeneous body of literature, we limited our selection to systematic reviews and meta-analyses. Third, we selected the most appropriate cognitive tests in relation to the GP's assessment of the likelihood of cognitive impairment. At last, we incorporated the cognitive tests in a practical diagnostic algorithm and completed this algorithm using current guidelines and consensus documents to determine the key points that should be addressed in the first steps of the diagnostic procedure.

Required test features

For all three likelihoods of cognitive impairment we identified the cognitive tests of which appropriate cut-off scores had been reported in at least two independent studies.

Cognitive impairment not likely

When a patient complains but the GP considers cognitive impairment to be not likely, the prior probability that this patient has cognitive impairment is low and the chance this patient has dementia will be even lower [4]. The main objective of a cognitive test in this situation is to rule out cognitive impairment, in particular MCI. A test should have a high negative predictive value (NPV) and should preferably be brief. A high positive predictive value (PPV) is less relevant if one aims to rule out a condition, as a low PPV can be amended by performing an additional test in case of a positive test result. For this situation, we only considered tests that have been studied for MCI.

Cognitive impairment possible

This is the most challenging diagnostic situation, the "grey zone". When the GP considers cognitive impairment to be possible, but ADL appears to be preserved, the prior probability that the patient has MCI, or possibly even dementia is substantial [4]. The main objective of a cognitive test in this situation is to distinguish between presence or absence of cognitive impairment. A cognitive test in this situation should therefore be able to detect MCI and dementia in a population with a moderately high prevalence of cognitive impairment. We may assume that a test validated for MCI with an adequate NPV, will also detect dementia. Therefore, we considered tests that have been studied for MCI only, or MCI and dementia. We prioritised a high NPV above a high PPV to avoid false reassurance.

Cognitive impairment likely

When the GP considers the likelihood of cognitive impairment to be high and ADL appears to be affected, the prior probability that this patient has dementia is high [4]. A cognitive test in this situation should therefore be able to detect dementia in a population with a high prevalence of cognitive impairment. For this situation, we only considered tests that have been studied for dementia. The main objective of a test in this situation is to confirm that the patient has dementia; a test with a high PPV for dementia is therefore preferred.

Results

We critically appraised ten systematic reviews and two meta-analyses [5–16]. Only one review, which is based on the comprehensive research report produced by Kaiser Permanente Research Affiliates Evidence-based Practice Center, provided sufficient details to assess the value of cognitive tests for our algorithm [17]. It includes a dual independent review of studies on brief (i.e. administered within 10 min or self-administered within 20 min) cognitive tests conducted in a primary care setting.

Selecting cognitive tests

Cognitive impairment not likely

As shown in Table 1, both the clock-drawing test [18] and the Montreal cognitive assessment (MoCA) [19] have a high (≥ 89%) NPV and a moderate PPV (≤50%) in populations with relatively low prevalence rates of MCI (14–24%). Taking into account their comparable diagnostic accuracy, the short administration time of the clock-drawing test (1–3 min) relatively to the MoCA (10 min), we selected the clock-drawing test for our algorithm. The clock-drawing test assesses multiple aspects of cognitive functioning, in particular visuospatial and praxis abilities. In contrast, the MoCA contains multiple subtests that tap into different cognitive domains and can thus provide some more information on the actual nature of the cognitive impairment.

Table 1 Evidence summary [17] of cognitive tests for MCI (MCI versus normal cognition, dementia not included)

Test	Studies (n)	Test time (min)	Cut-off score	Study population, % MCI	Number of participants analysed	Sens (95% CI)	Spec (95% CI)	PPV (95% CI)	NPV (95% CI)
CDT	3	1–3	≤ 9	48	465	41 (34, 47)	83 (78, 88)	69 (60, 77)	60 (55, 65)
			≤ 9	15	3198	58 (54, 63)	57 (55, 59)	19 (17, 22)	89 (87, 90)
			≤ 9	14	428	69 (56, 81)	63 (58, 68)	23 (17, 30)	93 (89, 96)
MMSE	2	7–10	< 28	84	91	47 (36, 59)	73 (45, 92)	90 (76, 97)	22 (11, 35)
			< 28	44	524	45 (39, 52)	80 (75, 84)	64 (56, 71)	66 (60,70)
MoCA	2	10	< 26	24	152	100 (91, 100)	50 (41,59)	39 (29, 50)	100 (94, 100)
			< 26	20	99	80 (56, 94)	76 (65, 85)	46 (29, 63)	94 (85, 98)

Only the studies reporting a cut-off score that was studied more than once are depicted in the table. *Abbreviations*: *CI*=Confidence Interval, *MCI* Mild Cognitive Impairment, *NR* Not Reported, *Sens* Sensitivity, *Spec* Specificity, *NPV* Negative Predictive Value, *PPV* Positive Predictive Value, *AUC* Area Under the Curve. Abbreviations cognitive tests: *CDT* ClockDrawing Test, *MMSE* Mini Mental State Examination, *MoCA* Montreal Cognitive Assessment

Cognitive impairment possible

As shown in Tables 1 and 2, all tests that have been studied for MCI only, or cognitive impairment, have limited PPVs (≤71%), with the exception of study populations in which MCI or cognitive impairment is highly prevalent (≥50%). The MoCA has the most favorable NPV (≥ 94%) for both MCI and cognitive impairment overall and was therefore selected for our algorithm.

Cognitive impairment likely

Table 3 demonstrates that the Mental Status Questionnaire, the Short Portable Mental Status Questionnaire and the Memory Impairment Screen were only investigated in study populations with a prevalence of dementia ≤18% and it is therefore unclear if they are suitable in a situation with a high prior probability of dementia. The Abbreviated Mental Test and the Mini-Cog were both studied twice, once in a population with a very low prevalence of dementia (3% and 4% respectively) and once in a population with a high prevalence of dementia (29% and 40% respectively). In populations with a high prevalence of dementia the PPV of both tests was 71%. The MMSE (cut-off <24) has a comparable PPV (73%) in a population with a dementia prevalence of 28%. The NPV of all tests - with the exception of the Abbreviated Mental Test - was above 90%. In conclusion, both the Mini-cog and the MMSE with a cut-off <24 have favourable test features for this situation. Since the MMSE [20] is most frequently studied and well known, we selected this test as most suitable for our algorithm.

Proposed algorithm for a cognitive evaluation

Cognitive complaints

The starting point of the algorithm (1.1) is cognitive complaints expressed by the patient or a relative, or suspicion of cognitive impairment by the GP. In the evaluation of cognitive complaints, the mode of onset (1.2) provides essential guidance. In MCI and dementia, which is mostly caused by neurodegenerative or vascular pathologies, cognitive impairment is acquired and has a slowly progressive onset. This algorithm is not applicable to cognitive symptoms that develop within days or weeks. In that situation, other diagnoses such as a delirium or other neurological conditions are more likely.

History taking and informant interview

History taking and an informant interview are fundamental in a cognitive evaluation [2]. Concerns expressed by a close informant are generally even more predictive

Table 2 Evidence summary [17] of cognitive tests for cognitive impairment (dementia and MCI versus normal cognition)

Test	Studies (n)	Test time (min)	Cut-off score	Study population, % dementia / % MCI	Number of participants analysed	Sens (95% CI)	Spec (95% CI)	PPV (95% CI)	NPV (95% CI)
MoCA	1	10	< 26	8/19	107	86 (67, 96)	76 (65, 85)	56 (40, 71)	94 (85, 98)
Mini-Cog	2	3–4	2/3	40/12	371	84 (79, 89)	88 (81, 93)	92 (87, 95)	77 (70, 83)
			2/3	3/39	630	39 (34, 45)	78 (73, 82)	57 (49, 64)	63 (59, 68)
MMSE	3	7–10	23/24	4/26	269	53 (43, 64)	92 (88, 95)	71 (59, 81)	85 (78, 89)
			23/24	9/47	160	77 (67, 85)	70 (58, 80)	77 (67, 85)	70 (56, 80)
			23/24	4/5	1115	72 (62, 81)	89 (65, 99)	39 (32, 47)	97 (96, 98)

Only the studies reporting a cut-off score that was studied more than once are depicted in the table. *Abbreviations*: *CI* Confidence Interval, *MCI* Mild Cognitive Impairment, *NR* Not Reported, *Sens* Sensitivity, *Spec* Specificity, *NPV* Negative Predictive Value, *PPV* Positive Predictive Value, *AUC* Area Under the Curve. Abbreviations cognitive tests: *MoCA* Montreal Cognitive Assessment, *MMSE* Mini Mental State Examination

Table 3 Evidence summary [17] of cognitive tests for dementia (dementia versus no dementia)

Test	Studies (n)	Test time (min)	Cut-off score	Study population, % dementia	Number of participants analysed	Sens (95% CI)	Spec (95% CI)	PPV (95% CI)	NPV (95% CI)
AMT	2		7/8	29	269	42 (31, 53)	93 (89, 96)	71 (56, 83)	80 (74, 85)
			7/8	4	358	92 (64, 100)	95 (93, 97)	43 (25, 63)	100 (98, 100)
Mini-Cog	2	3–4	2/3	40	371	97 (93, 99)	71 (65, 77)	71 (64, 77)	97 (93, 99)
			2/3	3	630	76 (54, 90)	73 (69, 76)	9 (5, 14)	99 (97,100)
MIS	3	4	4	10	483	80 (66, 90)	96 (94, 98)	70 (57, 82)	98 (96, 99)
			4	18	318	76 (42, 100)	73 (56, 96)	38 (29, 47)	94 (89, 97)
			4	12	240	86 (67, 96)	97 (94, 99)	80 (61, 92)	98 (95, 100)
MMSE	5	7–10	23/24	4	1115	91 (78, 98)	87 (85, 89)	23 (17, 29)	100 (99, 100)
			23/24	1	709	87 (78, 95)	89 (86, 92)	52 (44, 60)	98 (96, 99)
			23/24	4	358	77 (46, 95)	97 (94,98)	46 (24, 68)	99 (97, 100)
			23/24	6	648	88 (74, 96)	88 (85, 90)	32 (24, 42)	99 (98, 100)
			23/24	28	360	84 (75, 90)	88 (84, 92)	73 (64, 81)	94 (90, 96)
MMSE	4	7–10	24/25	29	283	81 (70, 88)	76 (70, 82)	57 (48, 67)	90 (85, 95)
			24/25	4	269	98 (78, 100)	84 (79, 87)	21 (13, 33)	100 (99, 100)
			24/25	14	274	85 (70, 94)	81 (75, 86)	42 (31, 54)	97 (94, 99)
			24/25	19	449	84 (75, 91)	83 (79, 87)	55 (46, 63)	96 (93, 98)
MSQ	2	4	7/8	16	164	100 (87, 100)	84 (76, 89)	54 (39, 69)	100 (97, 100)
			7/8	4	358	92 (64, 100)	98 (96, 99)	67 (41, 87)	100 (98, 100)
SPMSQ	2	3–4	7/8	3	119	100 (29, 100)	100 (97, 100)	100 (29, 100)	100 (97, 100)
			7/8	4	358	100 (75, 100)	97 (94, 98)	54 (33, 75)	100 (99, 100)

Only the studies reporting a cut-off score that was studied more than once are depicted in the table. *Abbreviations*: *CI* Confidence Interval, *MCI* Mild Cognitive Impairment, *NR* Not Reported; *Sens* Sensitivity, *Spec* Specificity, *NPV* Negative Predictive Value, *PPV* Positive Predictive Value, *AUC* Area Under the Curve. Abbreviations cognitive tests: *AMT* Abbreviated Mental Test, *MIS* Memory Impairment Screen, *MMSE* Mini Mental State Examination, *MSQ* Mental Status Questionnaire, *SPMSQ* Short Portable Mental Status Questionnaire

of cognitive impairment than self-reported symptoms [2]. An informant interview is preferably performed with a close informant separately from the patient. If an informant is not available and diagnostic uncertainty persists after the initial visit, the patient should bring an informant to a follow-up visit. The following topics should be addressed:

Nature and course of the symptoms The GP should ascertain when and how symptoms started and how these developed over time. Memory problems are typically one of the first symptoms of cognitive impairment, but other cognitive domains may also be affected (Table 4) [21].

Personality and behavioural changes Changes in personality and behaviour are common in people with cognitive impairment and can cause considerable distress for both the patient and relatives. The Neuropsychiatric Inventory Questionnaire is frequently recommended to assess severity and impact of behavioural changes [22, 23]. The score of this 12-item informant questionnaire ranges from 0 to 36 with higher scores indicating more behavioural disturbance [24].

Depressive symptoms GPs should be alert for depressive symptoms in patients with suspected cognitive impairment [25]. Depression can be a prodromal symptom of dementia but depressive symptoms can also follow cognitive decline. In addition, depressive symptoms can influence cognitive testing. If a depression is likely, focus should be on diagnosing and treating depression first. For his, a depression scale, such as the 15-item Geriatric Depression Scale, can be used [26]. Cognitive symptoms should always be re-evaluated after the depression is treated.

Risk factors Age is the most important predisposing risk factor for cognitive impairment with estimated prevalence rates around 1% at the age of 60 and 30–60% in individuals of ≥90 years [27]. Lower intelligence, education and occupational attainment are associated with a

Table 4 Signs and symptoms to discuss during history taking and to help signalling cognitive impairment [21]

Memory impairment

- Repeating questions or conversations
- Hesitations, inconsistencies, omissions or confabulations
- Head turning sign (to verify answers with a caregiver)
- Misplacing personal belongings
- Forgetting events or appointments
- Getting lost on a familiar route

Aphasia

- Difficulty thinking of common words while speaking or using incorrect words
- No fluent production of words

Apraxia

- Difficulties in performing or imitating simple tasks (such as combing hair or brushing teeth) with intact comprehension, motor skills and perception

Agnosia

- Impaired ability to recognise faces or common objects or to find objects in direct view despite good acuity (visual agnosia)
- Impaired ability to recognise or identify objects by touch alone (tactile agnosia)

Disturbance in executive functioning

- Not correcting mistakes
- Difficulty learning how to use a new gadget or machine around the house
- Inability to manage finances
- Loss of abstract thinking, logical reasoning and/or visuoconstruction (e.g. drawing a clock)
- Lack of insight in own functioning
- Loss of initiative, increased impulsivity or uninhibited behaviour

higher risk of developing cognitive impairment [28]. Additional risk factors are a positive family history (especially early-onset cases) and head trauma [29]. Diabetes and cardiovascular risk factors, such as smoking and hypertension are other predisposing factors [30].

Daily functioning Daily functioning comprises ADL and instrumental ADL (IADL). ADLs are basic daily self-care activities including feeding, bathing, dressing, mobility, toileting and continence. IADLs are more advanced activities including telephone use, shopping, food preparation, housekeeping, laundry, transportation, responsibility for medication and handling finances. In patients with MCI, ADLs are preserved while there can be minimal impairment in IADLs [31]. In patients with dementia (I)ADLs are affected by definition [32]. It should be noticed that the boundaries between "normal" and "impaired" daily functioning are not always evident and are influenced by pre-existent activity levels. The Katz ADL [33] and the Lawton IADL [34] scales are frequently recommended to assess (I)ADL. Both scales can be completed by the patient or an informant.

Is cognitive impairment not likely, possible or likely?

Based on the previous steps the GP can estimate the likelihood that the patient has cognitive impairment and choose the most suitable cognitive test (Fig. 1). If according to the GP the likelihood that the patients has cognitive impairment is very low or very high, it may well be that none of the cognitive tests are of added value. Not using any cognitive test could then be a good option.

What if the cognitive test result does not match the GPs expectations?

The steps in the proposed algorithm will guide the GP towards the most probable diagnosis (Fig. 1). However, if there is a mismatch between the findings of history taking and the test, the results need to be reconsidered. It is important to perform an informant interview if not done previously and to consider alternative diagnoses. If uncertainty persists, the GP may decide to re-evaluate the patient in 6–12 months or to refer to a specialist for a more comprehensive cognitive assessment.

Discussion

Current guidelines and guidance articles about which, when and how to use cognitive test during a cognitive evaluation in primary care are diverse. Most often the same cognitive test(s) are recommended for *all* patients who consult the GP with cognitive complaints regardless of the prior probability of cognitive impairment [21–23, 35–41]. The MMSE is most frequently recommended, followed by the MoCA, the clock-drawing test and the Mini-Cog. The choices of the cognitive tests in our algorithm are therefore consistent with current recommendations. However, we recommend the use of three different tests in three different situations to make the diagnostic procedure more efficient and tailored to the individual patient.

To our knowledge, this is the first time that a diagnostic algorithm is presented where the choice of cognitive tests is guided by the prior probability that the patient has cognitive impairment. This allows the GP to take into account the true value of a test, in addition to information that has already been gathered. For example, the short and sensitive clock-drawing test will have no added value in patients who visit the GP with typical signs and symptoms of dementia and the added value of a normal MMSE score is limited in patients with only mild symptoms of cognitive impairment. It can therefore be expected that our algorithm is more efficient, although its true value should still be established.

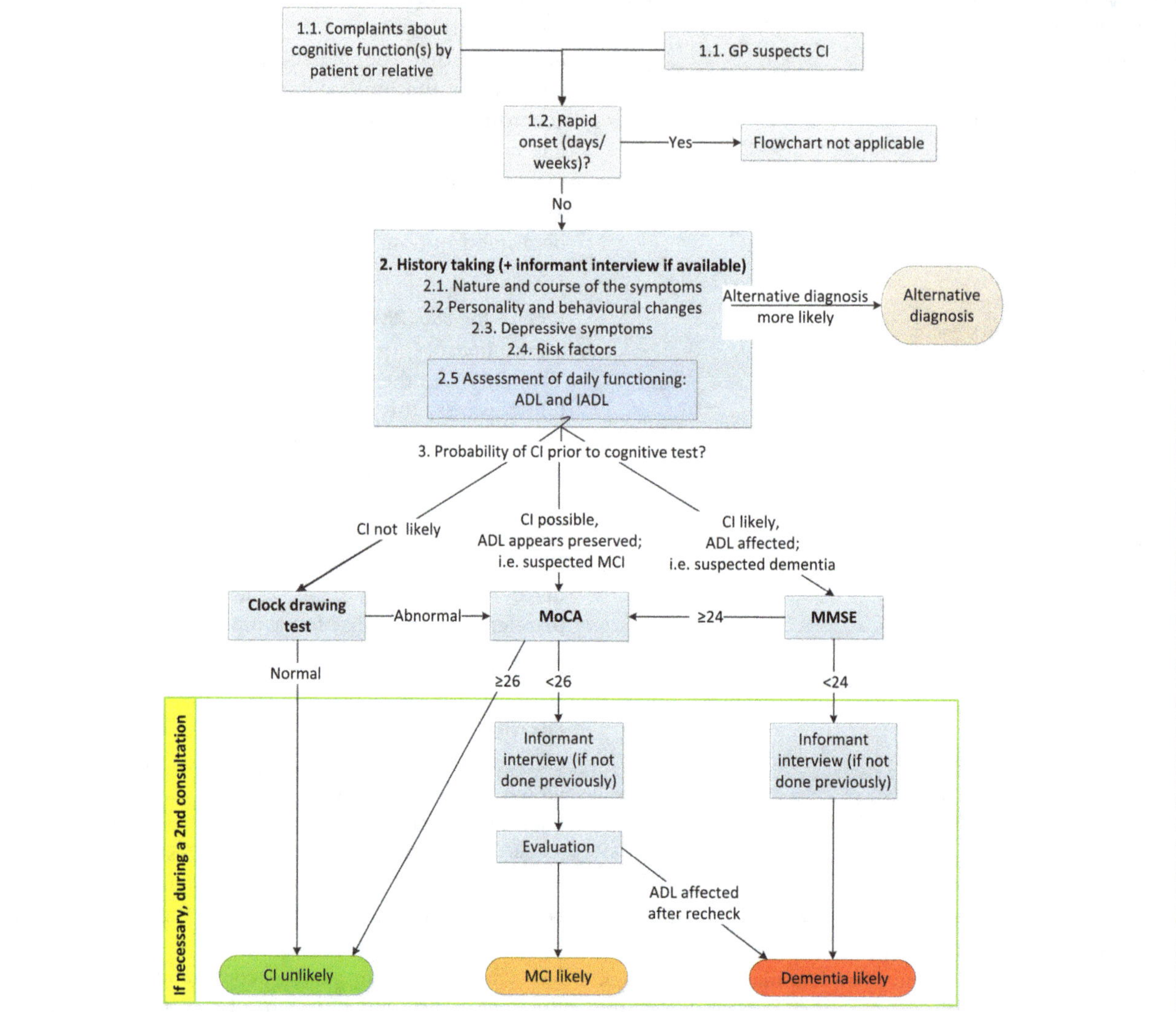

Fig. 1 Diagnostic algorithm for the evaluation of cognitive complaints in primary care

Several limitations of our approach in constructing the algorithm should be considered. The information on test characteristics of many tests was limited. Only a few tests have been studied in more than one fair or good quality study that included specific cut-off values. Hence, at present the available evidence to select suitable cognitive tests for the diagnostic algorithm was limited. Prioritising test characteristics is to a certain extent subjective, we tried to avoid subjectivity as much as possible by means of pre-defined criteria based on expert opinion and consensus; however, other opinions are possible and could lead to the selection of other cognitive tests. In addition, we had to make assumptions about the pre-test probability in each of the three situations we distinguished. Further study is needed to validate and evaluate this diagnostic algorithm.

Conclusions

In conclusion, the 'one-size-fits-all' approach for patients with cognitive complaints appears obsolete. The prior probability that the patient has cognitive impairment should be taken into account when choosing a cognitive test. The algorithm reflected in Fig. 1 may guide GPs during this diagnostic procedure.

Abbreviations

ADL: Activities of daily living; CI: Cognitive impairment (includes MCI and dementia); GP: General practitioner; IADL: Instrumental activities of daily living; MCI: Mild cognitive impairment; MMSE: Mini mental state examination; MoCA: Montreal cognitive assessment; NPV: Negative predictive value; PPV: Positive predictive value

Acknowledgements

Not applicable

Funding
This research received no grant from any funding agency in the public, commercial or not-for-profit sectors.

Authors' contributions
JJ, PSK, EPMvC, JLK, GJB and GEHMR all contributed to the conception of the work and discussed the diagnostic algorithm on several occasions. JJ searched for and selected references. JJ and PSK drafted the first manuscript. EPMvC, JLK, GJB and GEHMR critically revised the manuscript. All authors read and approved the final manuscript.

Consent for publication
Not applicable.

Competing interests
The authors declare that they have no competing interests.

Author details
[1]Julius Centre for Health Sciences and Primary Care, University Medical Centre Utrecht, Utrecht, The Netherlands. [2]Department of Neurology, Brain Centre Rudolf Magnus, University Medical Centre Utrecht, Utrecht, The Netherlands. [3]Department of General Practice, Academic Medical Centre, Amsterdam, The Netherlands.

References
1. Bradford A, Kunik ME, Schulz P, Williams SP, Singh H. Missed and delayed diagnosis of dementia in primary care: prevalence and contributing factors. Alzheimer Dis Assoc Disord. 2009;23:306–14.
2. Olazarán J, Torrero P, Cruz I, Aparicio E, Sanz A, Mula N, et al. Mild cognitive impairment and dementia in primary care: the value of medical history. Fam Pract. 2011;28:385–92.
3. Grobbee D, Hoes A. Clinical epidemiology: principles, methods, and applications for clinical research. London: Jones and Bartlett; 2014.
4. van den Dungen P, Moll van Charante EP, van de Ven PM, et al. Dutch family physicians' awareness of cognitive impairment among the elderly. BMC Geriatr. 2015;15:105.
5. Brodaty H, Low LF, Gibson L, Burns K. What is the best dementia screening instrument for general practitioners to use? Am J Geriatr Psychiatry. 2006;14: 391–400.
6. Cullen B, O'Neill B, Evans JJ, Coen RF, Lawlor BA. A review of screening tests for cognitive impairment. J Neurol Neurosurg Psychiatry. 2007;78:790–9.
7. Harvan JR, Cotter V. An evaluation of dementia screening in the primary care setting. J Am Acad Nurse Pract. 2006;18:351–60.
8. Ismail Z, Rajji TK, Shulman KI. Brief cognitive screening instruments: an update. Int J Geriatr Psychiatry. 2010;25:111–20.
9. Lin JS, O'Connor E, Rossom RC, Perdue LA, Eckstrom E. Screening for cognitive impairment in older adults: A systematic review for the U.S. Preventive Services Task Force. Ann Intern Med. 2013; doi:https://doi.org/10.7326/0003-4819-159-9-201311050-00730.
10. Lorentz WJ, Scanlan JM, Borson S. Brief screening tests for dementia. Can J Psychiatry. 2002; doi:https://doi.org/10.1177/070674370204700803.
11. Kansagara D, Freeman M. A systematic Evidence Review of the Signs and Symptoms of Dementia and Brief Cognitive Tests Available in VA. 2010 Apr. Available from: https://www.ncbi.nlm.nih.gov/books/NBK49021/
12. Milne A, Culverwell A, Guss R, Tuppen J, Whelton R. Screening for dementia in primary care: a review of the use, efficacy and quality of measures. Int Psychogeriatr. 2008;20:911–26.
13. Mitchell AJ, Malladi S. Screening and case finding tools for the detection of dementia. Part I: evidence-based meta-analysis of multidomain tests. Am J Geriatr Psychiatry. 2010;18:759–82.
14. Mitchell AJ, Malladi S. Screening and case-finding tools for the detection of dementia. Part II: evidence-based meta-analysis of single-domain tests. Am J Geriatr Psychiatry. 2010;18:783–800.
15. Woodford HJ, George J. Cognitive assessment in the elderly: a review of clinical methods. QJM. 2007;100:469–84.
16. Yokomizo JE, Simon SS, Bottino CM. Cognitive screening for dementia in primary care: a systematic review. Int Psychogeriatr. 2014; doi: https://doi.org/10.1017/S1041610214001082.
17. Lin J, O'Connor E, Rossom R, Perdue L, Burda B, Thompson M, et al. Screening for Cognitive Impairment in Older Adults: An Evidence Update for the U.S. Preventive Services Task Force. Rockville (MD): Agency for Healthcare Research and Quality (US); 2013 Nov. (Evidence Syntheses, No. 107.) https://www.ncbi.nlm.nih.gov/books/NBK174643/. Accessed 10 August 2017.
18. Shulman KI. Clock-drawing: is it the ideal cognitive screening test? Int J Geriatr Psychiatry. 2000;15:548–61.
19. Nasreddine ZS, Phillips NA, Bedirian V, Charbonneau S, Whitehead V, Collin I, et al. The Montreal cognitive assessment, MoCA: a brief screening tool for mild cognitive impairment. J Am Geriatr Soc. 2005;53:695–9.
20. Folstein MF, Folstein SE, McHugh PR. "Mini-Mental State". A practical method for grading the cognitive state of patients for the clinician. JPsychiatr Res. 1975;12:189–98.
21. Moll van Charante EP. Dementia guideline of the Dutch College of General Practitioners. Huisarts Wet. 2012;55:306–17.
22. Cummings JL, Frank JC, Cherry D, et al. Guidelines for managing Alzheimer's disease: part I. Assessment Am Fam Physician. 2002;65(11):2263–72.
23. Galvin JE, Sadowsky CH. Practical guidelines for the recognition and diagnosis of dementia. J Am Board Fam Med. 2012;25:367–82.
24. Kaufer DI, Cummings JL, Ketchel P, Smith V, MacMillan A, Shelley T, et al. Validation of the NPI-Q, a brief clinical form of the neuropsychiatric inventory. J Neuropsychiatry Clin Neurosci. 2000;12:233–9.
25. Thorpe L. Depression vs Dementia: How Do We Assess? The Canadian Review of Alzheimer's Disease and Other Dementias. 2009; 17–21. http://www.alzheimer.ca/~/media/Files/national/Articles-lit-review/article_Depression_vs_Dementia_2009_e.pdf. Accessed 24 November 2016.
26. Yesavage JA, Brink TL, Rose TL, Lum O, Huang V, Adey M, et al. Development and validation of a geriatric depression screening scale: a preliminary report. J Psychiatr Res. 1982;17:37–49.
27. Prince M, Bryce R, Albanese E, Wimo A, Ribeiro W, Ferri CP. The global prevalence of dementia: a systematic review and metaanalysis. Alzheimers Dement. 2013;9:63–75.
28. Meng X, D'Arcy C. Education and dementia in the context of the cognitive reserve hypothesis: a systematic review with meta-analyses and qualitative analyses. PLoS One. 2012;7:e38268.
29. Stephan BC, Brayne C. Risk factors and screening methods for detecting dementia: a narrative review. J Alzheimers Dis. 2014; doi:https://doi.org/10.3233/JAD-141413.
30. Exalto LG, Quesenberry CP, Barnes D, Kivipelto M, Biessels GJ, Whitmer RA. Midlife risk score for the prediction of dementia four decades later. Alzheimers Dement. 2014;10:562–70.
31. Winblad B, Palmer K, Kivipelto M, Jelic V, Fratiglioni L, Wahlund LO, et al. Mild cognitive impairment–beyond controversies, towards a consensus: report of the international working group on mild cognitive impairment. J Intern Med. 2004;256:240–6.
32. American Psychiatric Association. Diagnostic and statistical manual of mental disorders. 4th ed. Washington, DC: American Psychiatric Association; 2000.
33. Katz S, Akpom CA. 12. Index of ADL. Med Care. 1976;14:116–8.
34. Graf C. The Lawton instrumental activities of daily living scale. Am J Nurs. 2008;108:52–62.
35. Adelman AM, Daly MP. Initial evaluation of the patient with suspected dementia. Am Fam Physician. 2005;71(9):1745–50.
36. Feldman HH, Jacova C, Robillard A, Garcia A, Chow T, Borrie M, et al. Diagnosis and treatment of dementia: 2. Diagnosis CMAJ. 2008;178:825–36.
37. Geldmacher DS, Kerwin DR. Practical diagnosis and Management of Dementia due to Alzheimer's disease in the primary care setting: an evidence-based approach. Prim Care Companion CNS Disord. 2013;15
38. Lee L, Weston WW, Heckman G, Gagnon M, Lee FJ, Sloka S. Structured approach to patients with memory difficulties in family practice. Can Fam Physician. 2013;59(3):249–54.
39. Fairbairn A, Gould N, Kendall T, Ashley P, Bainbridge I, Bower, L, et al. National Institute for Health and Clinical Excellence. Dementia: Supporting people with

dementia and their carers in health and social care. Published 2006, Last updated September 2016. https://www.nice.org.uk/guidance/cg42/resources/dementia-supporting-people-with-dementia-and-their-carers-in-health-and-social-care-pdf-975443665093. Accessed 17 November 2016.

40. Dyer SM, Laver K, Pond CD, Cumming RG, Whitehead C, Crotty M. Clinical practice guidelines and principles of care for people with dementia in Australia. Aust Fam Physician. 2016;45(12):884–9.
41. Connelly P, Archibald C, Backett S, Brockie J, Carnon A, Cooper G, et al. Scottish Intercollegiate Guidelines Network. Managment of patients with dementia: A national clinical guideline. 2006. http://umh1946.edu.umh.es/wp-content/uploads/sites/172/2015/04/Management-of-patients-with-dementia-NHS.pdf. Accessed 17 November 2016.

7

Factors associated with low patient satisfaction in out-of-hours primary care in Denmark

Mette Tranberg[1*], Peter Vedsted[2], Bodil Hammer Bech[3], Morten Bondo Christensen[2], Søren Birkeland[4] and Grete Moth[2]

Abstract

Background: Low patient satisfaction with the quality of out-of-hours primary care (OOH-PC) has been linked with several individual and organizational factors. However, findings have been ambiguous and may not apply to the Danish out-of-hours (OOH) setting in which general practitioners (GPs) perform the initial telephone triage. This study aimed to identify patient-related, GP-related and organizational factors associated with low patient satisfaction.

Methods: The study was based on data from a 1-year population-based survey of OOH-PC (LV-KOS) in the Central Denmark Region in 2010–2011. GPs on OOH duty completed an electronic questionnaire in the OOH computer system, and the registered patients received a subsequent postal questionnaire focusing on contact evaluation, waiting time, demographic characteristics and general self-perceived health. Associations were analysed using multivariable logistic regression with dissatisfaction as the dependent variable.

Results: The patient response rate was 50.6%. For all contact types, 82.5% of the patients were satisfied with the OOH-PC service. More patients were dissatisfied with telephone consultations than with clinic consultations or home visits (8.5% vs. 6.0% and 4.3%, respectively). Contacts assessed by the GP as 'not severe' were associated with dissatisfaction for telephone consultations and home visits. Poor general self-perceived health was associated with dissatisfaction for all contact types. Living in urban areas was associated with dissatisfaction for telephone consultations, while unacceptable waiting time was associated with dissatisfaction for all contact types.

Conclusions: We found a high level of patient satisfaction with the OOH-PC service. The only factors affecting patient satisfaction across all contact types were unacceptable waiting time and poor general self-perceived health. For the other investigated factors, patient satisfaction depended on the type of contact. Generally, patients contacting for GP-assessed non-severe health problem and patients living in urban areas were more dissatisfied.

Keywords: Out-of-hours care, General practice, Denmark, Patient satisfaction, Delivery of health care

* Correspondence: mettrani@rm.dk
[1]Department of Public Health Programmes, Randers Regional Hospital, Østervangsvej 68, 8930 Randers NØ, Denmark
Full list of author information is available at the end of the article

Background

General practitioners (GPs) form the first line in the Danish healthcare system and are gatekeepers to specialist care. All citizens have free access to medical advice and health care [1, 2], including out-of-hours (OOH) services, which is run by GPs on a rota basis. In four out of the five existing region-based out-of-hours primary care (OOH-PC) cooperatives, GPs are responsible for providing health care for the citizens (0.6–1.8 million inhabitants) from 4 p.m. to 8 a.m. on weekdays and throughout weekends and public holidays [1, 3]. Unlike the OOH-PC settings in many other countries [3], all patient calls are answered and triaged by GPs [4]. They provide advice, write prescriptions, order home visits or refer to clinic consultations or directly to hospital. Most calls (59%) are terminated as telephone consultations [4].

The patient-perceived quality is a crucial element when assessing the provided OOH health care as identified factors associated with low patient evaluation may provide useful information in a quality improvement context [5, 6]. Previous studies of patient satisfaction in the United Kingdom [7–10], the Netherlands [11, 12] and Denmark [1, 13, 14] show that patients are generally satisfied with the OOH-PC service. Yet, the degree of satisfaction is lower for patients who receive telephone consultations than for patients who receive clinic consultations or home visits [1, 9, 11, 13, 15, 16].

Patient-related factors such as socio-economic status [17, 18], age [4, 8–10, 18], gender [4, 9], chronic disease [6] and self-perceived health [17, 19] are related to patient satisfaction. The same is the case for GP-related factors (e.g. age, gender and GP-assessed severity of the health problem) [4, 20, 21] and organizational factors (e.g. waiting time before consultation) [9–11, 16]. However, many of these findings are ambiguous [7, 8, 10, 17, 18] and may not be representative in a Danish OOH-PC setting.

We aimed to identify patient-related, GP-related and organizational factors associated with low patient satisfaction with telephone consultations, clinic consultations and home visits in the Danish OOH-PC service.

Methods

Design and setting

This cross-sectional study was based on data from a 1-year population-based survey of OOH-PC, *'Kontakt-og sygdomsmønster i lægevagten (LV-KOS)*, which was conducted on 1 June 2010–31 May 2011 in the Central Denmark Region, which is the largest of the four Danish region with a primary care-based OOH service (approximately 1.3 million citizens) [22]. The LV-KOS study has been described in detail elsewhere [22]

Data collection

A "pop-up" questionnaire, which was integrated into the existing electronic patient record system, appeared for the participating GPs after termination of every 10th telephone contact, every 3rd clinic consultation and every home visit. This sampling method was chosen to ensure sufficient numbers of registered clinic consultations and home visits to make valid estimates and yet avoid a considerable increase in the GP workload [22]. The questionnaire covered a range of items, e.g. about the patient's reasons for contacting and the GP-assessed severity of the presented health problem. Two to five days after the OOH-PC contact, the GP-registered patients received a postal questionnaire about their experience with the OOH-PC service, including general self-perceived health and general satisfaction with the contact. Only patients older than 18 years were asked about their general self-perceived health. Questionnaires regarding contact with children below 18 years of age were sent to the parents [22]. A reminder was sent in case of no response after two weeks [22]. Details of the GP and patient questionnaires are reported elsewhere [22].

Study population

In total, 18,267 patient contacts (telephone consultations, clinic consultations and home visits) were systematically registered by GPs. A total of 4015 (22%) were excluded from the patient survey, and these patients received no questionnaire. Reasons for exclusion were: protection against research participation (n = 2417 (60.2%)), previous inclusion of same patient (n = 863 (21.5%)), unknown postal address (n = 102 (2.5%)), sensitive matters (e.g. attempted suicide or terminal illness) (n = 377 (9.4%)) and death (n = 256 (6.4%)).

Data management

We included the following patient-related factors: patient age and gender, general self-perceived health, chronic disease, residence and employment status. We defined GP age, GP gender and GP-assessed severity of the health problem as GP-related factors. Finally, we included the patient-perceived waiting time before the received service as an organisation-related factor. The electronic OOH-PC database provided data on date and type of contact, GP age and gender, patient age and gender, and patient name and postal address [22]. Patient age was categorized into five groups: 0–4 years, 5–18 years, 19–50 years, 51–75 years and >75 years. This categorization was chosen based on the pattern of disease and the density of contacts to the OOH-PC service; patients aged 0–4 years were considered a special group and was analysed separately. The GP questionnaire also included information on GP-assessed severity of the health problem; the original five response categories were: "Severe", "Potentially severe and the patient needs to be seen", "Not severe", "Not ill" and "Don't know". When used for logistic regression analyses, this variable was dichotomised into "Potentially severe" (combining "Severe" and "Potentially severe and the patient needs to be seen") and "Not severe" (combining "Not severe" and "Not ill"). The answer "Don't know" was not included in the analyses ($n = 2$). We included a question on general self-perceived health inspired by the Short Form-12 (SF-12) questionnaire [23]. The five options for answers were: "Excellent", "Very good", "Good", "Less good" and "Poor". In the logistic regression analyses, these were dichotomised into "Good" (combining "Excellent", "Very good" and "Good") and "Poor" (combining "Less good" and "Poor") when included in the logistic regression analysis, as done in another study [24]. The patients were asked whether they had chronic disease(s) and whether they found the waiting time (before their consultation) acceptable. The original four answers were: "Yes", "No", "Neutral" and "Don't know". In the logistic regression analyses, the latter variable was dichotomised into "Acceptable waiting time" ("Yes") and "Unacceptable waiting time" ("No"). The answers "Neutral" and "Don't know" were not included in the analyses because answering "Neutral" or "Don't know" is not comparable with experiencing acceptable or unacceptable waiting time. In total, 93 and 870 patients answered "Don't know" or "Neutral", respectively, corresponding to 1.3% and 12.1% of the study population. Supplementary analyses showed that findings largely remained unchanged when including, for example, neutral respondents in the acceptable waiting group (data not shown).

The overall satisfaction with the contact was rated by the patient through selection of one of six response options: "Very satisfied", "Satisfied", "Dissatisfied", "Very dissatisfied", "Neutral" and "Don't know". These were dichotomised into "Satisfied" (combining "Very satisfied" and "Satisfied") and "Dissatisfied" (combining "Dissatisfied" and "Very dissatisfied") when used in the logistic regression analyses. The answers "Neutral" and "Don't know" were not included in the analyses. The rationale for not including these answers is that answering "Neutral" or "Don't know" cannot be unambiguously classified in any of the two categories. A total of 655 patients answered "Neutral", corresponding to 9.1% of the study population. However, supplementary analyses showed that findings largely remained unchanged when including, for example, neutral respondents in the satisfied group (data not shown). Additionally, only a small proportion of patients answered "Don't know", corresponding to 0.8% of the study population. English translations of the used questions are presented in Additional file 1.

Patient residence was grouped into "Urban area" (≥34,000 inhabitants) and "Rural area" (<34,000 inhabitants) based on the patient's postal code. Patients living outside the Central Denmark Region were scored as "unknown". Distance to emergency departments may affect the patient's consumption of OOH-PC services. As the distance is longer in rural areas and shorter in urban areas, we considered population density to be the most appropriate basis for classification of the patients' residence. Patients living outside the Central Denmark Region were excluded (e.g. tourists) because our evaluation focused on the experience of the OOH-PC service among ordinary patients.

The Danish Register for Evaluation of Marginalization (DREAM) provided information on the patient's employment status [25]. This variable was used as a proxy measurement for socio-economic status [25]. Based on the DREAM code for the week of the OOH-PC contact, employment status was categorized as "Self-supporting" (coded with receipt of no benefit in DREAM; maternity leave or student), "Pensioners and retirees" (coded with receipt of benefits related to old age or early retirement) and "Not self-supporting" (coded with receipt of partial or full disability pension, social assistance or sick leave).

Statistical analyses

The chi-square test was used to test differences between respondents and non-respondents in terms of age, gender and residence. Descriptive statistics were used to summarize patient characteristics for each type of contact. Logistic regression was used to estimate crude and adjusted odds ratios (ORs) for overall dissatisfaction with the OOH-PC service in terms of patient-related, GP-related and organizational factors. Unadjusted analyses were performed for each independent variable. These analyses were followed by analyses adjusted for statistically significant variables ($p < 0.01$) from the univariate analyses. This led us to include residence, general self-perceived health, self-reported chronic disease, employment status, GP age, GP-assessed severity of contact and patient-perceived waiting time before contact in the adjusted analyses. We also included patient age [4, 8–10, 18], patient gender [4, 9] and GP gender [20, 21] in the adjusted analyses because they were found to be important confounding variables in the literature.

Patient age was entered as a continuous variable. The small number of dissatisfied patients made it impossible for us to include all variables in the models. Therefore, we made different models, i.e. included different numbers of confounding variables in the analyses, because we had to prioritise and include only the most important confounding variables in our models to avoid getting an unstable model with wide confidence intervals. The selection of confounding variables in the models was based on excluding any variable that did not fulfil the criteria to be considered as a valid confounder in the exact model (i.e. not associated with the exposure) and thus was expected to have little effect on the OR estimate. To evaluate the robustness of our assumptions, the excluded variables were initially included in the models. If including the variable did not affect the results, this variable was not retained in the adjusted model. In total, four different adjusted models were used to measure the associations between the patient-related factors and dissatisfaction. Model 1: Associations between the patient's residence and dissatisfaction included patient's gender, age, general self-perceived health, self-reported chronic disease, employment status and GP-assessed severity of contact as confounding variables. The variable patient-perceived waiting time before contact was excluded. Model 2: Associations between the patient's general self-perceived health and dissatisfaction included patient's gender, age, residence, self-reported chronic disease, patient-perceived waiting time before contact and GP-assessed severity of contact as confounding variables. The variable employment status was excluded. Model 3: Associations between self-reported chronic disease and dissatisfaction included patient's gender, age, residence, general self-perceived health and GP-assessed severity of contact as confounding variables. The variables employment status and patient-perceived waiting time before contact were excluded. Model 4: Associations between the patient's employment status and dissatisfaction included patient's gender, age, residence, general self-perceived health, self-reported chronic disease and GP-assessed severity of contact as confounding variables. The variable patient-perceived waiting time before contact was excluded.

Three adjusted models were used to measure associations between GP and organizational-related factors and dissatisfaction. Model 1: Associations between GP gender and dissatisfaction and between GP age and dissatisfaction included the same confounding variables. These were patient's gender, age, general self-perceived health, patient-perceived waiting time before contact and GP-assessed severity of contact as confounding variables. The variables GP age, patient residence, self-reported chronic disease and employment status were excluded. Model 2: Associations between GP-assessed severity of contact and dissatisfaction included patient's gender, age, residence, general self-perceived health, self-reported chronic disease, patient-perceived waiting time before contact, GP age and gender as confounding variables. Employment status was excluded from the model. Model 3: Associations between patient-perceived waiting time before contact and dissatisfaction included patient's gender, age, residence, general self-perceived health, self-reported chronic disease and employment status as confounding variables. The variable GP-assessed severity of contact was excluded from the model.

As different patients may have been in contact with the same GP, we accounted for GP clustering by using robust standard errors in all unadjusted and adjusted models [26]. Due to the sampling method (one in ten telephone contacts, one in three clinical consultations and every home visit), all statistical analyses were performed separately for each contact type. *P*-values of 0.05 or less were considered statistically significant. All statistical analyses were conducted using Stata 11.0. (StataCorp LP, College Station, TX, USA).

Ethical approvals

The study was approved by the Danish Data Protection Agency (j.no. 2013–41-1594). Approval from the Danish National Committee on Health Research Ethics was not required as no biomedical intervention was performed in this study. According to Danish law, confidentiality aspects and associated bioethical issues in non-interventional health care research are managed by the Data Protection Agency and governed by the Danish Act on Processing of Personal Data. Informed consent from participants and GPs was obtained through their acceptance to fill out the questionnaires.

Results

In total, 14,252 (75.1%) patients received a postal questionnaire, and 7213 patients responded (50.6%). No statistically significant differences were found between respondents and non-respondents for gender, except for home visits for which a higher proportion of men responded ($p < 0.001$) (Table 1). Statistically significantly higher response rates were found for respondents in rural areas. Patients aged 19–50 years comprised the highest proportion of respondents for telephone consultations and clinic consultations, whereas patients aged 51–75 years formed the highest proportion of respondents for home visits.

The overall satisfaction and contact characteristics are shown in Table 2. For all contact types, 6.1% of the patients were dissatisfied and 82.5% were satisfied with the OOH-PC service. Patients receiving telephone consultations were more often dissatisfied than patients receiving clinic consultations or home visits ($p < 0.001$). The proportion of patients who found that they had experienced unacceptable waiting time was highest among patients receiving clinic consultations. Patients reporting to find the waiting time unacceptable were mostly women, aged 19–50 years and living in rural areas (data not shown).

Table 3 depicts associations between patient-related factors and dissatisfaction. Living in urban areas was statistically significantly associated with dissatisfaction among patients receiving a telephone consultation, but this association was not found for other contact types. Poor general self-perceived health was associated with

Table 1 Comparison between respondents (n = 7213) and non-respondents (n = 7039) in terms of gender, age group and residence

	Telephone consultations			Clinic consultations			Home visits		
	Non-respondents n = 1899 (100%) n (%)	Respondents n = 1789 (100%) n (%)	P-value[a]	Non-respondents n = 2521 (100%) n (%)	Respondents n = 3183 (100%) n (%)	P-value[a]	Non-respondents n = 2619 (100%) n (%)	Respondents n = 2241 (100%) n (%)	P-value[a]
Gender									
Male	888 (46.8)	825 (46.1)	0.679	1236 (49.0)	1541 (48.4)	0.645	1233 (47.0)	1124 (50.2)	<0.001
Female	1011 (53.2)	964 (53.9)		1285 (51.0)	1642 (51.6)		1386 (53.0)	1117 (49.8)	
Age groups (years)									
0–4	329 (17.3)	482 (26.9)	<0.001	580 (23.0)	931 (29.3)	<0.001	170 (6.5)	200 (8.9)	<0.001
5–18	257 (13.5)	298 (16.7)		439 (17.4)	679 (21.3)		140 (5.3)	155 (6.9)	
19–50	817 (43.0)	568 (31.8)		1180 (46.8)	947 (29.8)		583 (22.3)	405 (18.1)	
51–75	297 (15.6)	337 (18.6)		278 (11.0)	549 (17.3)		726 (27.8)	832 (37.1)	
> 75	199 (10.5)	104 (15.8)		44 (1.7)	77 (2.4)		1000 (38.2)	649 (29.0)	
Patient's residence									
Urban area	939 (49.4)	824 (46.1)	<0.001	1368 (54.3)	1523 (47.9)	<0.001	1178 (45.0)	871 (38.9)	<0.001
Rural area	893 (47.0)	918 (51.3)		1049 (41.6)	1569 (49.3)		1409 (53.8)	1357 (60.6)	
Missing data	67 (3.5)	47 (2.6)		104 (4.1)	91 (2.9)		32 (1.2)	57 (0.6)	

[a]Tested using a chi-square test

dissatisfaction for all three contact types. No statistically significant association was seen between self-reported chronic disease and dissatisfaction for any contact type in the adjusted models. No statistically significant association was found between employment status and dissatisfaction although 'not self-supporting' tended to be associated with dissatisfaction with clinic consultations.

Table 4 shows associations between GP-related and organizational factors and dissatisfaction. GP assessment of patient contact as non-severe was statically significantly associated with dissatisfaction among patients who received a telephone consultation or home visit. Contact with a GP aged >60 years was statically significantly associated with dissatisfaction among patients receiving a telephone consultation or home visit. For all contact types, patient-assessed unacceptable waiting time was associated with dissatisfaction, while no association was found between GP gender and dissatisfaction.

Discussion

Main findings

Overall, 6.1% of patients evaluated the OOH-PC encounter as dissatisfying, while 82.5% of patients were satisfied. Patients receiving a telephone consultation were significantly more dissatisfied than patients receiving a clinic consultation or home visit. Poor general self-perceived health was associated with dissatisfaction for all contact types, while GP-assessed non-severe contacts were associated with dissatisfaction among patients receiving a telephone consultation or home visit. However, having a chronic disease was not in itself associated with dissatisfaction. Patient-assessed unacceptable waiting time was associated with dissatisfaction for all types of contact. Higher GP age was associated with dissatisfaction with telephone consultations and home visits. These findings indicate that patients who perceive their general health as low and are triaged as non-severe contact or triaged by older GPs form a specific group of patients who tend to give negative evaluations of the OOH-PC service. Still, the strongest and most decisive factor for dissatisfaction was unacceptable waiting time.

Strengths and weaknesses

The study was based on a large sample of contacts to the OOH-PC service, and the large data set ensured high statistical precision. Furthermore, the participating GPs and the randomly included contacts have been demonstrated to be highly representative of all contacts in the OOH-PC service [22]. The core items of the questionnaires had low levels of missing data; this indicates that the relevance of the questions was accepted by the respondents.

The short time period between the contact with the OOH-PC service and the completion of the questionnaire reduced the risk of recall bias. Misclassification of the independent self-reported patient-related and organization-related factors is unlikely to depend on the level of dissatisfaction, so misclassification is not considered to have caused bias in our findings.

Likewise, the random recruitment of patients through electronic "pop-up" questionnaires combined with very high participation rates among GPs also limited selection

Table 2 Contact characteristics

	Telephone consultations		Clinic consultations		Home visits		*P*-value[a]
	n	(%)	n	(%)	n	(%)	
Number of patient contacts (n = 7213)	1789	(100)	3183	(100)	2241	(100)	
Overall satisfaction							
Satisfied	1379	(77.0)	2656	(83.4)	1916	(85.5)	<0.001
Dissatisfied	152	(8.5)	192	(6.0)	98	(4.3)	
Neutral	214	(12.0)	301	(9.5)	140	(6.3)	
Don't know	17	(1.0)	11	(0.4)	28	(1.3)	
Missing data	27	(1.5)	23	(0.7)	59	(2.6)	
Organizational factor:							
Patient-perceived waiting time							
Acceptable waiting time	1325	(74.1)	2279	(71.8)	1647	(73.5)	<0.001
Unacceptable waiting time	174	(9.7)	459	(14.4)	258	(11.5)	
Neutral	231	(12.9)	387	(12.2)	252	(11.2)	
Don't know	31	(1.7)	24	(0.8)	38	(1.7)	
Missing data	28	(1.6)	34	(1.1)	46	(2.1)	
Patient-related factors:							
Age groups (years)							
0–4	482	(26.9)	931	(29.3)	200	(8.9)	<0.001
5–18	298	(16.7)	679	(21.3)	155	(7.0)	
19–50	568	(31.8)	947	(30.0)	405	(18.1)	
51–75	337	(18.8)	549	(17.3)	832	(37.3)	
> 75	104	(5.8)	77	(2.4)	649	(29.0)	
Gender							
Male	825	(46.1)	1541	(48.4)	1124	(50.2)	<0.001
Female	964	(53.8)	1642	(51.6)	1117	(49.8)	
Patient's residence							
Rural area	918	(51.3)	1569	(49.3)	1357	(60.6)	<0.001
Urban area	824	(46.1)	1523	(47.9)	871	(38.9)	
Unknown[b]	47	(2.6)	91	(2.9)	13	(0.6)	
Employment status							
Self-supporting	1287	(71.9)	2563	(80.5)	1140	(50.9)	<0.001
Pensioners and retirees	171	(9.6)	244	(7.7)	682	(30.4)	
Not self-supporting	247	(13.8)	325	(10.2)	373	(16.6)	
Missing data	84	(4.7)	51	(1.6)	46	(2.1)	
General self-perceived health[c]							
Excellent	112	(10.9)	179	(11.1)	72	(3.8)	<0.001
Very good	300	(29.3)	580	(36.1)	281	(14.8)	
Good	333	(32.5)	521	(32.4)	582	(30.7)	
Poor	186	(18.2)	244	(15.2)	626	(33.0)	
Very poor	66	(6.4)	50	(3.1)	252	(13.3)	
Missing data	28	(2.7)	34	(2.1)	84	(4.4)	
Self-reported chronic disease							
No chronic disease	1292	(72.2)	2491	(78.3)	1049	(46.8)	<0.001
Chronic disease[d]	497	(27.8)	692	(21.7)	1192	(53.2)	

Table 2 Contact characteristics *(Continued)*

	Telephone consultations		Clinic consultations		Home visits		*P*-value[a]
	n	(%)	n	(%)	n	(%)	
Number of patient contacts (*n* = 7213)	1789	(100)	3183	(100)	2241	(100)	
GP-related factors:							
GP-assessed severity of contact							
Potentially severe	236	(13.2)	1209	(38.0)	1161	(51.8)	<0.001
Not severe	1486	(83.0)	1937	(60.9)	1061	(47.3)	
Don't know	67	(3.8)	37	(1.2)	17	(0.8)	
Missing data	0	(0.0)	0	(0)	2	(0.1)	

[a]Tested using a chi-square test
[b]Patients living outside the Central Denmark Region
[c]Only patients aged >18 years
[d]See Additional file 1

bias [22]. The overall patient response rate is considered acceptable for a survey in a heterogeneous population [27, 28] and resembles the response rates for other surveys in this field [8, 11, 12, 17, 19]. However, non-respondents differed from respondents in terms of age and residence, whereas no gender differences were found, except for home visits. The fairly low response rate among parents of children aged 5–18 years is difficult to explain, but may be due to reluctance to complete time-consuming paper questionnaires. This group tended to be younger and in better health. They may, therefore, find the questionnaire less relevant than older patients. We found lower response rates among older patients (> 75 years). This finding is consistent with findings made in other studies. The lower response rate in the group of older patients is not surprising as they are generally less resourceful and more ill than younger patients [27]. However, we see no reason why the lower response rates among these groups should be associated with dissatisfaction with their contact to the

Table 3 Likelihood (OR) of dissatisfaction with different contact types according to patient-related factors

	Telephone consultations		Clinic consultations		Home visits	
	Crude OR (95% CI) *n* = 1,321[a]	Adjusted OR (95% CI) n= 698[a]	Crude OR (95% CI) *n* = 1,397[a]	Adjusted OR (95% CI) n = 1,158[a]	Crude OR (95% CI) n = 1,637[a]	Adjusted OR (95% CI) n = 1,394[a]
Residence						
Rural area (ref)	1	1	1	1	1	1
Urban area	**1.58 (1.10–2.27)**	**1.65 (1.09–2.50)[b]**	1.16 (0.87–1.53)	1.09 (0.73–1.64)[b]	1.46 (0.92–2.30)	1.42 (0.81–2.50)[b]
General self-perceived health						
Good health (ref)	1	1	1	1	1	1
Poor health	**3.22 (2.13–4.88)**	**3.35 (1.78–6.31)[c]**	1.35 (0.85–2.14)	**1.76 (1.02–3.04)[c]**	**2.16 (1.36–3.42)**	**2.45 (1.33–4.50)[c]**
Self-reported chronic disease						
No chronic disease (ref)	1	1	1	1	1	1
Chronic disease[f]	**2.26 (1.67–3.07)**	1.31 (0.81–2.01)[d]	0.88 (0.60–1.29)	0.78 (0.47–1.30)[d]	1.28 (0.85–1.94)	1.35 (0.74–2.46)[d]
Employment status						
Self-supporting (ref)	1	1	1	1	1	1
Pensioners and retirees	1.07 (0.57–1.99)	0.75 (0.34–1.67)[e]	0.51(0.25-1.07)	1.25 (0.47–3.34)[e]	**0.51 (0.29–0.90)**	0.60 (0.29–1.24)[e]
Not self-supporting	**2.27 (1.50–3.44)**	1.02 (0.59–1.76)[e]	1.37 (0.82–2.03)	1.53 (0.93–2.52)[e]	**1.64 (1.08–2.49)**	1.07 (0.57–2.00)[e]

Statistically significant estimates are shown in bold
[a]The lowest amount of observations in the models
[b]Adjusted for patient's gender, age, general self-perceived health, self-reported chronic disease, employment status and GP-assessed severity of contact. Including patient-perceived waiting time in the model did not affect the results, and the variable was not retained in the adjusted model
[c]Adjusted for patient's gender, age, residence, self-reported chronic disease, patient-perceived waiting time and GP-assessed severity of contact. Including employment status in the model did not affect the results, and the variable was not retained in the adjusted model
[d]Adjusted for patient's gender, age, residence, general self-perceived health and GP-assessed severity of contact. Including employment status and patient-perceived waiting time in the model did not affect the results, and the variables were not retained in the adjusted model
[e]Adjusted for patient's gender, age, residence, general self-perceived health, self-reported chronic disease and GP-assessed severity of contact. Including patient-perceived waiting time in the model did not affect the results, and the variable was not retained in the adjusted model
[f]See Additional file 1

Table 4 Likelihood (OR) of dissatisfaction with different contact types according to GP-related and organizational factors

	Telephone consultations		Clinic consultations		Home visits	
	Crude OR (95% CI) n = 1,321[a]	Adjusted OR (95% CI) n= 698[a]	Crude OR (95% CI) n = 2,467[a]	Adjusted OR (95% CI) n = 1,157[a]	Crude OR (95% CI) n = 1,749[a]	Adjusted OR (95% CI) n = 1,395[a]
GP-related factors:						
GP gender						
Male (ref)	1	1	1	1	1	1
Female	1.23 (0.84–1.82)	1.14 (0.67–1.94)[b]	0.99 (0.67–1.47)	1.18 (0.73–1.92)[b]	0.68 (0.41–1.11)	0.70 (0.41–1.20)[b]
GP age (years)						
< 41 (ref)	1	1	1	1	1	1
41–50	1.51 (0.94–2.43)	1.25 (0.59–2.63)[b]	**2.16 (1.39–3.37)**	1.03 (0.53–2.00)[b]	1.06 (0.58–1.94)	1.00 (0.48–2.05)[b]
51–60	0.99 (0.65–1.51)	1.30 (0.68–2.50)[b]	**2.01 (1.31–3.07)**	1.33 (0.78–2.29)[b]	1.31 (0.78–2.21)	1.16 (0.60–2.27)[b]
> 60	1.52 (1.00–2.31)	**1.96 (1.04–3.68)**[b]	1.46 (0.78–2.74)	1.12 (0.51–2.45)[b]	**2.26 (1.03–4.98)**	**2.82 (1.24–6.40)**[b]
GP-assessed severity of contact						
Potentially severe (ref)	1	1	1	1	1	1
Not severe	**2.41 (1.27–4.58)**	**7.15 (2.49-20.6)**[c]	1.47 (1.00–2.10)	1.28 (0.79–2.09)[c]	**2.69 (1.72–4.02)**	**2.41 (1.38–4.21)**[c]
Organizational factor:						
Patient-perceived waiting time						
Acceptable waiting time (ref)	1	1	1	1	1	1
Unacceptable waiting time	**3.28 (2.00–5.35)**	**3.25 (1.85–5.72)**[d]	**2.75 (1.98–3.83)**	**3.21 (2.03–5.06)**[d]	**4.08 (2.47–6.74)**	**3.83 (2.11–6.96)**[d]

Statistically significant estimates are shown in bold
[a]The lowest amount of observations in the models
[b]Adjusted for patient's gender, age, general self-perceived health, patient-perceived waiting time, GP-assessed severity of contact. Including GP age, patient residence, self-reported chronic disease and employment status in the model did not affect the results, and the variables were not retained in the adjusted model
[c]Adjusted for patient's gender, age, residence, general self-perceived health, self-reported chronic disease, patient-perceived waiting time, GP age and gender. Including employment status in the model did not affect the results, and the variable was not retained in the adjusted model
[d]Adjusted for patient's gender, age, residence, general self-perceived health, self-reported chronic disease and employment status. Including GP-assessed severity of contact in the model did not affect the results, and the variable was not retained in the adjusted model

OOH-PC service; selection bias is thus unlikely to explain our results. This argument is supported by a systematic review of the literature on patient satisfaction, which shows that older respondents and healthier respondents generally report higher levels of satisfaction [29].

If the excluded patients (22%) were more dissatisfied than the included patients, we cannot exclude selection bias. However, the choice to exclude specific patients was based on ethical concerns and logistical issues, e.g. unknown address, and is thus unrelated to the patient's experience of the contact. Therefore, this exclusion should not have influenced the reported ORs.

Other studies have reported that dissatisfied patients are less likely to participate than satisfied patients [30], and the level of dissatisfaction in our study may thus be underestimated. Further, residual confounding cannot be excluded as some factors, e.g. education level, marital status and ethnicity, have been shown to be related to dissatisfaction in previous studies [9, 19]. Using the OR as a measure may overestimate associations if the prevalence of the outcome measure is high [31]. However, the level of overestimation in our study is considered negligible due to a low prevalence of the outcome measure (less than 7% of the patients were dissatisfied).

As the organization of OOH-PC in Denmark is fairly homogenous, the results of the present study can be generalized to other regions in Denmark [1, 3]. Despite differences between the OOH-PC services provided in Denmark and in other countries, the patient-related findings are likely to be generalizable to other countries with comparable OOH-PC settings that include telephone triage by health professionals.

Comparison with other studies

Telephone consultations were more often associated with dissatisfaction than clinic consultations and home visits. This finding is in accordance with previous studies conducted in countries with other ways of organizing the OOH-PC service [1, 9, 11, 12, 15]. We do not know the reason for this, but the result is most likely related to variances in patient populations and GP triage [17]. The variance in dissatisfaction scores for different types of contacts should be further investigated in future studies. Our study found that poor general self-perceived health, but not chronic disease, was related to dissatisfaction, which is in line with the findings in other studies [6, 17, 19]. It has been suggested that patients with poor general self-perceived health might be more vulnerable to the physician's attitude and behaviour [17, 32], and this is likely to be associated with expectations. Previous studies have suggested that a mismatch between the patient's expectations and the service received has a major impact on the level of satisfaction with the OOH-PC service [7, 16, 18]. This may explain the association found between GP-assessed non-severity of the contact and high level of patient dissatisfaction. Thus, some patients may be particularly dissatisfied with telephone consultations if they expected that they would be offered more comprehensive treatment (clinic consultation or home visit) and/or that the triage GP would rate their health problem as more severe.

Residence in urban areas was statistically significantly associated with more dissatisfaction with telephone consultations. The observed association may, to some extent, be explained by a lower threshold for contacting the OOH-PC service in urban areas, which can lead to a mismatch between expected and received service [7]. Alternatively, this finding might reflect differences in access to general practice as suggested by Wilson et al. [18]. However, the present study is unable to investigate this further. Our finding that higher GP age was associated with dissatisfaction with telephone consultations and home visits is in line with the findings of a previous study, which shows that patients tend to rate younger GPs more positively than older GPs [20, 21]. This might also reflect that older GPs are more experienced and thus may provide a different type of telephone consultation (e.g. shorter consultations and fewer referrals to face-to-face contacts).

In consistence with previous findings, unacceptable waiting time was strongly associated with increased dissatisfaction [9–11, 16]. Measuring the actual (rather than the perceived) waiting time might add relevant information as to whether it would be realistic to address this patient-perceived problem. Patients who found the waiting time unacceptable were often women aged 19–50 years and living in rural areas (data not shown).

In contrast to findings in previous studies, our results showed no association between employment status (i.e. socio-economic status) and dissatisfaction [17, 18]. A possible explanation for this finding may be different categorizations of socio-economic factors in different studies.

Conclusions and implications

In general, a high level of patient satisfaction with the OOH-PC service was observed. However, we found lower patient satisfaction with the OOH-PC service among patients who received a telephone consultation. Across all contact types, unacceptable waiting time (organizational factor) and poor general self-perceived health (patient factor) were the only factors associated with dissatisfaction. For the other investigated factors, patient satisfaction depended on the type of contact. Generally, patients living in urban areas and patients with GP-assessed non-severe contact were more dissatisfied. Our findings suggest that a multifaceted approach is required if we intend to increase the satisfaction in all patient groups. GPs could be more aware of the expectations and needs in some patient groups. Patients who contacted the OOH-PC with health problems that were assessed by the triage GP as less appropriate for this setting were more often less satisfied with the service provided; this indicates a mismatch between patient expectations and the actual purpose of OOH-PC. Initiatives that may help adjust the patient-perceived waiting times could be an expedient strategy for achieving higher patient satisfaction.

Abbreviations

DREAM: The Danish Register for Evaluation of Marginalization; GP: General Practitioners; LV KOS: In Danish: *Kontakt-og sygdomsmønster i lægevagten*; OOH: Out-Of-Hours; OOH-PC: Out-of-hours primary care

Acknowledgements

We would like to thank statistician Anders Helles Carlsen from the Research Unit for General Practice, Department of Public Health, Aarhus University, Denmark, for help with the statistical analyses.

Funding

We would like to thank the Danish foundation TrygFonden for financial support.

Authors´ contributions

MT had the primary responsibility for all data and statistical analyses, and she drafted the manuscript. GM contributed to the research design, data collection and drafting of manuscript. BHB contributed to drafting of the manuscript, MBC contributed to research design and drafting of the manuscript. SB contributed to drafting of the manuscript. PV contributed to research design and drafting of the manuscript. All authors read and approved the final manuscript.

Consent for publication

Not applicable.

Competing interests

The authors declare that they have no competing interests.

Author details

[1]Department of Public Health Programmes, Randers Regional Hospital, Østervangsvej 68, 8930 Randers NØ, Denmark. [2]Research Unit for General Practice, Department of Public Health, Aarhus University, Bartholins Allé 2, 8000 Aarhus C, Denmark. [3]Section for Epidemiology, Department of Public Health, Aarhus University, Bartholins Allé 2, 8000 Aarhus C, Denmark. [4]Department of Psychology, Faculty of Health Sciences, University of Southern Denmark, Campusvej 55, 5230 Odense M, Denmark.

References

1. Danish Health and Medicines Authority. Kvaliteten i den danske lægevagtsordning [Quality of the Danish out-of-hours primary care service]. First ed.: Danish Health and Medicines Authority; 2009.
2. Pedersen KM, Andersen JS, Søndergaard J. General practice and primary health care in Denmark. The Journal of the American Board of Family Medicine. 2012;25(Suppl 1):S34–8.
3. Flarup L, Moth G, Christensen MB, Vedsted P, Olesen F. Den danske lægevagtsordning i internationalt perspektiv- en sammenlignende undersøgelse af lægevagten i Danmark, England, Holland, Norge og Sverige [The Danish out-of-hours primary care service in an international perspective - a comparative study of out-of-hours primary care service in Denmark, England, Netherlands, Norway and Sweden]. First ed.: The Research Unit for General Practice, Aarhus University; 2010.
4. Moth, G., Flarup L, Christensen B.M, Olsen F., Vedsted P. Forskningsenheden for almen praksis. Kontakt- og sygdomsmønsteret i lægevagten, LV-KOS 2011 [A survey on reasons for encounter and disease patterns in the Danish out-of hours primary care service, LV-KOS]. First ed.: The Research Unit for General Practice, Aarhus University; 2012.
5. Mainz J, Bartels P, Bek T, Møller Pedersen K, Krøll V, Rhode P editors. Kvalitetsudvikling i praksis[Quality improvement in practice]. First ed. Copenhagen.: Munksgaard Danmark; 2011.
6. Heje,H.N., Olsen F, Vedsted P. Patienternes vurdering af de praktiserende læger-overordnede resultater fra DanPEP-projektet [patient evaluations of general practitioners- results from the DanPEP- study]. Ugeskr Laeger 2010; 172(15):1105–1112.
7. McKinley RK, Stevenson K, Adams S, Manku-Scott TK. Meeting patient expectations of care: the major determinant of satisfaction with out-of-hours primary medical care? Fam Pract. 2002;19(4):333–8.
8. Shipman C, Payne F, Hooper R, Dale J. Patient satisfaction with out-of-hours services how do GP co-operatives compare with deputizing and practice-based arrangements? J Public Health Med 2000 /;22(2):149–154.
9. Salisbury C. Postal survey of patients' satisfaction with a general practice out of hours cooperative. BMJ 1997:31;314(7094):1594–1598.
10. McKinley RK, Roberts C. Patient satisfaction with out of hours primary medical care. Qual Health Care 2001 03;10(1):23–28.
11. van Uden CJ, Ament AJ, Hobma SO, Zwietering PJ, Crebolder HF. Patient satisfaction with out-of-hours primary care in the Netherlands. BMC Health Serv Res. 2005 Jan 15;5(1):6.
12. Moll van Charante E, Giesen P, Mokkink H, Oort F, Grol R, Klazinga N, et al. Patient satisfaction with large-scale out-of-hours primary health care in The Netherlands: development of a postal questionnaire. Fam Pract. 2006;23(4): 437–43.
13. Hansen BL, Munck A. Out-of-hours service in Denmark: the effect of a structural change. Br J Gen Pract. 1998;48(433):1497.
14. Christensen M, Skafte-Holm P, Nielsen E, Greibe J, Moos A, Andersen D, et al. Hvad er din mening om lægevagten? [what is your opinion about the out-of-hours primary care service?]. Ugeskr Laeger. 2000;162:3508–12.
15. Leibowitz R, Day S, Dunt DA. Systematic review of the effect of different models of after-hours primary medical care services on clinical outcome, medical workload, and patient and GP satisfaction. Fam Pract. 2003;20(3): 311–7.
16. Christensen MB, Thomsen L, Oestergaard J, Skafte-Holm P. Fokus på lægevagten[focus on the out-of-hours primary care service]. Ugeskr Laeger. 1999;161:1812–6.
17. Glynn L, Byrne M, Newell J, Murphy A. The effect of health status on patients' satisfaction with out-of-hours care provided by a family doctor co-operative. Fam Pract. 2004;21(6):677–83.
18. Wilson P, McConnachie A, O'Donnell CA, Ross S, Moffat KJ, Drummond N. Assessing dissatisfaction with an out of hours service: reasons and remedies. Health Bull (Edinb). 2001 Jan;59(1):37–44.
19. Danielsen K, Bjertnaes O, Garratt A, Forland O, Iversen H, Hunskaar S. The association between demographic factors, user reported experiences and user satisfaction: results from three casualty clinics in Norway. BMC Fam Pract. 2010;11(1):73.
20. Baker R. Characteristics of practices, general practitioners and patients related to levels of patients' satisfaction with consultations. Br J Gen Pract. 1996;46(411):601–5.
21. Heje HN, Vedsted P, Sokolowski I, Olesen F. Doctor and practice characteristics associated with differences in patient evaluations of general practice. BMC Health Serv Res. 2007;7(1):46.
22. Flarup L, Moth G, Christensen MB, Vestergaard M, Olesen F, Vedsted P. A feasible method to study the Danish out-of-hours primary care service. Dan Med J. 2014;61(5):A4847.
23. Riddle DL, Lee KT, Stratford PW. Use of SF-36 and SF-12 health status measures: a quantitative comparison for groups versus individual patients. Med Care. 2001;39(8):867–78.
24. Holmgren K, Dahlin-Ivanoff S, Björkelund C, Hensing G. The prevalence of work-related stress, and its association with self-perceived health and sick-leave, in a population of employed Swedish women. BMC Public Health. 2009;9(1):1.
25. Hjollund NH, Larsen FB, Andersen JH. Register-based follow-up of social benefits and other transfer payments: accuracy and degree of completeness in a Danish interdepartmental administrative database compared with a population-based survey. Scand J Public Health. 2007;35(5):497–502.
26. Donner A, Klar N. Design and analysis of cluster randomization trials in Health Research: London Arnold Publishers; 2000.
27. Millar MM, Dillman DA. Improving response to web and mixed-mode surveys. Public Opin Q. 2011;75(2):249–69.
28. Murphy CA. Increasing the response rates of reluctant professionals to mail surveys. Appl Nurs Res. 1993;6(3):137–41.
29. Crow R, Gage H, Hampson S, Hart J, Kimber A, Storey L, et al. The measurement of satisfaction with healthcare: implications for practice from a systematic review of the literature. Health Technol Assess. 2002;6(32)
30. Vedsted P, Mainz J, Olsen F. Betydning af påmindelser og lægens engagement ved en spørgeskemaundersøgelse i almen praksis [the significance of reminders and the engagement of GPs in a questionnaire survey in general practice]. Ugeskr Laeger. 2001;163(40):5529–32.
31. Barros AJ, Hirakata VN. Alternatives for logistic regression in cross-sectional studies: an empirical comparison of models that directly estimate the prevalence ratio. BMC Med Res Methodol. 2003;3(1):21.
32. Hall JA, Milburn MA, Epstein AMA. Causal model of health status and satisfaction with medical care. Med Care. 1993:84–94.

8

Perceptions of insulin use in type 2 diabetes in primary care

Kathy Ellis[*], Henrietta Mulnier and Angus Forbes

Abstract

Background: Increasing numbers of patients with type 2 diabetes mellitus are progressing to insulin therapy, and despite its potency many such individuals still have suboptimal glycaemic control. Insulin initiation and intensification is now often conducted by Practice Nurses and General Practitioners in many parts of the UK. Therefore, gaining insight into perspectives of patients and primary care clinicians is important in determining self-management and engagement with insulin. A thematic synthesis of studies was conducted exploring the views and experiences of people with type 2 diabetes and of healthcare professionals on insulin use and management in the context of primary care.

Methods: Protocol based systematic searches of electronic databases (CINAHL, Cochrane Library, EMBASE, MEDLINE, PsycINFO, and Web of Science) were performed on 1 October 2014 and updated on 31 March 2015, to identify studies that identified the views and experiences of adults with type 2 diabetes or primary care clinicians on the use of insulin in the management of type 2 diabetes. Studies meeting the review inclusion criteria were critically appraised using the CASP qualitative research checklist or Barley's checklist for survey designs. A thematic synthesis was then conducted of the collected studies.

Results: Thirty-four studies were selected. Of these, 12 used qualitative interviews (nine with patients and three with healthcare professionals) and 22 were survey based (14 with patients, three with healthcare professionals, and five with both). Twelve key themes were identified and formed three domains, patient perceptions, healthcare professional perceptions, and health professional-patient relationships. The patient-centred themes were: insulin-related beliefs, social influences, psychological factors, hypoglycaemia, and therapy barriers. The clinician-related themes were: insulin skills of general practitioners, healthcare integration, healthcare professional-perceived barriers, hypoglycaemia, and explanations for adherence. Healthcare professional-patient relationship themes were drawn from the perspectives of patients and from clinicians.

Conclusions: This review reveals multiple barriers to optimal insulin use in primary care at both the patient and healthcare professional levels. These barriers indicate the need for multimodal interventions to: improve the knowledge and competencies of primary care professionals in insulin use; provide more effective patient education and self-management support; and introduce integrated insulin support systems.

Keywords: Insulin, Type 2 diabetes, Patients, General practice, Primary care, Perceptions

* Correspondence: kathy.ellis@kcl.ac.uk
Florence Nightingale Faculty of Nursing, Midwifery and Palliative Care, King's College London, 57 Waterloo Road, London SE1 8WA, UK

Background

Many patients living with type 2 diabetes mellitus (T2DM) require insulin as an adjunct to lifestyle interventions and oral hypoglycaemic agents [1–3]. As the population of people affected by T2DM increases, the number of those requiring insulin therapy also increases. While insulin therapy was traditionally managed by specialist diabetes services it is now largely managed in primary care by Practice Nurses (PNs) and General Practitioners (GPs) [4–7].

While insulin is a very effective glucose lowering therapy, it has been shown that many people with insulin treated T2DM have poor glycaemic control (8, 9, 10). There are a number of factors that may explain this problem. Firstly, that there may be some clinical inertia in introducing insulin, as it is often introduced after patients have had poor glycaemic control for some time. Secondly, it has been suggested that both patients and clinicians are reluctant to start insulin due to what has been termed psychological insulin resistance [4, 8, 9]. There is a perception that insulin: represents the last line of treatment and is associated with failure; increases the patient's self-management burden; and imposes hazards such as hypoglycaemia and weight gain [10]. Hence, despite improvements in insulin delivery and support systems, insulin is often not used optimally in primary care settings, increasing the patients risks of complications. [1, 11, 12]. Therefore, developing a better understanding as to what factors influence insulin use in primary care is important to shape interventions to enhance insulin management in this setting.

While previous reviews have explored some of the factors related to why insulin use often fails to deliver good outcomes [10, 13–18], these factors have not been considered systematically in the context of the management of T2DM in primary care from both the patient and healthcare professional perspectives collectively. In this paper, we present a synthesis of the views of patients already established on insulin treatment, and health professionals within primary care, to elicit mechanisms that may explain the use of the therapy and to consider how these may be addressed through more optimal strategies for insulin management in this population.

The aim of the review was to identify and synthesise studies exploring the views and experiences of people with insulin treated T2DM and healthcare professionals (HCPs) within the context of primary care on insulin use to elicit the factors that contribute to sub-optimal insulin use in primary care. The review addressed the following questions:

1. What are the perceptions and experiences of people with T2DM in relation to insulin treatment and use?
2. What are the perceptions and experiences of primary care HCPs on insulin treatment use in people with T2DM?
3. What potential patient-professional interactions impact on insulin use in T2DM?

Methods

Thematic synthesis is a process of identifying new insights by integrating data from original studies and is one of a range of methods available for synthesizing diverse forms of evidence [13, 19–26]. Thematic synthesis generally refers to the integration of findings from qualitative studies, but it has also been used to integrate quantitative and qualitative research; including studies using descriptive or interpretive phenomenological approaches [20, 24, 27–29]. While integrating findings derived from different methods can be challenging and subject to criticism [20, 23, 26, 30], the approach can allow a more expansive interpretation of what is known about the studied phenomena. In this review a narrative synthesis was used to identify the key themes, as an established method for integrating across study types [20, 21, 23–25, 27–29]. Thomas & Harden's [26] approach was observed as a framework for the analysis, but with the inclusion of quantitative in addition to qualitative studies. This progressed in three steps.

Step 1. Identification of studies

Reports of qualitative and quantitative studies addressing the review questions were identified from peer-reviewed journals, conference reports and theses.

Inclusion criteria

Papers were required to report on studies of insulin-related experiences and/or perceptions in either adults aged ≥18 years with insulin treated T2DM or of primary care HCPs. It was also required that the study should focus on patients already receiving insulin therapy, and not on insulin initiation. Study design eligibility included qualitative and descriptive quantitative studies such as surveys and included those with lower or unreported response rates (which may not be apparent especially in web-based surveys).

Search strategy

A protocol-based search was performed by KE on 1 October 2014 and updated on 31 March 2015, to retrieve articles from electronic databases including CINAHL, Cochrane Library, EMBASE, MEDLINE, PsycINFO and Web of Science. The search was structured by terms for T2DM; insulin therapy; and primary care. Discrete searches were also performed with terms for primary care HCPs. The electronic database search strategy can be viewed in Additional file 1. There was no limit to the year of publication but they were required to be published in English. The search was supplemented with: open web-based searches (Google Scholar and EthOs); citation and key author searching; and hand searches of journals. Using EndNote X7 bibliography software, titles and abstracts were screened for inclusion. Full-text articles of the remaining reports were then fully assessed for eligibility by KE before the final selection. To help ensure lack of bias, AF and HM reviewed the search strategy, studies generated, and the final selection; and agreement was reached between the reviewers. In the absence of a standard guideline for reporting thematic syntheses with combined qualitative and quantitative studies [27], the principles of ENTREQ and PRISMA were applied and their study reporting checklists used [31, 32].

Step 2. Content extraction and appraisal

Data were extracted by KE using standardized extraction tools [33, 34], one for qualitative designs and one for surveys. Methodological quality and risk of bias for studies with qualitative designs were assessed using the Critical Appraisal Skills Programme (CASP) qualitative research checklist [35] whilst the survey studies were assessed with Barley et al.'s tool [28]. A score of one was given where the study answered most parts of the appraisal tools' questions.

Step 3. Synthesis of the extracted content

The included studies were subjected to a thematic synthesis by KE, and reviewed by HM and AF until agreement was reached. This was undertaken in 3 stages.

Stage 1 Findings of the qualitative studies were scrutinized for concepts, themes and authors' interpretations relating to managing insulin treated T2DM. Themes were developed inductively, and the text was then coded manually. Next, the main themes from the quantitative studies were identified, and categorized separately.

Stage 2 Descriptive themes and sub-themes from the qualitative studies were inductively developed from the coded text and organized into two primary thematic frameworks one for patients and the other for HCPs. The main finding clusters (including thematic analysis of survey comments) from the quantitative studies were then mapped onto these frameworks, to integrate themes from the different data sources.

Stage 3 Analytical themes were then generated from the descriptive themes for patients and HCPs, to further address the aims of the review, and to identify areas for further research.

Results

Summary of the selected studies

The search strategy identified 147 papers for screening, 70 of which were fully appraised for eligibility. Though the numbers retrieved were lower than anticipated, this was attributed to the inclusion criteria with its focus on experiences and perceptions of T2DM participants already established on insulin and primary care HCPs. Thirty-four of the screened studies fulfilled the inclusion criteria with 36 being rejected with reasons (see Table 1.). Of the included studies, 12 were qualitative [36–47] (nine with patient participants and three with HCPs) and 22 were surveys [48–69] (14 with patient participants, three with HCPs and five with both patients and HCPs). Five of the surveys were discrete reports from two larger studies.

The qualitative studies included data from 173 patients with insulin treated T2DM, aged 23–90 years. The HCP studies included: GPs (n = 65); endocrinologists (n = 2), PNs (n = 8), diabetes nurse educators (n = 3) and pharmacist (n = 1). Their methodologies varied and included focus groups; and in-depth and semi-structured interviews conducted mainly face-to-face, with one study using both telephone interviews and focus groups. The majority of these studies used a thematic, descriptive approach, with some using other methods such as grounded theory, theoretical frameworks, and interpretative phenomenological methods of inquiry.

The quantitative studies were survey-based with mainly cross-sectional designs and included: 13,476 patients with T2DM receiving insulin, aged 41–99 years; GPs (n = 4,176); diabetes consultants (2,192); general physicians (n = 166); general nurses (n = 51); Diabetes Specialist Nurses (DSNs) (n = 50); and diabetes educators (n = 100). The majority of the surveys were web-based with some being undertaken as face-to-face questionnaires or by telephone.

A number of studies took place in multiple sites and in two or more countries. The qualitative research sites included: Asia (n = 4), Australia (n = 1), Europe (n = 7), New Zealand (n = 1), and North America (n = 1). Those of the quantitative studies included: Asia (n = 7), Australia (n = 1), Europe (n = 15), North America (n = 12), South America (n = 2), and South Africa (n = 1).

The methodology and reporting quality of the qualitative studies was generally good with scores ranging from 8 to 10; the quantitative studies were of moderate strength with scores ranging from 3 to 7. Tables 2, 3, 4. present an overview of the included studies, and the selection process is shown in a PRISMA flow chart in Fig. 1. The appraisal scores are presented in Additional file 2. Where available, the survey response-rate has been entered although this was not available in many of the surveys which were reported

Table 1 Rejected Studies with Reasons

Author & Reference	Year	Reason for Rejection
Aloumanis [83]	2013	The focus is on clinical outcomes rather than perceptions and experiences.
Bahrmann [9]	2014	The focus is on psychological insulin resistance in insulin naïve patients compared to those established on insulin.
Balkau [84]	2012	The patient participants are insulin naïve.
Beresford [85]	2011	Insufficient data specific to insulin treated T2DM.
Beverly [86]	2012	Insufficient data specific to insulin treated T2DM.
Brod [87]	2013b	It was not possible to differentiate data specific to insulin treated T2DM.
Carbone [88]	2007	It was not possible to differentiate data specific to insulin treated T2DM.
Chai [89]	2012	Conference abstract only. No other data available.
Chai [90]	2013	Conference poster only. No other data available.
Chai [91]	2014	Conference abstract only. No other data available.
Chan [92]	2014	The patient participants are insulin naïve.
Choudhury [93]	2014	It was not possible to differentiate data specific to insulin treated T2DM.
Cramer & Pugh [94]	2005	The focus is on insulin prescriptions issued and not on perceptions or experiences.
Gaborit [95]	2011	The focus is on knowledge rather than experiences of insulin adjustment.
Hermanns [96]	2010	The focus is on comparing barriers of insulin naïve patients.
Hinder & Greenhalgh [97]	2012	Insufficient data specific to insulin treated T2DM.
Frei [98]	2012	The focus is on clinical characteristics and demographics.
Hunt [99]	1998	Insufficient data specific to insulin treated T2DM.
Khattab [100]	2010	The focus is on clinical characteristics and demographics.
Lai [101]	2007	It was not possible to differentiate data specific to insulin treated T2DM.
Lakkis [102]	2013	The focus is on attitudes of clinicians towards initiating insulin.
Mollem [103]	1996	It was not possible to differentiate data specific to insulin treated T2DM.
Morris [104]	2005	Patients only recently initiated with insulin therapy.
Munro [73]	2013	There is no information specific to insulin treated T2DM.
Oliveria [105]	2007	The focus is on patients who did not start or continue insulin therapy.
Peyrot [106]	2005	Patient participants are insulin naïve. Perceptions of clinicians relate to insulin initiation.
Peyrot [107]	2006	Insufficient data specific to insulin treated T2DM.
Peyrot [108]	2013	Insufficient data specific to insulin treated T2DM.
Pooley [109]	2001	No data specific to insulin treated T2DM.
Ritholz [72]	2011	Insufficient data specific to insulin treated T2DM
Shiu & Wong [110]	2000	It was not possible to differentiate data specific to insulin treated T2DM.
Thomson [111]	1991	The focus is on knowledge rather than experiences or perceptions of hypoglycaemia.
Wendel [112]	2014	The focus is on incidence of hypoglycaemia and prescribing behaviour rather than perceptions of hypoglycaemia
Wong [113]	2011	Patients were insulin naïve.
Yoshioka [74]	2014	The focus is on insulin initiation.
Zafar [8]	2015	Insufficient data specific to insulin treated T2DM.

online. Survey limitations include pharmaceutical company support, recruitment bias with sampling from research panels and self-selection in online surveys; and self-reporting of clinical data. However, it was decided to include the surveys because of their contribution to the overall themes of the synthesis.

In total, 12 themes with 46 sub-themes from the patient studies; and 14 themes with 54 sub-themes from the HCP studies were included in the primary thematic frameworks.

Integrated themes

The synthesis integrated the two thematic frameworks to form 12 primary themes expressed in three domains: patient perceptions, HCP perceptions, and HCP-patient relationships (see Fig. 2.). The themes

Table 2 Overview of the Included Qualitative Studies with Patient Participants

Author & Reference	Year	Country	Diabetes Type	Aim	Sample and Setting	Data Collection	Data Analysis
Abu Hassan [36]	2013	Malaysia	Insulin T2DM	To explore patients' reasons for accepting insulin and their initial barriers.	Patients with insulin T2DM ($n = 21$) Primary Care Clinic	In-depth interviews Focus groups	Thematic analysis
Brod [37]	2014	Canada, China & Germany	T1DM & Insulin T2DM	To examine unintentional insulin dosing and injection irregularities due to forgetting among people with diabetes.	Patients with T1DM ($n = 22$) Insulin T2DM ($n = 42$) At least twice in the last three months of forgetting injection, or time/amount taken, or questioning if insulin was taken. Research recruitment databases	Telephone interviews Focus groups	Thematic analysis with grounded theory
Brown [38]	2007	UK	Insulin T2DM & Non-Insulin T2DM	To gain an understanding of how health beliefs influence how African-Caribbeans manage their T2DM.	T2DM adults (n = 16) Insulin T2DM (n = 6) Self-help groups and GP practices Inner-city African-Caribbean community	In-depth interviews	Thematic analysis
Browne [39]	2013	Australia	Insulin T2DM & Non-Insulin T2DM	To explore the social experiences of adults with T2DM, focusing on the perception & experience of diabetes- related stigma.	T2DM adults ($n = 25$) Insulin T2DM (n = 5) State diabetes organisation	Semi-structured interviews	Inductive thematic analysis
Hortensius [40]	2012	Netherlands	T1DM & Insulin T2DM	To investigate patients' perspectives of SMBG & all relevant aspects influencing SMBG.	Insulin treated DM patients ($n = 28$) T1DM ($n = 13$) T2DM ($n = 15$) Outpatient clinic (T1DM) GP practices (T2DM)	In-depth interviews	Thematic analysis with grounded theory.
Janes [41]	2013	New Zealand	Insulin T2DM	To better understand barriers to glycaemic control from the patient's perspective.	Insulin treated patients T2DM (n = 15) Diabetes clinic	Semi-structured interviews.	Thematic analysis with a patient-centred framework. Interpretative phenomenological method of inquiry
Jenkins [42]	2011	UK and Ireland	Insulin T2DM	To explore participants' experiences of intensifying insulin therapy during the Treating to Target in T2DM (4-T) trial.	T2DM patients ($n = 41$) Whose insulin was intensified in 4-T trial. Primary care	In-depth interviews	Thematic analysis with grounded theory.
Ong [43]	2014	Malaysia	Insulin T2DM	To explore the barriers and facilitators to SMBG, in insulin T2DM patients.	Insulin treated T2DM patients (n = 15) Primary care clinic	Semi-structured interviews	Inductive thematic analysis
Vinter-Repalust [44]	2004	Croatia	Insulin T2DM & Non-insulin T2DM	To explore patients' attitudes, thoughts, & fears connected with their illness; expectations of the healthcare system; and problems while adhering to the therapeutic regime.	Patients with T2DM ($n = 49$) Insulin T2DM (n = 13) General practice	Focus group discussions.	Inductive thematic analysis

Key: *DSN* **diabetes specialist nurse,** *PN* **practice nurse,** *GP* **general practitioner,** *HCP* **health care professional,** *OHAs* **oral hypoglycaemic agents,** *PCPs* **primary care physicians,** *QOL* **quality of life,** *SMBG* **self-monitoring of blood glucose,** *T1DM* **type 1 diabetes mellitus,** *T2DM* **type 2 diabetes mellitus,** *Insulin T2DM* **insulin treated type 2 diabetes mellitus**

Table 3 Overview of the Included Qualitative Studies with HCP Participants

Author & Reference	Year	Country	Aim	Sample and Setting	Data Collection	Data Analysis
Goderis [45]	2009	Belgium	To evaluate barriers and facilitators to high quality diabetes care by GPs participating in a quality improvement programme promoting compliance with international guidance.	GPs participating in the programme (n = 20) General Practice.	Semi-structured interviews	Thematic analysis with an implementation and behavioural change model.
Jeavons [46]	2006	UK	To determine doctors' and nurses' attitudes and beliefs on treating T2DM with less than ideal control.	GPs (*n* = 15) Practice Nurses (n = 8) General Practice	Focus groups.	Thematic analysis with grounded theory.
Lee [47]	2013	Malaysia	To explore the views of Malaysian healthcare professionals on the barriers faced by patients using insulin.	Primary care doctors (*n* = 20) Family medicine specialists (*n* = 10) Policymakers (n = 5) Diabetes educators (*n* = 3) Endocrinologists (n = 2) Pharmacist (n = 1) Primary & secondary care	In-depth interviews Focus group discussions	Inductive thematic analysis

Key: *DSN* diabetes specialist nurse, *PN* practice nurse, *GP* general practitioner, *HCP* health care professional, *OHAs* oral hypoglycaemic agents, *PCPs* primary care physicians, *QOL* quality of life, *SMBG* self-monitoring of blood glucose, *T1DM* type 1 diabetes mellitus, *T2DM* type 2 diabetes mellitus, *Insulin T2DM* insulin treated type 2 diabetes mellitus

for each domain are described below with linkage to the source data from qualitative studies (with participant comments) and surveys (which are identified). A summary of the survey findings will then follow. There were more themes relating to barriers than to facilitators to managing insulin.

Domain 1. Patient perceptions

In this domain five themes relating to patient perceptions of insulin emerged from the synthesis: insulin-related beliefs, social influences, psychological factors, hypoglycaemia, and therapy barriers.

Theme 1. Insulin-related beliefs

The data showed that a patient's beliefs about insulin can mediate their orientation to using insulin. These beliefs include: illness severity; cultural beliefs; and insulin specific beliefs. Many patients reported how when insulin was first suggested, they believed it meant their diabetes had suddenly become very serious [36, 38, 41, 62].

> *"...I felt like once you hit insulin you are on a slide to ... you know [death]."* [Participant 13] [41]

Survey respondents also reported their perceived seriousness of the condition [62].

Cultural beliefs can influence insulin adherence negatively, particularly when cultural traditions conflicted with the underlying constructions about what insulin was and how diabetes should be treated [36, 38, 41]. One patient from a UK African-Caribbean community said:

> *"I'm telling you I've known people take insulin here and they go back to the Caribbean and don't take insulin.... they don't have the pollution that you have here, your body perspires more so all the impurities or all the stuff that it retains in your body keeps coming out .."* [Interview 16] [38]

Janes et al. described how cultural beliefs could be in direct conflict with using drugs [41]. One individual relied on traditional Maori beliefs and medicinal plants for healing:

> *"The body is tapu [restricted]... it makes me not like poking holes in it* [with needles]*"* [Participant 13]

Theme 2. Social influences

Social factors included stigma, family and friends, economics, work and social activities. Perceived stigma relating to injecting in public was associated with insulin adherence [36, 39, 41–43, 59]. For some this stigma was reflected in the belief that others perceived injecting insulin as being associated with drug addiction [36, 41, 42].

> *"Our society is quite ignorant of insulin therapy and they might associate insulin injection with drug addicts"* [2 years of insulin use/ 5 years of having diabetes] [36]

Table 4 Overview of the Included Quantitative Studies with Patients, HCPs, or Patients and HCPs

Author & Reference	Year	Country	Diabetes Type Patients or HCPs	Aim	Sample and Recruitment	Data Collection
Ary [48]	1986	USA	Insulin T2DM & Non-insulin T2DM Patients only	To assess levels of regime adherence and reasons for non-adherence in T1DM and T2DM	Patients with T1DM (n = 24) Non-insulin T2DM (n = 125) Insulin T2DM (n = 59) Recruited by doctors, newspaper adverts & American Diabetes Association meetings	Face-to-face Questionnaire
Brod [49]	2012a	USA, Canada, Japan, Germany, UK and Denmark	Insulin T2DM Patients and HCPs	To estimate the prevalence of self-treated hypoglycaemia in patients using basal analogues. To identify demographic treatment-related and behavioural risk factors. To describe patient and physician responses to these in the Global Attitude of Patients and Physicians 2 (GAPP2) study.	T2DM Patients using basal insulin analogues (n = 3,042) Physicians (n = 1,222): Specialists (45%) PCPs (55%) Online research panel	Cross-sectional online questionnaire
Brod [50].	2012b	USA, Canada, Japan, Germany, UK and Denmark	Insulin T2DM Patients and HCPs	To describe basal insulin analogue dosing irregularities; the effect on patient functioning, well-being and management; and the identification of patients most at risk in the GAPP2 study.	T2DM Patients using basal insulin analogues (n = 3,042) Physicians (n = 1,222): Specialists (45%) PCPs (55%) Online research panel	Cross-sectional online questionnaire
Brod [51]	2012c	USA, UK, Germany and France	T1DM, Insulin T2DM & Non-insulin T2DM Patients only	To determine how non-severe nocturnal hypoglycaemic events (NSNHEs) affect diabetes management, sleep quality, functioning, and to assess if these impacts differ by diabetes type or country.	T1DM and T2DM patients (n = 1086) who experienced NSNHE in the last month: T1DM (n = 676) Non-Insulin T2DM (n = 124) Insulin T2DM (n = 286) Online venues	Web-based survey
Brod [52]	2013a	USA, UK, Germany, Canada, France, Italy, Spain, Netherlands and Sweden	T1DM, Insulin T2DM & Non-insulin T2DM Patients only	To explore the burden and impact of NSNHEs on diabetes management, patient monitoring and well-being to better understand the role NSNHEs play in caring for people with diabetes and to facilitate optimal diabetes treatment strategies.	Patients (n = 2,108) with: T1DM or T2DM. T1DM (n = 692) Non-insulin T2DM (n = 543) Insulin T2DM (n = 873) Online venues	Web based survey
Cefalu [53]	2008	USA, Mexico, UK, France, Germany, Spain and Brazil	Insulin T2DM & Non-Insulin T2DM Patients only	To understand patients' perspectives to achieving good glycaemic control and determine how their perceptions of insulin may affect their decisions to initiate or intensify insulin.	T2DM adults (n = 1,444) of which: Insulin T2DM (n = 469) Online databases	Structured online and telephone survey.
Cuddihy [54]	2011	Germany, Japan, Spain, Turkey, UK and USA	HCPs Only	To investigate the opinions of PCPs and diabetes specialists on their perceived role in tackling T2DM and the challenges they face, particularly to insulin intensification.	Diabetes specialist physicians (n = 300) PCPs (n = 300) Recruited by telephone and online panels	Online survey

Table 4 Overview of the Included Quantitative Studies with Patients, HCPs, or Patients and HCPs *(Continued)*

Author & Reference	Year	Country	Diabetes Type Patients or HCPs	Aim	Sample and Recruitment	Data Collection
Diago-Cabezudo [55]	2013	Europe	T1DM & Insulin T2DM Patients only	To evaluate the effects of hypoglycaemia on the lives of patients with DM and determine if SMBG to prevent hypoglycaemic is an appealing and widely accepted concept.	Insulin treated patients (n = 1,848) T1DM (n = 924) Insulin T2DM (n = 924) Online databases	Online survey
Fulcher [56]	2014	Argentina, Australia, Brazil, Israel, Mexico and South Africa	T1DM, Insulin T2DM & Non-insulin T2DM Patients only	To understand the impact of nocturnal and daytime non-severe hypoglycaemic events on healthcare systems, work productivity & QOL in T1DM or T2DM.	T1DM (n = 64) Non-insulin T2DM (n = 76) Insulin T2DM (n = 160) Recruited from online panels and by HCPs	Online and face-to-face surveys
Leiter [57]	2005	Canada	T1DM & Insulin T2DM Patients only	To assess impact of mild, moderate and severe hypoglycaemia and fear of future episodes on patients with T1DM or insulin-treated T2DM	Adults with insulin treated T2DM (n = 335) T1DM (n = 202) insulin T2DM (n = 133) Diabetes Clinics	Self-administered questionnaire
Leiter [58]	2014	Canada	Insulin T2DM Patients and HCPs	To assess the frequency and impact of dosing irregularities and self-treated hypoglycaemia in T2DM patients treated with insulin analogues in the GAPP2 study.	Patients with Insulin treated T2DM (n = 156) Physicians (n = 202) Of which: PCPs (n = 160) Specialists (n = 42) Online panels and HCP registers	Online survey
Mehmet [59]	2015	UK	T1DM & Insulin T2DM Patients only	To determine if patients report problems with injecting insulin/ SMBG in front of others and explore reasons why.	Insulin T2DM (n = 27) T1DM (n = 49) Hospital Clinic	Self-completed questionnaire
Mitchell [60]	2013	UK	Insulin T2DM & Non-insulin T2DM Patients only	To characterize hypoglycaemic events in T2DM and assess the relationship between the experiences and health outcomes.	T2DM adults (n = 1,329) of which: Insulin T2DM (n = 301) Research survey panel	Longitudinal online survey
Mollema [61]	2001	Netherlands	T1DM & Insulin T2DM Patients only	To examine functioning and self-management of insulin treated patients suffering from extreme fear of self-injecting and/or fear of self-testing.	Patients with insulin treated diabetes (n = 1,275) of which: T1DM (n = 740) T2DM (n = 535) Randomly drawn from the Dutch Diabetes Association	Cross-sectional postal questionnaire
Mosnier-Pudar [62]	2009	France	Insulin T2DM & Non-insulin T2DM Patients only	To describe T2DM from the patient's standpoint in a representative French panel in 2008.	T2DM Patients (n = 1,092) of which: Non-Insulin (n = 885) Insulin T2DM (n = 207) From a polling institute in France	Postal questionnaire
Peyrot [63]	2012a	China, Japan, USA, Germany, Spain, France, Turkey & UK	T1DM & Insulin T2DM Patients only	To examine factors associated with insulin injection omission/ non-	Insulin treated DM adults (n = 1,530) of which: T1DM (n = 110)	Cross-sectional telephone survey

Table 4 Overview of the Included Quantitative Studies with Patients, HCPs, or Patients and HCPs *(Continued)*

Author & Reference	Year	Country	Diabetes Type Patients or HCPs	Aim	Sample and Recruitment	Data Collection
				adherence in the Global Attitude of Patients and Physicians (GAPP) Study.	T2DM (n = 1,420) Research panels	
Peyrot [64]	2012b	China, Japan, USA, Germany, Spain, France, Turkey & UK	T1DM & Insulin T2DM Patients and HCPs	To examine patient and physician beliefs regarding insulin therapy and degree to which patients adhere to insulin regimes in the GAPP Study.	Insulin treated DM adults (n = 1,530) of which: T1DM (n = 180) T2DM (n = 1,350) Physicians (n = 1,250) of which Specialists (n = 600) PCPs (n = 650) Research panels	Cross-sectional telephone survey
Rubin [65]	2009	USA	T1DM & Insulin T2DM Patients and HCPs	To compare patients' perceptions of injection-related problems with clinicians' estimates of those problems.	Insulin treated adults (n = 501) of which T2DM (n = 385) PCPs (n = 101) Endocrinologists (n = 100) Diabetes Educators (n = 100) Chronic illness panel, Medical Register and Research database.	Online survey
Shiu [66]	2004	Hong Kong	Insulin T2DM Patients only	To examine the relationship between a sense of coherence, fear of hypoglycaemia and metabolic control to identify whether other variables including age, hypoglycaemic experience and adherence to self-care practice, confounded the findings from two Swedish studies.	Insulin treated T2DM adults (n = 72) Diabetes Centre	Cross-sectional face-to-face questionnaire
Siminerio [67]	2007	USA	HCPs only	To examine nurse and physician perceptions of nurse involvement in diabetes care.	General Nurses(n = 51) DSNs (n = 50) Generalist Physicians (n = 166) Diabetes Specialist Physicians (n = 50) Professional directories and listing	Cross-sectional survey conducted face-to-face or by telephone.
Van Avendonk [68]	2009	Netherlands	HCPs only	To investigate the organisation of insulin therapy in general practice and assess factors associated with providing insulin in T2DM patients.	Dutch GPs (n = 1,621) University Medical Centre database.	Postal questionnaire
Zambanini [69]	1999	UK	T1DM & Insulin T2DM Patients only	To assess: prevalence of phobia and anxiety-related to insulin injections; association between insulin injection anxiety symptoms with level of general anxiety in the study group; and evaluate their influence of, on glycaemic control.	Insulin treated patients (n = 115) of which: T1DM (n = 80) and Insulin T2DM (n = 35) Hospital diabetes clinic.	Questionnaire administered by HCPs

Key: *DSN* diabetes specialist nurse, *PN* practice nurse, *GP* general practitioner, *HCP* health care professional, *OHAs* oral hypoglycaemic agents, *PCPs* primary care physicians, *QOL* quality of life, *SMBG* self-monitoring of blood glucose, *T1DM* type 1 diabetes mellitus, *T2DM* type 2 diabetes mellitus, *Insulin T2DM* insulin treated type 2 diabetes mellitus

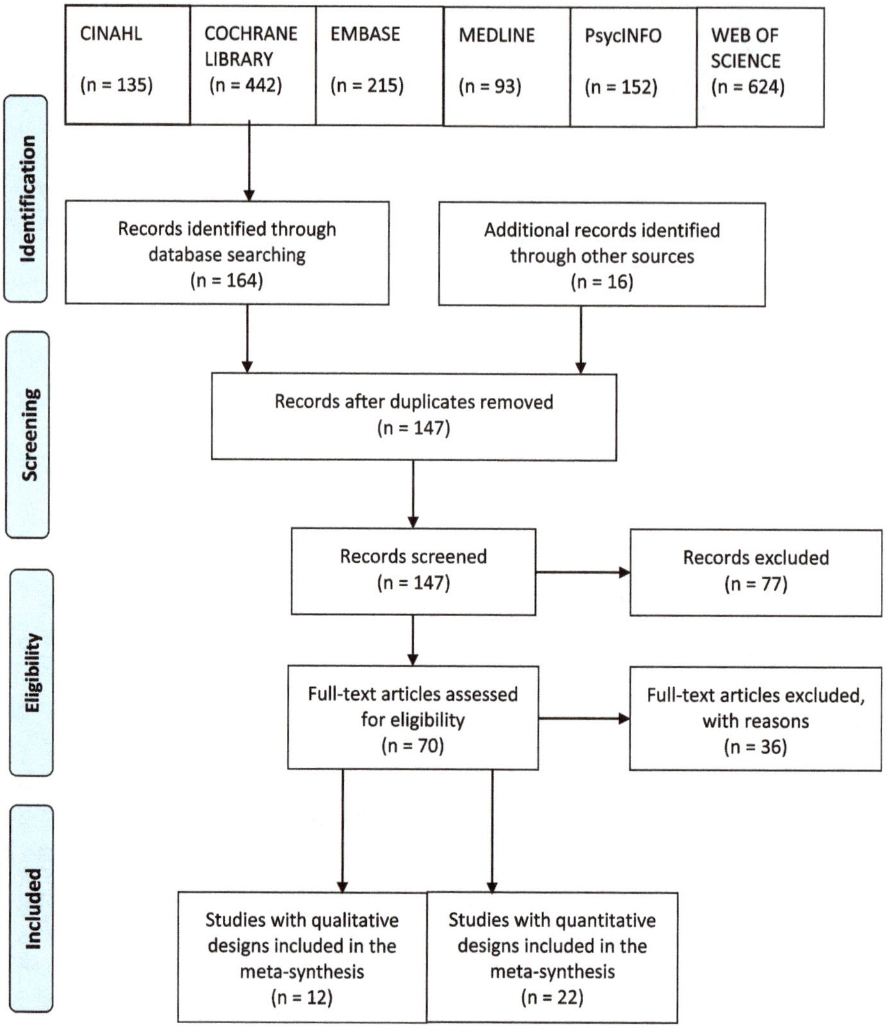

Fig. 1 PRISMA Flow Diagram Illustrating the Selection Process

Of the T2DM patients (n = 27) in Mehmet et al.'s survey [59] the majority (n = 20) also experienced problems injecting in public, the main reason being worry about upsetting or offending others.

Patients developed various strategies to adjust for this stigma adding to the complexity of insulin use:

> *"If I go out with anybody I always go and do it (inject) in the toilet. I won't ever do it outside."* [Participant 26] [42]

Patients were influenced by family and friends in managing their insulin [36, 41, 43, 44]. For some this created barriers to insulin use, as they had to observe the requirements and routines of the family over mealtimes impacting on their insulin behaviours. However, others identified the potentially positive influence of family support [36]:

> *"I always refer to these two 'specialists' (my father and older brother who are on insulin) when it comes to insulin"* [6 years of insulin use/ 10 years of having diabetes]

> *"I gained a lot of knowledge from self-reading and relatives who are on insulin"* [2 years of insulin use/ 5 years of having diabetes]

Economic factors (such as the cost of blood-testing strips and loss of earnings) and employment disruption were both identified as socially specific mediators of insulin use [41, 43, 44]:

> *"Cost is a problem. If I went to the doctor plus medication, that was my week's pay gone."* [Participant 15] [41]

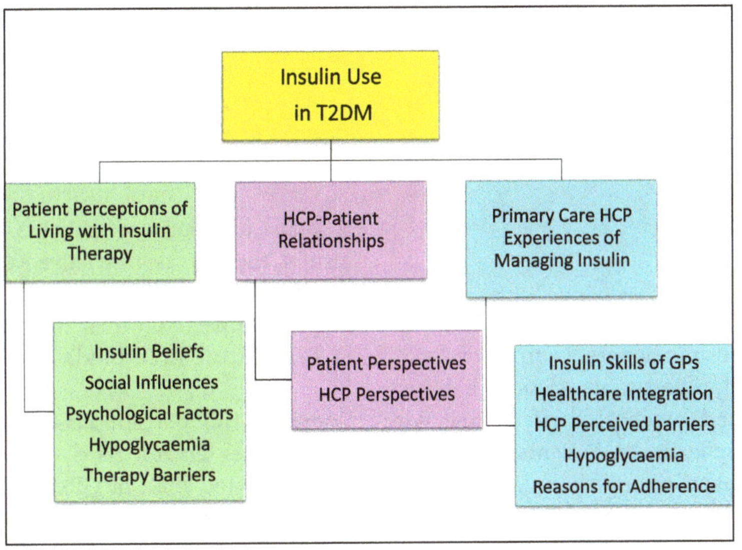

Fig. 2 Twelve Primary Themes formed from the Thematic Frameworks. Key: HCP = Healthcare Professional; T2DM = type 2 diabetes mellitus

> *"I would come off an '18 hour' and the day shift boss would ring me up, says 'hey, can you come in and do a couple of hours, bro.'... Insulin was not easy to take and you would pop it in, but no, I had to wait between shifts.."* [Participant 11] [41]

Others, however, felt supported at work [36].

The impact of insulin use on travel, leisure, and social activities was perceived negatively by patients [36, 38–41], as it restricted their social interactions and influenced their insulin injecting behaviours when in social settings:

> *"I wouldn't go out to lunch with them [friends] and in the end, I had to tell them why. I said, 'I can't. I have got to have insulin. And I am not going to go into a toilet'."* [Participant 23] [42]

Theme 3. Psychological factors

Psychological factors related to fear and anxiety, shame and depression. Fear and anxiety about hypoglycaemia (see Theme 4), injection pain, and weight gain were perceived by many participants as significant mediators in insulin utilisation [36–38, 40, 41, 43, 44] and included survey participants [53, 61, 65, 69].

> *"I am scared of needle.. you know, the poking itself, it is painful.. using needle some more, and you poke yourself... it is painful"* [3 years of insulin use/ 6 years of having diabetes] [36]

Feelings of shame and self-blame were evident in the participant accounts of some studies [38, 41]. These feelings were linked to the perceptions that they had somehow caused their disease and that their need for insulin was because they had not properly controlled their diabetes:

> *A good diabetic is one who controls their diabetes ...I am not a good diabetic.* [Participant 7] [41]

Negative emotions such depression also had an impact on insulin use. In one large survey depression was the strongest predictor of the severity of fear of self-injecting [61]. In the qualitative studies, negative emotions were often identified in the context of low patient activation in relation to self-management:

> *"In that period of depression I was just happy when I felt good and that things were moving again, and that I could do my job again ...and for me that was enough. The diabetes just wasn't that important for me."* [Participant] [40]

Theme 4. Hypoglycaemia

Hypoglycaemia was identified in survey participants as a key barrier and concern for patients with impact on their emotional state, daily functioning and engagement with their insulin [45, 49, 51, 52, 55–58, 60, 66]. In consequence patients reported injecting smaller doses to keep their blood glucose elevated. The survey studies identified that a fear of hypoglycaemia is common and is associated with reduced adherence [49, 51, 57]. The patient accounts in the qualitative studies gave many examples of these behavioural responses to hypoglycaemia:

"When I am hypoglycaemic, I feel wretched. ... I don't really have a problem with high sugar levels, but the low ones are quite bothersome." [Participant] [40]

"to avoid hypos... I won't have my insulin" [Participant 4] [41]

Theme 5. Therapy barriers

The inherent complexities of managing insulin, was often an impediment to insulin adherence in several surveys [48, 50, 62, 63] which reported associations between insulin non-adherence and practical barriers, injection difficulties and regimen inflexibility. Patients remembering whether they had taken their insulin was another factor, with people omitting injections if they were unsure whether they had taken it or not:

"I am type 2 and when I forget my insulin in the morning, then I skip it and take my next insulin with my next meal." [Germany, Male] [37]

The challenges associated with sustaining regular self-monitoring of blood glucose (SMBG) were also identified as impeding insulin behaviours [40, 43]:

"Beginning [SMBG] yes, beginning very keen, now no. I'm just simply lazy to do it." [P06, 69-year-old female retiree, diabetes for 15 years] [43]

While some patients found SMBG to be helpful in achieving better glycaemic control and in detecting hypoglycaemia, others perceived it as a burden [40]. Some patients reduced SMBG once they established a dose they felt was right for them, such that they could not monitor any changes in their insulin requirement [43].

A further area of therapy complexity was in the titration of the insulin dose. Five qualitative studies [37, 40, 42–44] and several surveys [50, 52, 53, 58], reported that patients struggled with titration, often ignoring instructions, or adopting their own approach. There was some divergence between patients as to whether they wanted the HCP to make insulin changes or whether they preferred to control it themselves:

"I never change the therapy my doctor prescribed! I trust him, that's his job, not mine!" [67-year-old woman] [44]

One patient became more confident after receiving appropriate HCP support:

"At first I was very afraid about changing my dosage of insulin. But then my doctor explained to me how... In the beginning, I used to call him, but now I frequently change the dosage on the basis of my own physical activity, diet, and sugar levels." [55-year-old woman] [44]

Whilst a majority of patients and physicians regarded insulin therapy as restrictive in one survey [64], more patients saw insulin treatment as having positive than negative impacts on their life though this trend was less in T2DM than T1DM individuals.

Domain 2. HCP perceptions

Five themes emerged in relation to HCP perceptions: insulin-related skills of GPs, healthcare integration, HCP perceptions of patient-related barriers, hypoglycaemia, and HCP explanations for insulin adherence.

Theme 1. Insulin-related skills

This theme relates to the skills required by primary care HCPs to initiate and intensify insulin therapy, and to provide ongoing support for patients. While many HCPs were positive about helping patients to manage insulin, others felt they lacked the skills to do so effectively [45, 46]. They believed insulin-related training was important, but they also wanted ongoing support from a diabetes specialist. GP attitudes seemed to modify when they had acquired insulin-related skills, increasing their motivation and confidence in supporting patients:

"My attitude about insulin therapy onset has changed. Before the start of Of the project, I tried too long oral anti diabetics, but the courses have changed my attitude. I became confident in starting insulin therapy, whereas before I would never initiate insulin therapy." [GP12-S3] [45]

However, some felt excluded, believing that specialists wanted to continue to manage insulin treated patients themselves:

"Specialists gain too much control of referred patients and often exclude GPs from direct patient care. This is especially true of patients on insulin who get free instructions and monitoring kits at the diabetes centres, unlike patients in primary care. So, it's nearly impossible for GPs to hold on to patients on insulin." [GP1-S2] [45]

In one survey [54], there was disagreement regarding who was responsible for intensification but the majority of both diabetes specialists and primary care physicians agreed that doctors in primary care should become more involved in managing insulin. In another [67] nurses and physicians agree that nurses should take a larger role in managing diabetes.

Theme 2. Healthcare integration

The level of integration between the different components of the health system was identified as having a key role in how patients were supported in using insulin [45, 47] as illustrated by this GP:

> *"This is a big change from the usual 'let us do our work; after all we are the specialists and you may help a little bit'. We collaborate as one team – there's mutual support! We're on the same wavelength and feel we work together toward the same objectives."* [GP13-S4] [45]

Better collaboration between primary and secondary care was considered by most physicians in Cuddihy et al. 's survey [57] as one of the most important factors in improving insulin treatment of T2DM.

The systems in which primary care HCPs work influenced how involved they are in starting and/or managing insulin therapy. GPs and PNs identified that a lack of resources and familiarity with starting and managing insulin impacted negatively on the insulin support they could provide [46]. One large Dutch survey observed that the more structured practices employing a PN and with a designated diabetes clinic were more likely to manage insulin therapy themselves [68].

Theme 3. HCP perceptions of patient barriers

HCPs reported that patient-level factors heavily influenced insulin use, echoing many of those voiced by the patients, including: beliefs, culture, economics and psychological barriers. In addition, they believed patient education impacted positively on insulin use [45–47]. They felt, that for patients, insulin treatment represented failure and a more serious stage of the illness:

> *"I think probably they think it's the end, that's it, there's nothing else they can have after that."* [HCP] [46]

They also identified that patients often altered their insulin behaviours subjectively based on how they felt, rather than by following their targets [47]. Some found it challenging when dealing with patients from different ethnic backgrounds [46]. They reported how some cultural beliefs created barriers to insulin use:

> *"We see patients twice a year and the family and friends are there all the time, you know, I mean, we are supposed to be more powerful figures, but I mean, it's quite difficult to overcome very different beliefs within the family."* [HCP] [46]

HCPs perceived that SMBG for insulin optimisation was moderated by fear and in some countries cost:

> *"Those who can afford also don't see that it's important to invest on the glucometer ... When we talk about meter and everything, you have to talk about fear of pricking. That's another barrier."* [Family medicine specialist, public health clinic] [47]

> *"How come when we [public health clinics] give all [insulin and pens], we provide everything free, but the glucometer is not given, test strips are not given, and how are they [patients] monitoring the blood glucose?"* [GP, private general practice] [47]

The psychological factors identified by the HCPs again reflected the insulin-related fears and anxieties reported by patients, such as: hypoglycaemia, concerns about weight gain, and fear of injection pain.

> *"Surely, one of the biggest barriers is this fear of going onto needles for the rest of your life. I think the effect of getting older is that they hate the idea of hypoglycaemia as well. They get very frightened of that."* [HCP] [46]

HCPs believed patients had insufficient understanding of diabetes and needed much more input in relation to insulin titration and dose adjustment if they were going to use insulin effectively [46, 47]:

> *"So ... the most common thing, what happen is, people start insulin, but after that, they don't optimize and specify the regime. The patient who started just on one regime for, like, many years and nobody have actually taught the patient how to do the self-titration of the insulin too ...."* [Family medicine specialist, public health clinic] [47]

Theme 4. Hypoglycaemia

HCPs identified fear of hypoglycaemia as a significant issue in optimal insulin use in surveys [54, 58, 64] and interviews [46, 47].

> *"I think the effect of getting older is that they hate the idea of hypoglycaemia as well. They get very frightened of that."* [HCP] [46]

Theme 5. Explanations for insulin adherence

HCP explanations for low insulin adherence included: being too busy; travelling; the timing of meals; stress or emotional problems; public embarrassment; and the patient's perception of their diabetes control:

> *"....so it depends how their [patients'] lifestyle... It depends on their work also ... how's their working and meal times. Their mealtimes also ... they will tell us."* [Family medicine specialist, public health clinic] [47]

> *"Maybe they [patients] will continue [using insulin] for a while, they will get better, they said, No, I don't want injection anymore."* [R1, GP, private general practice] [47]

> *"They said 'I am better, so I can stop now.'"* [R2, GP, private general practice] [47]

HCPs in surveys [50, 64] reported that their typical patient did not take their insulin as prescribed citing similar reasons as patients [64]. Prescribers did not routinely discuss basal adherence patterns with their basal-bolus patients [50].

Domain 3. HCP-patient relationships

This domain identifies the role of the HCP-Patient relationship, with regard to insulin therapy utilisation. For patients, communication and relational care were important in shaping their insulin views and behaviours. From the HCPs perspective, their interactions with patients were influenced by their personal confidence in using insulin therapy. The domain is comprised of two themes.

Theme 1. Patient perspectives of relational care

The quality of the relationship and communication with HCPs was valued by patients. In many of the qualitative studies it was identified as an important factor contributing to their adherence to insulin [36, 38, 40, 44] and in surveys [52, 62]. The nature of the relationship could contribute positively or negatively on the patient's insulin behaviours depending. Key factors that influenced the quality of the relationship were: how the HCP communicated insulin-related information; whether they elicited and responded to patient concerns; the time available for the consultation; and how accessible and relevant the support provided was to the patient:

> *"I have got a good doctor... but they are busy, real busy, and I suppose you have not got time to talk."* [Patient 8] [41]

> *"..we discussed about the issues of insulin, my worries and thoughts about insulin. I became less apprehensive and was ready to start on insulin therapy"* [2 years of insulin use/ 5 years of having diabetes] [36]

Another aspect of the relationship was reflected in the divergent agenda of the HCP and the patient. While HCPs tended to focus on tightening glycaemic control, patients were more concerned with their wider life needs and their quality of life (QOL). This was reflected in the ways patients moderated their behaviour to try and appease the HCPs:

> *"I have been using it [SMBG] every day because I know I have got an appointment coming up, so I better behave [participant giggled]. So that I can tell the doctor, you know, I want to bring down the insulin dose."* [P01, 57-year-old female clerk] [43]

Theme 2. HCP perspectives

HCP perceptions of their relationship with patients included the impact of integrated care working, the time available for providing insulin-related support, their own ambivalence about insulin therapy, and whether they had the required skills [45–47] and included surveyed HCPs [67, 68]. It was perceived that the relationship between GPs and patients was enhanced when the GPs were equipped with insulin-related skills with good support from diabetes specialist services:

> *"Diabetes patients themselves feel much more appreciated; because of that, the link between us and our patients has strengthened."* [GP17-S4] [45]

When the HCP adopted a patient-centred approach in their relationship, this could enhance insulin use:

> *"...Because when we negotiate, you know, some, they said okay, after negotiating, then they're okay. Then they try to follow."* [Family medicine specialist] [47]

Summary of the survey findings

The surveys reported a number of factors that might mediate insulin use. In the patient based surveys (n = 14) these included: hypoglycaemia [49, 52, 55–57, 60, 66] glycaemic control [66], injecting in public [59], problems with injections [61, 69], insulin intensification [53], insulin adherence [48, 63], and perceptions of T2DM [62]. Studies with both patients and HCPs (n = 5), identified hypoglycaemia [49, 58], dosing irregularities [50, 58], insulin adherence [64], and injection-related problems [65].

HCP surveys (n = 3) included: insulin intensification [54], HCP perceptions of nurse involvement in T2DM [67], and insulin management in general practice [68]. A table of the findings and key topics can be viewed in Additional file 3.

Patient-related themes

Hypoglycaemia Hypoglycaemic events associated with insulin, particularly nocturnal hypoglycaemia, were reported as having a disrupting effect on: diabetes self-management; sleep quality and next-day functioning; work performance and driving; and personal well-being [49, 52]. It was also reported that many patients with T2DM had no warning signs of hypoglycaemia [55]. Some studies reported that hypoglycaemia had negative financial consequences and impact on QOL [49, 56, 66]. Severe hypoglycaemic episodes led people to fear future events [57] with subsequent worse self-reported glycaemic control [60]. Exposure to insulin-related hypoglycaemia was reported to lead to poor insulin adherence and omission [48, 49, 58, 63, 66].

Injection-related problems Patients in Mehmet et al.'s [59] study reported problems injecting in front of others, most commonly because they worried about upsetting or offending them. Others experienced anxiety and fear of injections [61]. Zambanini et al. [69] found insulin injections were avoided in 14% of participants because of related anxiety.

Adherence to insulin Insulin non-adherence was common taking the form of dosing irregularities and insulin omission [50, 58, 64, 65]. Factors contributing to insulin adherence, included: being in a public place or travelling; fear of hypoglycaemia; and therapy complexity [48, 63].

The majority of patients surveyed by Cefalu et al. [53]; wished there was another way to take insulin whether they were using insulin (n = 371;79%) or not (n = 782; 80%). Non-adherence was also associated with dosing irregularities, reduced doses, and mistimed doses [50, 58, 64, 65].

HCP-related themes

Adherence to insulin Physicians (55% from primary care and 45% specialists) reported that glucose control was negatively impacted by the level of insulin adherence, with missed, mistimed, or reduced insulin doses being identified [50]. Despite acknowledging the clinical relevance of irregular dosing, 32% of physicians reported not routinely discussing these with their basal insulin patients and 29% with their basal-bolus patients.

Hypoglycaemia was identified by HCPs as having an effect on insulin adherence [49, 58]. In Peyrot et al.'s study [64], patients and physicians agreed the five most common reasons for insulin omission or non-adherence was being too busy; travelling; skipped meals; stress or emotional problems; and public embarrassment. Rubin et al. [65] reported 50% of their patients would be more likely to take insulin regularly if the pain of injecting could be ameliorated.

Insulin-related role Cuddihy et al. [54] surveyed 600 physicians (50% from primary care and 50% specialists) and found that notable proportions of primary care physicians never initiate or modify insulin and never or rarely intensify it mainly because of lack of experience and lack of time to educate patients. There was also disagreement regarding who was responsible for intensification. However, 86% of all the physicians agreed that primary care physicians should become more involved in managing insulin. In another study [67] nurses and physicians agreed, nurses should take a larger role in managing diabetes. Finally, in a survey by Van Avendonk et al. [68] of Dutch GPs (n = 1621) 67% started and managed insulin therapy in T2DM. Associated factors were being male, above age 40 years, working in a health centre, and working together with a Practice Nurse.

Analytical themes

Four analytical themes, the equivalent of third-order interpretations in meta-ethnography [19, 26], were then generated from the integrated themes. These interpretations provided new perspectives to identify modifiable mechanisms that could be manipulated to enhance insulin use and adherence. The themes are interrelated as expressed in the model outlined in Fig. 3.

Theme 1. Understanding and attending to patient barriers

It is evident that there are multiple barriers to insulin uptake and utilisation in patients with T2DM. These barriers are common and are multi-levelled, with major factors being: psychological issues such as fear or hypoglycaemia and negative beliefs about insulin; and social factors such as external prejudice, stigma and life disruption/constraints. Despite being aware of these patient level barriers to insulin adherence, the primary care HCP accounts did not identify strategies for addressing them. If these barriers are to be overcome a multi-modal approach providing targeted support to patients and enhancing the primary care HCP's skills in overcoming these are required, with key components being: patient centred education and self-management support addressing patient level barriers; training for primary care HCPs to enhance their confidence in using insulin and in being able to elicit and respond to patient needs in relation to insulin self-management.

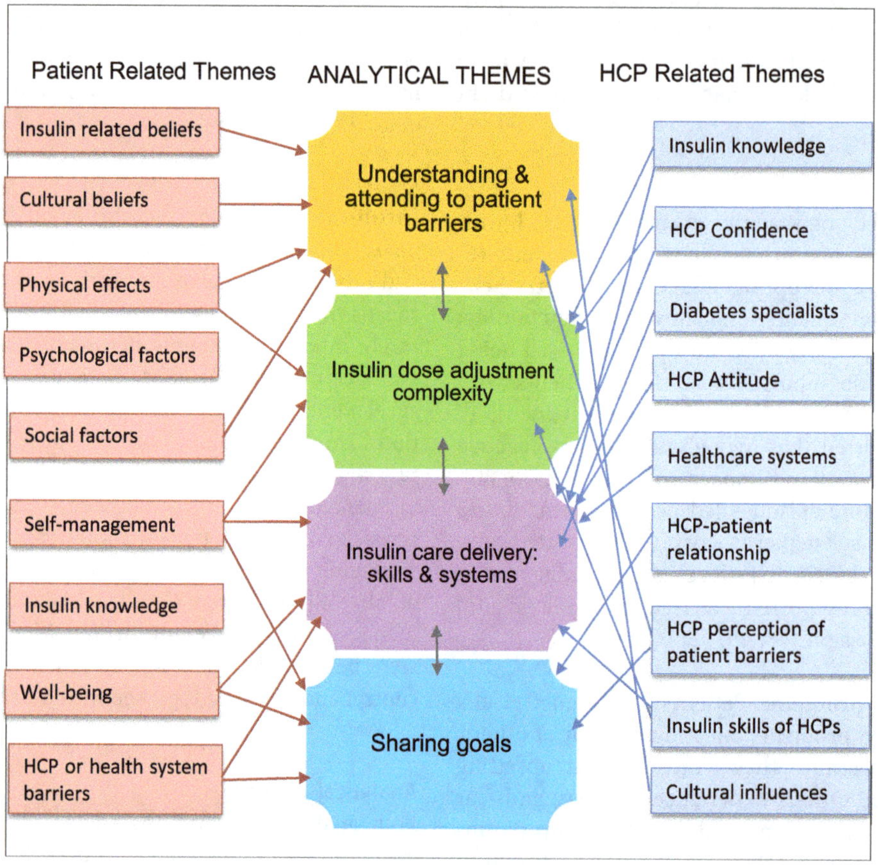

Fig. 3 Analytical Model and the Interrelated Themes. Key: HCP = Healthcare Professional

Theme 2. Insulin dose adjustment complexity

The collected data suggests that current methods of insulin dose titration are not always systematic but are often suboptimal with poor adherence. Dose adjustment seems to be further complicated by patient perceptions on insulin use which can be subjective and are influenced by factors such as avoiding hypoglycaemia and the management of wider aspects of their social and working lives. Hence, if insulin dose adjustment is to be more optimally managed then there is a need for a simpler patient centred approach. This approach again needs to attend to potential behavioural confounders and ensure that patients have a clear perspective on the process, its importance and what they hope to achieve.

Theme 3. Sharing goals

The data identified that there may be some divergence between the patient's blood glucose goals and those of their HCPs. Patients identified that HCPs focussed more on achieving a glycaemic target whereas subjectively they may feel better with higher glucose levels. Hence, insulin use may be enhanced if there is a stronger connectivity between the patient and the HCP in setting and agreeing therapy goals.

Theme 4. Insulin care delivery: Skills and systems

The insulin-related skills and attitudes of primary care HCPs may be significant in determining the use of insulin and the outcomes achieved. The skills are not isolated to the individual HCP, as the data suggest that the context of practice is important too, placing an emphasis on systemic factors including care integration and teamwork. This emphasis is further reinforced by the data highlighting continuity and consistency in the support provided to patients. There were also data suggesting the need to integrate specialist support within the system to help primary care professionals optimise care delivery. Where available, the specialist support could also be provided by those practices already experienced and skilled in insulin initiation/intensification. Therefore, if insulin therapy is going to be better delivered within primary care not only will the HCPs need better training, they will also need to develop support systems that are internally (a team approach) and externally integrated (specialist support).

Discussion

This synthesis has identified a wide range of factors that modify the use of insulin in people with T2DM. These factors can be broadly divided into three interrelated levels, the patient, the HCP and the care system. The use of data derived from both patients and HCPs enhances the analytical potential of the synthesis to consider the interactive components expressed from these different perspectives. These generated the potential development of newer services for patient benefit.

Patients

The findings of the review have identified a wide range of factors that drive patients' behaviours in relation to insulin use. These factors include: underlying beliefs about insulin; psychosocial factors; the self-management skills and knowledge of the patient; and their experiences in using insulin. It is also clear from the review that many of these factors are interactive. While many of these factors have been reported in previous reviews [10, 13, 16, 70] this review has considered how these factors are expressed and interact in the experiences of patients with the added perspective of how they relate to the views and behaviours of health professionals. This latter element is important as it is the interaction between patients and health professionals where many of the challenges and barriers for effective insulin use in patients with T2DM reside. The review has also highlighted the problems and issues that affect patients' use of insulin. Addressing these issues is important and they need to be considered in the patient education and self-management support provided to patients. The findings suggest that as well as the technical aspect of self-management, the support provided needs to consider the patients' underlying beliefs, their psychological orientation to insulin and the influence of wider social factors. Addressing the problem of clinical and psychological inertia of the intensification of insulin therapy is key part of the process [8, 12, 71]. Given that factors such as perceived stigma in their use of insulin restricts how they use it, it may be important to help patients develop strategies to ameliorate those feelings. Wider factors such as family dynamics also need to be considered. Therefore, if patients are going to supported in using insulin effectively the barriers and factors highlighted in the review need to be incorporated into the insulin assessment process and attended to in the self-management support provided. It is also necessary to establish whether or not a patient wishes or is able to self-manage their insulin titration as some patients may prefer to be led by their HCP as was apparent in this synthesis [42, 44],

HCPs

The HCPs accounts utilised within the review were predominantly those of primary care physicians. While these accounts were derived from studies undertaken in different healthcare systems, they shared similar perspectives on insulin management. The two key factors that governed the delivery of insulin care were the skills of the HCP and the time available. The former would suggest that there is a need for professional education. Given the findings of the patient accounts, this education needs to offer more than the technical aspects of insulin and should include an understanding of the psychosocial factors that may influence insulin use. In relation to time, it may be important to identify the role of other team members in delivering insulin support such as primary care nurses or diabetes specialist nurses supporting the primary care team. These benefits were highlighted in a study by Ritholz et al. [72] but the physician participants stressed the necessity of regular and ongoing communication among team members to ensure patients received consistent information. The review has also identified that the interactions between HCPs and patients are pivotal in determining whether insulin is used effectively. The relational aspect of care and continuity of support seem to be particularly important. In keeping with other studies [73, 74], the review identified that patients and HCPs can sometimes have divergent views in some areas, in particular glycaemic targets, highlighting the need for agreeing blood glucose goals in a collaborative way when supporting patents to adjust their insulin. Serrano et al. [75] illustrated some effective approaches to shared-decision making to enhance patient understanding of choices in diabetes management. Therefore, primary care HCPs can have a very important contribution to make in using insulin effectively provided they have the appropriate training, the time needed to deliver care and supportive health systems.

Healthcare systems

The evidence presented in this thematic synthesis revealed how integrated healthcare systems, teamwork, the way GP practices were organised, and in one study, the presence of a Practice Nurse [68], all facilitated the role of general practice in insulin treated T2DM. Diabetes specialists also shared this view. The thematic synthesis identified that the support of diabetes specialist teams, can help primary care HCPs to deliver insulin support. Therefore, to ensure that insulin is used optimally in primary care, the findings of the review indicate that the care system needs to be designed to ensure that patients are assessed and followed up by an appropriately trained HCP, who can provide continuity in their care experience. The system also needs to consider how to integrate specialist diabetes support to help the primary care teams in their clinical decision making and in building the resources that patients will need to support their insulin use.

Limitations

This review has a number of limitations. The principle one is the reliance on the quality of the data from the primary studies, as most of the studies were not exclusive to T2DM patients, and not all based only in primary care. The latter was addressed by only including data from participants with T2DM in primary care. Another limitation was that many of the studies were biased toward the perspectives of primary care physicians, and identifying more accounts from other team members would have enhanced the review findings. From a UK perspective, more accounts of the contribution from PNs would have been desirable. It was also noted that while it was possible to elicit barriers to effective insulin utilisation, there were few studies that identified potential facilitators of insulin management, although the review was able to theorise these based on the nature of the identified barriers. Another potential source of bias was that some of the surveys were supported by insulin-related companies, although no evidence of such bias and the nature of the surveys were not related to product evaluation. The inclusion of both qualitative and quantitative designed studies is a further weakness, particularly with the variety of qualitative approaches, incorporating interpretive and descriptive approaches. However, this integration could also be viewed as a strength as identifying common themes in the different data sources adds to the likely generalisability of the findings. Finally, the literature search was completed in March 2015 and further studies have since been identified. These include a patient survey of frequency of self-treated hypoglycaemia [76], a focus group study of insulin treated T2DM patients to identify fear of hypoglycaemia [77], interviews and focus groups of patients and HCPs to ascertain their perspectives on psychological insulin resistance [78], semi-structured interviews of patients to establish barriers to and enablers of insulin self-titration [79], and finally interviews of patients with insulin treated T2DM to detect their reasons for poor glycaemic control [80].

Despite these limitations, the synthesis has provided some novel insights into the collective factors impacting on insulin treated patients in primary care. These will be a helpful reference for further exploratory studies in developing new interventions.

Conclusions

Insulin use is often poor in people with T2DM, and associated with sub-optimal long-glycaemic control, with risk of complications and increased mortality [10–12, 81, 82]. This review reveals the burden experienced by T2DM patients receiving insulin and the skills needed to equip primary care HCPs to support them. Integrated healthcare systems with appropriate resources could help facilitate this but patient-centred care by appropriately skilled GPs and PNs is also required.

Abbreviations

CASP: Critical appraisal skills programme; DSN: Diabetes Specialist Nurse; GP: General Practitioner; HCP: Healthcare professional; OHAs: Oral hypoglycaemic agents; PCP: Primary Care Physician; PN: Practice Nurse; QOL: Quality of life; RR: Response-rate; SMBG: Self-monitoring of blood glucose; T1DM: Type 1 diabetes mellitus; T2DM: Type 2 diabetes mellitus

Acknowledgements

KE received a Band Trust Research Scholarship from the Florence Nightingale Foundation; and a PhD fee support award from the National Institute for Health Research (NIHR) Collaboration for Leadership in Applied Health Research & Care, South London at King's College London.

Authors' contributions

KE conducted and wrote up the synthesis. HM Reviewed and edited the manuscript. AF made a significant contribution to the design and write up of the report. All the authors have read and approved the manuscript.

Authors' information

KE is a PhD student at King's College London.
HM is a lecturer at King's College London.
AF is Chair of Clinical Diabetes Nursing at King's College London

Competing interests

The authors declare that they have no competing interests.

References

1. Diabetes UK. Diabetes: facts and stats. 2016; https://www.diabetes.org.uk/. Accessed 19 Dec 2017.
2. Evans ML, Sharplin P, Owens DR, Chamberlain GH, Longman AJ, McEwan P. Insulin usage in type 2 diabetes mellitus patients in UK clinical practice: a retrospective cohort-based analysis using the THIN database. British J Diab Vasc Dis. 2010;10(4):178–82.
3. Mulnier H, Seaman H, Lovell D, Lawrenson R. The increasing proportion of patients with type 2 diabetes converting to insulin therapy. Practical Diabetes International. 2005;22(6):202–6.
4. Dale J, Martin S, Gadsby R. Insulin initiation in primary care for patients with type 2 diabetes: 3-year follow-up study. Primary Care Diabetes. 2010;4(2):85–9.
5. Burden ML, Burden AC. Attitudes to starting insulin in primary care. Practical Diabetes International. 2007;24(7):346–50.
6. Chadder L. An evaluation of insulin training for GPs and practice nurses. Journal of Diabetes Nursing. 2013;17(4):141–7.
7. Ellis K, Pinnock H, Apampa B. Insulin initiation in a general practice clinic: a questionnaire-based study. Diabetes & Prim Care. 2011;13(3):181–9.
8. Zafar A, Stone MA, Davies MJ, Khunti K. Acknowledging and allocating responsibility for clinical inertia in the management of type 2 diabetes in primary care: a qualitative study. Diabet Med. 2015;32(3):407–13.
9. Bahrmann A, Abel A, Zeyfang A, Petrak F, Kubiak T, Hummel J, Oster P, Bahrmann P. Psychological insulin resistance in geriatric patients with diabetes mellitus. Patient Educ Couns. 2014;94(3):417–22.
10. Davies MJ, Gagliardino JJ, Gray LJ, Khunti K, Mohan V, Hughes R. Real-world factors affecting adherence to insulin therapy in patients with type 1 or type 2 diabetes mellitus: a systematic review. Diabet Med. 2013;30(5):512–24.
11. Holman RR, Paul SK, Bethel MA, Matthews DR, Haw N. 10-year follow-up of intensive glucose control in type 2 diabetes. N Engl J Med. 2008;359(15):1577–89.
12. Paul SK, Klein K, Thorsted BL, Wolden ML, Khunti K. Delay in treatment intensification increases the risks of cardiovascular events in patients with type 2 diabetes. Cardiovasc Diabetol. 2015;14(1):1–10.
13. Barendse S, Singh H, Frier BM, Speight J. The impact of hypoglycaemia on quality of life and related patient reported outcomes in type 2 diabetes: a narrative review. Diabet Med. 2012;29(3):293–302.

14. Campbell R, Pound P, Pope C, Britten N, Pill R, Morgan M, Donovan J. Evaluating meta-ethnography: a synthesis of qualitative research on lay experiences of diabetes and diabetes care. Soc Sci Med. 2003;56(4):671–84.
15. Khunti K, Davies M, Kalra S. Self-titration of insulin in the management of people with type 2 diabetes: a practical solution to improve management in primary care. Diabetes. Obes Metab. 2013;15(8):690–700.
16. Gherman A, Veresiu IA, Sassu RA, Schnur JB, Scheckner BL, Montgomery GH. Psychological insulin resistance: a critical review of the literature. Practical Diabetes International. 2011;28(3):125–8.
17. Lustman PJ, Clouse RE. Depression in diabetic patients: the relationship between mood and glycemic control. J Diabetes Complicat. 2005;19(2):113–22.
18. Pontiroli AE, Miele L, Morabito A. Increase of body weight during the first year of intensive insulin treatment in type 2 diabetes: systematic review and meta-analysis. Diabetes. Obes Metab. 2011;13(11):1008–19.
19. Britten N, Campbell R, Pope C, Donovan J, Morgan M, Pill R. Using meta ethnography to synthesise qualitative research: a worked example. J. Health Serv. Res. Policy. 2002;7(4):209–15.
20. Dixon-Woods M, Agarwal S, Jones D, Young B, Sutton A. Synthesising qualitative and quantitative evidence: a review of possible methods. Journal of Health Service Research and Policy. 2005;10(1):45–53.
21. Forbes A, Griffiths P. Methodological strategies for the identification and synthesis of 'evidence' to support decision-making in relation to complex healthcare systems and practices. Nurs Inq. 2002;9(3):141–55.
22. Mohammed MA, Moles RJ, Chen TF. Meta-synthesis of qualitative research: the challenges and opportunities. Int J Clin Pharm. 2016;38(3):695–704.
23. Noblit GW, Hare RD. Meta-ethnography: synthesizing qualitative studies. London: Sage; 1988.
24. Pedersen VH, Dagenais P, Lehoux P. Multi-source synthesis of data to inform health policy. Int J Technol Assess Health Care. 2011;27(3):238–46.
25. Walsh D, Downe S. Meta-synthesis method for qualitative research: a literature review. J Adv Nurs. 2005;50(2):204–11.
26. Thomas J, Harden A. Methods for the thematic synthesis of qualitative research in systematic reviews. BMC Med Res Methodol. 2008;8:45.
27. Carroll C. Qualitative evidence synthesis to improve implementation of clinical guidelines. Br Med J. 2017;356:108–10.
28. Barley EA, Murray J, Walters P, Tylee A. Managing depression in primary care: a meta-synthesis of qualitative and quantitative research from the UK to identify barriers and facilitators. BMC Fam Pract. 2011;12:47.
29. Mold F, Forbes A. Patients' and professionals' experiences and perspectives of obesity in health-care settings: a synthesis of current research. Health Expect. 2013;16(2):119–42.
30. Lopez KA, Willis DG. Descriptive versus interpretive phenomenology: their contributions to nursing knowledge. Qual Health Res. 2004;14(5):726–35.
31. Moher D, Liberati A, Tetzlaff J, Altman DG. Preferred reporting items for systematic reviews and Meta-analyses: the PRISMA statement. Ann Intern Med. 2009;151(4):264–9.
32. Tong A, Flemming K, McInnes E, Oliver S, Craig J. Enhancing transparency in reporting the synthesis of qualitative research: ENTREQ. BMC Med Res Methodol. 2012;12:181.
33. Cronin P, Ryan F, Coughlan M. Undertaking a literature review: a step-by-step approach. Br J Nurs. 2008;17(1):38–43.
34. Whiting L. Systematic review protocols: an introduction. Nurse Res. 2009; 17(1):34–43.
35. Critical Appraisal Skills Programme (CASP) Qualitative checklist. 2013; https://casp-uk.net//. Accessed 13 Aug 2016.
36. Abu Hassan H, Tohid H, Mohd Amin R, Long Bidin MB, Muthupalaniappen L, Omar K. Factors influencing insulin acceptance among type 2 diabetes mellitus patients in a primary care clinic: a qualitative exploration. BMC Fam Pract. 2013;14:164.
37. Brod M, Pohlman B, Kongso JH. Insulin administration and the impacts of forgetting a dose. Patient. 2014;7:63–71.
38. Brown K, Avis M, Hubbard M. Health beliefs of African-Caribbean people with type 2 diabetes: a qualitative study. Br J Gen Pract. 2007;57(539):461–9.
39. Browne JL, Ventura A, Mosely K, Speight J. 'I call it the blame and shame disease': a qualitative study about perceptions of social stigma surrounding type 2 diabetes. BMJ Open. 2013;3:e003384. https://doi.org/10.1136/bmjopen-2013-003384.
40. Hortensius J, Kars MC, Wierenga WS, Kleefstra N, Bilo HJ, van der Bijl JJ. Perspectives of patients with type 1 or insulin-treated type 2 diabetes on self-monitoring of blood glucose: a qualitative study. BMC Public Health. 2012;12:167.
41. Janes R, Titchener J, Pere J, Pere R, Senior J. Understanding barriers to glycaemic control from the patient's perspective. Journal of Primary Health Care. 2013;5(2):114–22.
42. Jenkins N, Hallowell N, Farmer AJ, Holman RR, Lawton J. Participants' experiences of intensifying insulin therapy during the treating to target in Type2 diabetes (4-T) trial: qualitative interview study. Diabet Med. 2011; 28(5):543–8.
43. Ong WM, Chua SS, Ng CJ. Barriers and facilitators to self-monitoring of blood glucose in people with type 2 diabetes using insulin: a qualitative study. Patient Preference and Adherence. 2014;8:237–46.
44. Vinter-Repalust N, Petricek G, Katic M. Obstacles which patients with type 2 diabetes meet while adhering to the therapeutic regimen in everyday life: qualitative study. Croat. Med. J. 2004;45(5):630–6.
45. Goderis G, Borgermans L, Mathieu C, Van den Broeke C, Hannes K, Heyrman J, Grol. Barriers and facilitators to evidence based care of type 2 diabetes patients: experiences of general practitioners participating to a quality improvement program. Implement Sci. 2009;4:41.
46. Jeavons D, Hungin APS, Cornford CS. Patients with poorly controlled diabetes in primary care: healthcare clinicians' beliefs and attitudes. Postgrad Med J. 2006;82(967):347–50.
47. Lee YK, Ng CJ, Lee PY, Khoo EM, Abdullah KL, Low WY, Samad AA, Chen WS. What are the barriers faced by patients using insulin? A qualitative study of Malaysian health care professionals' views. Patient Preference and Adherence. 2013;7:103–9.
48. Ary DV, Toobert D, Wilson W, Glasgow RE. Patient perspective on factors contributing to nonadherence to diabetes regimen. Diabetes Care. 1986; 9(2):168–72.
49. Brod M, Rana A, Barnett AH. Impact of self-treated hypoglycaemia in type 2 diabetes: a multinational survey in patients and physicians. Curr Med Res Opin. 2012a;28(12):1947–58.
50. Brod M, Rana A, Barnett AH. Adherence patterns in patients with type 2 diabetes on basal insulin analogues: missed, mistimed and reduced doses. Curr Med Res Opin. 2012b;28(12):1933–46.
51. Brod M, Christensen T, Bushnell DM. Impact of nocturnal hypoglycemic events on diabetes management, sleep quality, and next-day function: results from a four-country survey. J Med Econ. 2012c;15(1):77–86.
52. Brod M, Wolden M, Christensen T, Bushnell DM. A nine country study of the burden of non-severe nocturnal hypoglycaemic events on diabetes management and daily function. Diabetes Obesity and Metabolism. 2013a; 15(6):546–57.
53. Cefalu WT, Mathieu C, Davidson J, Freemantle N, Gough S, Canovatchel W. Patients' perceptions of subcutaneous insulin in the OPTIMIZE study: a multicenter follow-up study. Diabetes Technol. Ther. 2008;10(1):25–38.
54. Cuddihy RM, Philis-Tsimikas A, Nazeri A. Type 2 diabetes care and insulin intensification: is a more multidisciplinary approach needed? Results from the modify survey. Diabetes Educator. 2011;37(1):111–23.
55. Diago-Cabezudo JI, Madec-Hily A, Aslam A. Perceptions of hypoglycemia and self-monitoring of blood glucose in insulin-treated diabetes patients: results from a European online survey. Diabetes Management. 2013;3(1):15–23.
56. Fulcher G, Singer J, Castañeda R, Fraige Filho F, Maffei L, Snyman J, Brod M. The psychosocial and financial impact of non-severe hypoglycemic events on people with diabetes: two international surveys. J Med Econ. 2014; 17(10):751–61.
57. Leiter LA, Yale J-F, Chiasson J-L, Harris S, Kleinstiver P, Sauriol L. Assessment of the impact of fear of hypoglycemic episodes on glycemic and hypoglycemia management. Can J Diabetes. 2005;29(3):186–92.
58. Leiter LA, Boras D, Woo VC. Dosing irregularities and self-treated hypoglycemia in type 2 diabetes: results from the Canadian cohort of an international survey of patients and healthcare professionals. Can J Diabetes. 2014;38:38–44.
59. Mehmet S, Hussey C, Ibrahim S. Patients' perceptions of injecting insulin and self-monitoring of blood glucose in the presence of others. Practical Diabetes. 2015;32(2):59–63.
60. Mitchell BD, Vietri J, Zagar A, Curtis B, Reaney M. Hypoglycaemic events in patients with type 2 diabetes in the United Kingdom: associations with patient-reported outcomes and self-reported HbA1c. BMC Endocr Disord. 2013;13:59.
61. Mollema E, Snoek F, Ader HJ, Heine R, van der Ploeg H. Insulin-treated diabetes patients with fear of self-injecting or fear of self-testing: psychological comorbidity and general well-being. J Psychosom Res. 2001; 51(5):665–72.

62. Mosnier-Pudar H, Hochberg G, Eschwege E, Virally ML, Halimi S, Guillausseau PJ, Peixoto O, Touboul C, Dubois C, Dejager S. How do patients with type 2 diabetes perceive their disease? Insights from the French DIABASIS survey. Diabetes & Metabolism. 2009;35(3):220–7.
63. Peyrot M, Barnett AH, Meneghini LF, Schumm-Draeger PM. Factors associated with injection omission/non-adherence in the global attitudes of patients and physicians in insulin therapy study. Diabetes Obes. Metab. 2012a;14(12):1081–7.
64. Peyrot M, Barnett AH, Meneghini LF, Shumm-Draeger PM. Insulin adherence behaviours and barriers in th1e multinational global attitudes of patients and physicians in insulin therapy study. Diabet Med. 2012b;29(5):682–9.
65. Rubin RR, Peyrot M, Kruger DF, Travis LB. Barriers to insulin injection therapy: patient and health care provider perspectives. The Diabetes Educator. 2009; 35(6):1014–22.
66. Shiu AT. Sense of coherence amongst Hong Kong Chinese adults with insulin-treated type 2 diabetes. Int J Nurs Stud. 2004;41(4):387–96.
67. Siminerio LM, Funnell MM, Peyrot M, Rubin RR. US Nurses' perceptions of their role in diabetes care: results of the cross-national diabetes attitudes wishes and needs (DAWN) study. Diabetes Educ. 2007;33(1):152–62.
68. Van Avendonk MJ, Gorter KJ, van den Donk M, Rutten GE. Insulin therapy in type 2 diabetes is no longer a secondary care activity in the Netherlands. Primary Care Diabetes. 2009;3:23–8.
69. Zambanini A, Newson RB, Maisey M, Feher MD. Injection related anxiety in insulin-treated diabetes. Diabetes Research & Clinical Practice. 1999;46(3): 239–46.
70. Fu AZ, Qiu Y, Radican L. Impact of fear of insulin or fear of injection on treatment outcomes of patients with diabetes. Curr Med Res Opin. 2009; 25(5):1413–20.
71. Khunti K, Nikolajsen A, Thorsted BL, Andersen M, Davies MJ, Paul SK. Clinical inertia with regard to intensifying therapy in people with type 2 diabetes treated with basal insulin. Diabetes. Obes Metab. 2016;18(4):401–9.
72. Ritholz MD, Beverly EA, Abrahamson MJ, Brooks KM, Hultgren BA, Weinger K. Physicians' perceptions of the type 2 diabetes multidisciplinary treatment team a qualitative study. Diabetes Educator. 2011;37(6):794–800.
73. Munro N, Barnard KD, Brice R, Cummings M, Davies M, Hall G. Discordant perceptions regarding the interactions between people with diabetes and healthcare professionals in the UK: findings from the DAWN2 study, Research poster. 14th annual conference of the South Asian Health Foundation; 2013. p. 21–2. http://www.diabetesonthenet.com/. Accessed 7 Nov 2014.
74. Yoshioka N, Ishii H, Tajima N, Iwamoto Y. Differences in physician and patient perceptions about insulin therapy for management of type 2 diabetes: the DAWN Japan study. Curr Med Res Opin. 2014;30(2):177–83.
75. Serrano V, Rodriguez-Gutierrez R, Hargraves I, Gionfriddo MR, Tamhane S, Montori VM. Shared decision-making in the care of individuals with diabetes. Diabet Med. 2016;33(6):742–51.
76. Frier BM, Jensen MM, Chubb BD. Hypoglycaemia in adults with insulin-treated diabetes in the UK: self-reported frequency and effects. Diabet Med. 2016;33(8):1125–32.
77. Grammes J, Stock W, Mann CG, Flynn EM, Kubiak T. Focus group study to identify the central facets of fear of hypoglycaemia in people with type 2 diabetes mellitus. Diabet Med. 2017;34(12):1765–72.
78. Krall J, Gabbay R, Zickmund S, Hamm ME, Williams KR, Siminerio L. Current perspectives on psychological insulin resistance: primary care provider and patient views. Diabetes Technol Ther. 2015;17(4):268–74.
79. McBain H, Begum S, Rahman S, Mulligan K. Barriers to and enablers of insulin self-titration in adults with type 2 diabetes: a qualitative study. Diabet Med. 2016;34(2):253–61.
80. Tong WT, Vethakkan SR, Ng CJ. Why do some people with type 2 diabetes who are using insulin have poor glycaemic control? A qualitative study. BMJ Open. 2015;5(1) https://doi.org/10.1136/bmjopen-2014-006407.
81. Donnelly LA, Morris AD, Evans JMM. Adherence to insulin and its association with glycaemic control in patients with type 2 diabetes. QJ Med. 2007;100(6):345–50.
82. Ho PM, Rumsfeld JS, Masoudi FA, McClure DL, Plomondon ME, Steiner JF, Magid DJ. Effect of medication nonadherence on hospitalization and mortality among patients with diabetes mellitus. Arch Intern Med. 2006; 166(17):1836–41.
83. Aloumanis K, Benroubi M, Sourmeli S, Drossinos V. Clinical outcomes and costs for patients with type 2 diabetes mellitus initiating insulin therapy in Greece: two-year experience from the INSTIGATE study. Primary Care Diabetes. 2013;7(3):235–42.
84. Balkau B, Bouee S, Avignon A, Verges B, Chartier I, Amelineau E, Halimi S. Type 2 diabetes treatment intensification in general practice in France in 2008-2009: the DIAttitude study. Diabetes & Metabolism. 2012;38(Suppl 3):S29–35.
85. Beresford C. Patients' perspectives of type 2 diabetes care by practice nurses: a qualitative study. J Diabetes Nurs. 2011;15(10):391–7.
86. Beverly EA, Ritholz MD, Brooks KM, Hultgren BA, Lee Y, Abrahamson MJ, Weinger K. A qualitative study of perceived responsibility and self-blame in type 2 diabetes: reflections of physicians and patients. J Gen Intern Med. 2012;27(9):1180–7.
87. Brod M, Pohlman B, Wolden M, Christensen T. Non-severe nocturnal hypoglycaemic events: experience and impacts on patient functioning and well-being. Qual Life Res. 2013b;22(5):997–1004.
88. Carbone ET, Rosal MC, Torres MI, Goins KV, Bermudez OI. Diabetes self-management: perspectives of Latino patients and their health care providers. Patient Educ Couns. 2007;66(2):202–10.
89. Chai J, Anderson C, Wong KT, Hussein Z. Patients' lived-experience of insulin therapy for type 2 diabetes management. Conference abstract. Res Soc Adm Pharm. 2012;8:e29–30.
90. Chai J, Anderson C, Wong KT, Hussein Z. Injecting insulin? How TOUGH can it be? Research poster. RPS annual conference 8-9 September 2013, Birmingham UK. Int J Pharm Pract. 2013;21(Suppl 2):32–3.
91. Chai J, Anderson C, Wong KT, Hussein Z. Social stigma affecting non-adherence of insulin therapy for type 2 diabetes Management in Malaysia. Conference Abstract Res. Social Adm. Pharm. 2014;10:e53.
92. Chan CMF, Liau Wei F, Teo NHL, Toh MP, Chen S. Understanding the perception of patients with type 2 diabetes on insulin therapy at primary healthcare setting in Singapore. Singapore. Nurs J. 2014;41(2):23–8.
93. Choudhury S, Das S, Hazra A. Survey of knowledge-attitude-practice concerning insulin use in adult diabetic patients in eastern India. Indian J Pharmacol. 2014;46(4):425–9.
94. Cramer JA, Pugh MJ. The influence of insulin use on Glycaemic control. How well do adults follow prescriptions for insulin? Diabetes Care. 2005; 28(1):78–83.
95. Gaborit B, Dutour O, Ronsin O, Atlan C, Darmon P, Gharsalli R, Pradel V, Dadoun F, Dutour A. Ramadan fasting with diabetes: an interview study of inpatients' and general practitioners' attitudes in the south of France. Diabetes and. Metabolism. 2011;37(5):395–402.
96. Hermanns N, Mahr M, Kulzer B, Skovlund SE, Haak T. Barriers towards insulin therapy in type 2 diabetic patients: results of an observational longitudinal study. Health Qual Life Outcomes. 2010;8:113.
97. Hinder S, Greenhalgh T. This does my head in ethnographic study of self-management by people with diabetes. BMC Health Serv Res. 2012;12:83.
98. Frei A, Herzog S, Woitzek K, Held U, Senn O, Rosemann T, Chmiel C. Characteristics of poorly controlled type 2 diabetes patients in Swiss primary care. Cardiovasc Diabetol. 2012;11:70.
99. Hunt LM, Valenzuela MA, Pugh JA. Porque me Toco a mi? Mexican American diabetes patients' causal stories and their relationship to treatment behaviours. Soc Sci Med. 1998;46(8):959–69.
100. Khattab M, Khader YS, Al-Khawaldeh A, Ajlouni K. Factors associated with poor glycemic control among patients with type 2 diabetes. J Diabetes Complicat. 2010;24(2):84–9.
101. Lai WA, Chie WC, Lew-Ting CY. How diabetic patients' ideas of illness course affect non-adherent behaviour: a qualitative study. Br J Gen Pract. 2007; 57(537):296–302.
102. Lakkis NA, Maalouf GJ, Mahmassani DM, Hamadeh GN. Insulin therapy attitudes and beliefs of physicians in middle eastern Arab countries. Fam Pract. 2013;30(5):560–7.
103. Mollem ED, Snoek FJ, Heine RJ. Assessment of perceived barriers in self-care of insulin requiring diabetic patients. Patient Educ Couns. 1996;29(3):277–81.
104. Morris J, Povey R, Street C. Experiences of people with type 2 diabetes who have changed from oral medication to self-administered insulin injections. Pract Diabetes Int. 2005;22(7):239–43.
105. Oliveria SA, Menditto LA, Yood MU, Koo YH, Wells KE, McCarthy BD. Barriers to the initiation of, and persistence with, insulin therapy. Curr Med Res Opin. 2007;23(12):3105–12.

106. Peyrot M, Rubin RR, Lauritzen T, Skovlund SE, Snoek FJ, Matthews DR, Landgraf R, Kleinebreil L. Resistance to insulin therapy among patients and providers: results of the cross-national diabetes attitudes, wishes, and needs (DAWN) study. Diabetes Care. 2005;28(11):2673–9.
107. Peyrot M, Rubin RR, Lauritzen T, Skovlund SE, Snoek FJ, Matthews DR, Landgraf R. Patient and provider perceptions of care for diabetes: results of the cross-national DAWN study. Diabetologia. 2006;49(2):279–88.
108. Peyrot M, Burns KK, Davies M, Forbes A, Hermanns N, Holt R, Kalra S, Nicolucci A, Pouwer F, Wens J, Willaing I, Skovlund SE. Diabetes attitudes wishes and needs 2 (DAWN2): a multinational, multi-stakeholder study of psychosocial issues in diabetes and person-centred diabetes care. Diabetes Res Clin Pract. 2013;99(2):174–84.
109. Pooley CG, Gerrard C, Hollis S, Morton S, Astbury J. 'Oh it's a wonderful practice … you can talk to them': a qualitative study of patients' and health professionals' views on the management of type 2 diabetes. Health Soc. Care Community. 2001;9(5):318–26.
110. Shiu ATY, Wong RYM. Fear of hypoglycaemia among insulin-treated Hong Kong Chinese patients: implications for diabetes patient education. Patient Educ Couns. 2000;41(3):251–61.
111. Thomson FJ, Masson EA, Leeming JT, Boulton AJM. Lack of knowledge of symptoms of Hypoglycaemia by elderly diabetic patients. Age Ageing. 1991;20:404–6.
112. Wendel CS, Fotieo GG, Shah JH, Felicetta J, Curtis BH, Murata GH. Incidence of non-severe hypoglycaemia and intensity of treatment among veterans with type 2 diabetes in the USA: a prospective observational study. Diabet Med. 2014;31(12):1524–31.
113. Wong S, Lee J, Ko Y, Chong MF, Lam CK, Tang WE. Perceptions of insulin therapy amongst Asian patients with diabetes in Singapore. Diabet Med. 2011;28(2):206–11.

9

Influence of mental health and alcohol or other drug use risk on adolescent reported care received in primary care settings

Lisa S. Meredith[1,2*], Brett A. Ewing[1], Bradley D. Stein[3], William G. Shadel[3], Stephanie Brooks Holliday [1], Layla Parast[1] and Elizabeth J. D'Amico[1]

Abstract

Background: To describe patterns of alcohol and other drug (AOD) use risk and adolescent reported primary care (PC) screening and intervention, and examine associations of AOD risk and mental health with reported care received.

Methods: We analyzed data from cross-sectional surveys collected from April 3, 2013 to November 24, 2015 from 1279 diverse adolescents ages 12–18 who reported visiting a doctor at least once in the past year. Key measures were AOD risk using the Personal Experience Screening Questionnaire; mental health using the 5-item Mental Health Inventory; binary measures of adolescent-reported screening and intervention.

Results: Half (49.2%) of the adolescents reported past year AOD use. Of the 769 (60.1%) of adolescents that reported being asked by a medical provider in PC about AOD use, only 37.2% reported receiving screening/intervention. The odds of reported screening/intervention were significantly higher for adolescents with higher AOD risk and lower mental health scores.

Conclusions: Adolescents at risk for AOD use and poor mental health are most likely to benefit from brief intervention. These findings suggest that strategies are needed to facilitate medical providers identification of need for counseling of both AOD and mental health care for at risk youth.

Keywords: Screening and brief intervention, Adolescents, Primary care

Background

Rates of alcohol and other drug use (AOD) continue to be high [1] and adolescent AOD use is associated with significant health and social consequences [2–8]. AOD use also increases risk of having an AOD disorder as an adult [9], and is associated with high economic and societal costs [10, 11]. Because most adolescents seek care in a primary care (PC) setting at least once a year [12–14], early identification or treatment by PC clinic staff is a promising way to prevent or ameliorate AOD among adolescents [15], and multiple guidelines recommend such screening [16–18]. However, rates of screening and intervention for AOD in PC are low for adolescents [19–22]. Some of the reasons for low AOD screening rates are that providers are unsure of the importance of prevention and approval of alcohol screening [23], limited organizational support, lack of training, discomfort [24], and limited opportunity [25]. Other obstacles include lower provider perceived alcohol-management skills, and lower provider self-efficacy [23, 25].

National surveys on adolescent AOD use and mental health problems consistently find overlap between these disorders [26–28]. Adolescent reports of AOD use and mental health symptoms also co-occur [29]. To our knowledge, the potential additive or interactive effect of having poor mental health and risky AOD use on PC screening/intervention has not been examined. We

* Correspondence: lisa_meredith@rand.org
[1]RAND Corporation, 1776 Main Street, Santa Monica, CA 90407-2138, USA
[2]VA HSR&D Center for the Study of Healthcare Innovation, Implementation, and Policy, California, Los Angeles, USA
Full list of author information is available at the end of the article

address this gap in the literature, by examining the association between AOD use and adolescent-reported screening/intervention by medical providers in PC settings. Our research questions were: 1) Are adolescents with greater risk for AOD more likely to report being screened by a medical provider in PC for AOD use and followed up with intervention compared to adolescents with less risk for AOD use? 2) Does having poorer mental health in addition to higher AOD risk increase the odds that adolescents will report receiving an intervention in a PC setting to address AOD risk?

Methods

Study settings

The study sample was recruited from PC clinics providing care predominantly for ethnically and racially diverse and underserved adolescents in Pittsburgh, PA (3 clinics) and Los Angeles, CA (1 clinic). These sites offer longitudinal, continuity-based care and episode-based urgent care to their patients. Clinics in both areas have a large percentage of minority patients and low-income patients who are uninsured or underinsured (i.e., insured through Medicare and/or Medicaid).

Participants and procedures

Every adolescent between age 12 and 18 in the clinic waiting rooms with a scheduled appointment was asked to be part of the project. For interested adolescents, we obtained parental consent and assent (if under 18) or consent if 18. Youth were screened by project staff using the National Institute of Alcohol and Alcohol Abuse (NIAAA) screening guide, completed a survey via the web from April 2013 to November 2015, and were paid $25. We obtained a certificate of confidentiality; the Institutional Review Boards and the clinics approved procedures.

Approximately 3309 adolescents were approached to participate; 27% ($n = 892$) were ineligible because they were not 12–18 years old, not proficient in English, were not at the clinic for their own appointment, or were disabled, and 18.5% ($n = 614$) refused to participate (mostly because of adolescents' concerns that their parents would learn they were at the clinic for a family planning appointment or because of time constraints). After exclusions, 1803 adolescents enrolled or consented for study staff to contact them. Of the 1803 adolescents, 230 did not complete the baseline survey within the field period or had inaccurate contact information. This yielded a final sample of 1573 adolescents. The average age was 15.5; 42.5% were male; 51.4% were Hispanic, 26.7% black, 14.8% white, and 7.2% multiethnic or other. We focus on 1279 adolescents who reported visiting the doctor at least once in the past year and also had usable information to allow categorization into an AOD risk category.

Measures

We used items from a longitudinal national household survey to assess five main outcomes of self-reports of screening and intervention [30, 31]. Adolescents were asked, "In the past 12 months, did any medical provider (e.g., primary care physician, general internist, nurse, physician assistant, chiropractor, or health clinic): 1) ask about use of alcohol or drugs (screening), 2) suggest cutting down or stopping use of alcohol or drugs (education/advice intervention), 3) suggest seeing a specialist or special program for emotions, mental health, or alcohol or drug use (referral intervention), or 4) provide counseling about emotions, mental health, alcohol or drug use for at least 5 minutes (counseling intervention)." We created binary indicators for each of these outcomes plus a fifth indicator for receipt of screening plus at least one type of intervention.

We assessed AOD risk using the 18-item Problem Severity Scale of the Personal Experience Screening Questionnaire (PESQ-PS) [32] that is reliable and valid for use in a general adolescent population. The PESQ-PS consists of eight items about AOD use in different contexts, nine items about behaviors and consequences of AOD use, and a single item about selling drugs to pay for AOD use. Items were rated on a 4-point frequency scale (never, once or twice, sometimes, or often). We used validated cut-points on the summed score (ranging from 18 to 72; $\alpha = 0.93$) to stratify adolescents into risk groups. Low risk or green flag suggests no further assessment or referral is recommended because the individual has no problem with AOD use. Medium risk or yellow flag suggests that the individual has a mild or moderate problem with AOD use requiring brief intervention. High risk or red flag suggests abusive or dependent use of AOD requiring comprehensive evaluation to confirm severity of the problem with likely referral for substance abuse treatment. Cut-points by gender and age range were >23–24 for yellow flag and >30–35 for red flag.

We measured mental health using the well-validated 5-item Mental Health Inventory (MHI-5) [33]. Respondents indicated frequency for five feelings during the past month on a 1–6 scale (all of the time to none of the time). Item content included feeling nervous, calm and peaceful, downhearted and blue, happy, and down in the dumps. Relevant items were reversed so that a higher total score (transformed to range from 0 to 100; $\alpha = 0.73$) indicated better mental health.

We controlled for adolescent age, gender, indicators of race/ethnicity, and mother's education (less than college vs. at least some college). We imputed incomplete data for mother's education using an ordinal logistic regression model with race/ethnicity, city, and living in a two-parent household [34, 35].

Analysis

We first describe sample characteristics, patterns of, and rates of screening and intervention overall and by risk AOD groups by the PESQ-PS. We use multivariable logistic regression to estimate odds of receiving screening and each type of intervention as a function of AOD use risk and mental health, controlling for demographic characteristics (age, gender, race, and mother's education). To understand the independent effect of AOD risk, the effect of AOD risk after controlling for mental health, and the interactive effect of AOD risk and mental health, we ran three sets of models: (1) including only the main effect for AOD risk groups without the MHI-5, (2) adding the main effect for MHI-5, and (3) adding the interaction between AOD risk and MHI-5. We conducted analyses using standard statistical software (SAS 9.3). We adjusted for clustering of adolescents within clinics using fixed effects for clinics.

Results

Sample characteristics

This analysis sample ($n = 1279$) was similar to the full enrolled sample ($n = 1573$) (Table 1): average age of 15.6 years, 40.4% male, 26.3% Black, 52.0% Hispanic, and 6.6% multiethnic. Most mothers (67.1%) had no college education. The average score on the MHI-5 was 68.5. All characteristics differed significantly across PESQ-PS risk groups except for mothers' education. Adolescents at highest risk (red flag) were significantly older ($p < .01$), more likely to be female ($p < .001$), more likely to be Hispanic (p < .001), and reported lower mental health scores (p < .001).

Table 1 Adolescent Sample Characteristics by AOD Risk Groups on the PESQ

	Full Sample (n = 1279)	PESQ Risk Group		
		Green Flag (n = 886)	Yellow Flag (n = 195)	Red Flag (n = 221)
Age**	15.6 (0.2)	15.2 (0.2)	16.3 (0.1)	16.7 (0.1)
Gender***				
Male	40.4	42.1	40.9	33.2
Female	59.6	57.9	59.1	66.8
Race***				
White	15.0	14.8	16.6	14.5
Black	26.3	28.5	24.9	19.1
Hispanic	52.0	48.8	55.4	61.4
Multiethnic/Other	6.6	7.9	3.1	5.0
Mother's Education				
Less than college	67.1	65.2	67.9	73.4
At least some college	32.9	34.8	32.1	26.6
MHI-5 Score (0–100)***	68.5 (1.0)	69.9 (0.7)	70.3 (2.0)	61.5 (1.0)

AOD Alcohol or drug use, *PESQ* Personal Experience Screening Questionnaire; 228 cases were imputed for missing data on mother's education; Analyses are adjusted for clustering within clinic; **p < .01; ***p < .001

Patterns of screening and intervention

Figure 1 illustrates the flow of screening and interventions as reported by the 1279 adolescents who answered the question about care received (screening and intervention) in a past year doctor visit. Of the 769 adolescents who reported being asked about AOD use (e.g., any reported AOD screening), 72.8% ($n = 560$) reported being screened for AOD use by the doctor but received no further intervention, and 209 reported being screened and at least one type of intervention. Of those 769 adolescents, only 13.1% ($n = 101$) reported being asked to cut down or stop using AOD, 11.8% ($n = 91$) reported being referred to a mental health specialist or substance use program, and 17.7% (n = 136) reported receiving counseling for at least five minutes about mental health or AOD. Limited numbers of adolescents reported receiving multiple interventions, with only 27 receiving all three interventions. Almost 40% of adolescents reported that they were not screened about AOD use, and the 510 adolescents, the majority received no intervention 85.1% ($n = 434$). But, 7.2% ($n = 37$) of unscreened adolescents reported being asked to cut down or stop using AOD, 4.9% ($n = 25$) reported being referred to a mental health specialist or substance use program, and 8.6% ($n = 44$) reported receiving counseling for at least five minutes about mental health or AOD.

Rates of screening and intervention

Rates of screening and intervention as reported by adolescents were significantly higher with increased risk (omnibus test, $p < .001$ for all) (Fig. 2). Adolescents in the red flag group were 18% more likely to be screened for AOD use compared with the green flag group ($p <$ 0.001). For intervention, 25% more red flag adolescents reported being advised to cut down or stop use than were green flag adolescents ($p = 0.003$). This difference was 12% more for referral ($p = 0.016$) and 18% more for counseling ($p = 0.002$). Red flag adolescents were also 29% more likely to report screening plus intervention relative to green flag adolescents (p = 0.002).

Associations between AOD risk and mental health with screening and intervention

Table 2 shows the results for multivariable logistic regression models estimating the likelihood of adolescent

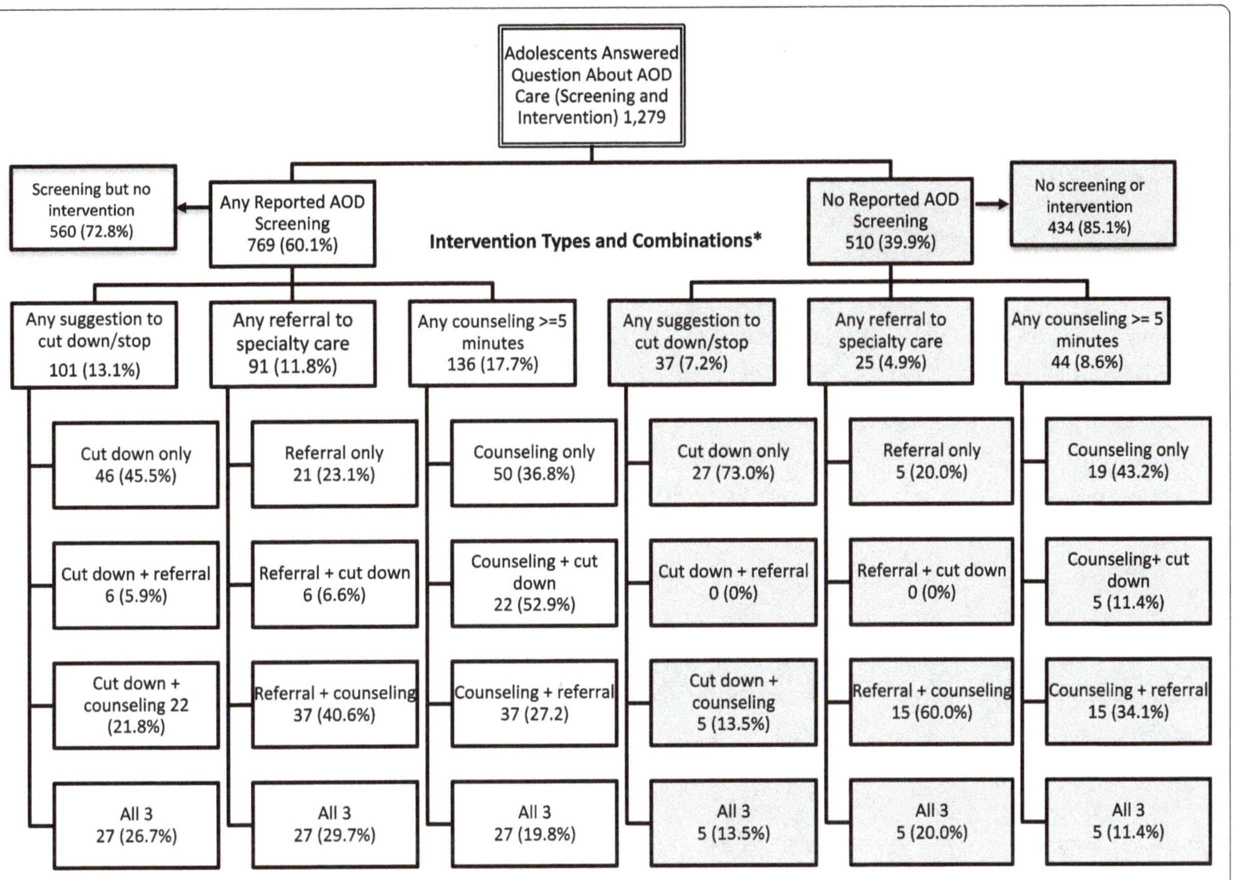

*Percentages for no intervention and any intervention combinations sum to more than 100% because of overlap across intervention types.

Fig. 1 Patterns of Past Year Adolescent Reported AOD Care (Screening and Intervention) Received by Medical Providers

reported screening and intervention received from medical providers after adjusting for clustering within clinic and demographic characteristics. Models include the main effects for both MHI-5 and AOD risk (without the interaction). Better mental health was not significantly associated with adolescents reporting being asked about AOD use or advice to cut down or stop using AOD, but was significantly associated with a slightly lower likelihood of reporting being referred, counseled, or getting screened and receiving any type of

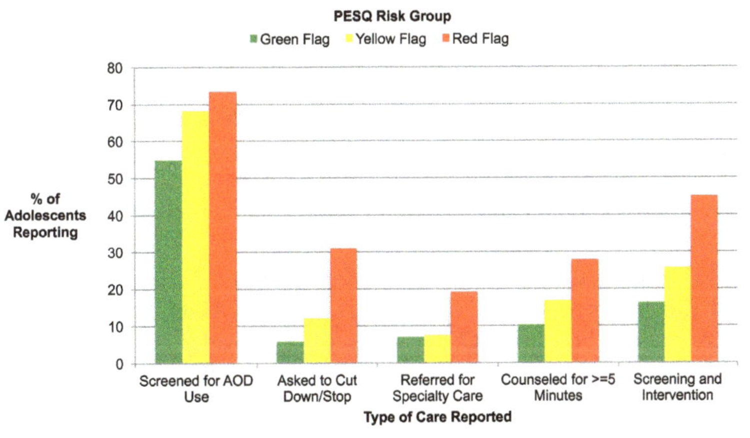

*Differences by PESQ risk group are significant at p<.001 (omnibus) for all five measures of care received.

Fig. 2 Adolescent Reported Care Received by AOD Risk Group*

Table 2 Odds Ratios for Adolescent Reported Screening or Intervention Received by Medical Providers in Primary Care

	Screening or Intervention (Dependent Variable)				
	Asked about AOD use	Suggested cutting down or stopping AOD use	Referred for specialty care	Counseled for > = 5 min	Asked and provided any treatment
Independent Variable	OR [95% CI]	OR [95% CI]	OR [95% CI]	OR [95% CI]	OR [95% CI]
MHI-5 Score (0–100)	1.01 [1.00–1.01]	1.01 [1.00–1.02]	0.97 [0.96–0.98]***	0.97 [0.97–0.98]***	0.98 [0.97–0.99]***
PESQ Risk Flags					
Red (vs. Green)	1.69 [1.19–2.40]**	8.89 [5.59–14.14]***	2.80 [1.73–4.54]***	3.48 [2.29–5.30]***	4.44 [3.11–6.36]***
Yellow (vs. Green)	1.36 [0.96–1.92]	2.37 [1.37–4.09]**	1.14 [0.61–2.14]	2.15 [1.35–3.42]***	2.03 [1.37–3.01]***
Age	1.25 [1.17–1.34]***	0.98 [0.88–1.11]	0.96 [0.85–1.08]	0.88 [0.80–0.97]*	0.93 [0.85–1.01]
Gender					
Female (vs. Male)	1.19 [0.93–1.52]	0.61 [0.41–0.91]*	0.81 [0.53–1.25]	0.93 [0.65–1.33]	0.81 [0.60–1.08]
Race					
Black (vs. White)	0.42 [0.27–0.66]***	1.03 [0.51–2.08]	1.00 [0.50–1.99]	0.91 [0.50–1.68]	0.80 [0.48–1.33]
Hispanic (vs. White)	0.40 [0.26–0.64]***	0.98 [0.49–1.97]	1.17 [0.58–2.33]	1.12 [0.62–2.01]	0.93 [0.57–1.54]
Multi/Other (vs. White)	0.56 [0.31–0.99]*	1.05 [0.41–2.69]	0.88 [0.32–2.38]	1.46 [0.69–3.10]	1.12 [0.58–2.13]
Mother's Education					
At least some college (vs. less than college)	1.07 [0.81–1.41]	0.93 [0.59–1.45]	1.10 [0.69–1.76]	1.31 [0.89–1.93]	1.22 [0.88–1.69]
Clinic					
Clinic A (vs. Clinic D)	0.80 [0.52–1.26]	1.53 [0.75–3.12]	1.45 [0.68–3.10]	1.25 [0.67–2.32]	1.36 [0.81–2.30]
Clinic B (vs. Clinic D)	0.66 [0.43–1.02]	1.08 [0.53–2.20]	1.86 [0.92–3.76]	1.36 [0.76–2.44]	1.26 [0.76–2.08]
Clinic C (vs. Clinic D)	0.87 [0.54–1.40]	0.98 [0.45–2.15]	1.79 [0.87–3.69]	0.79 [0.41–1.55]	0.98 [0.56–1.70]

228 cases were imputed for missing data on mother's education. OR = odds ratio; CI = confidence interval; AOD = alcohol or drug use; PESQ = Personal Experience Screening Questionnaire; Analyses are adjusted for clustering within clinic; *p < .05; **p < .01; ***p < .001

intervention (all OR = 0.97–0.98, $p < .001$). Higher AOD risk was significantly associated with increased likelihood of receiving screening and all types of intervention for red flag vs. green flag (all p < .001) and with suggesting cutting down ($p < .01$), counseling (p < .001), and screening plus any intervention (p < .001) for yellow flag vs. green flag. Compared to the green flag group, adolescents in the red flag group were 1.7 times more likely to report being screened, 8.9 times more likely to report being advised to cut down or stop AOD use, 2.8 times more likely to be referred, 3.5 times more likely to be counseled for at least five minutes, and 4.4 times more likely to have been both screened and received an intervention.

Compared with the set of models that excluded the main effect of MHI-5 (not shown), including MHI-5 in the model increased the associations between AOD risk and AOD screening (ΔOR = 0.06) and advice to cut-down or stop for red flag (ΔOR = 0.43), but decreased the associations for referral (ΔOR = −0.75), brief counseling (ΔOR = -0.67), and screening plus any intervention (ΔOR = −0.56) for red flag. However, the pattern of significance for the AOD risk associations was generally similar across the model specifications.

In terms of demographic associations with screening or intervention, being older was associated with higher odds of being screened (OR = 1.25, $p < .001$) but lower odds of being counseled (OR = 0.88, $p < .05$). Black (OR = 0.42, p < .001), Hispanic (OR = 0.40, $p < 0.001$) and Multiracial or other non-white race/ethnicity (OR = 0.56, $p < .01$) adolescents had lower odds of being screened. We found no significant interactions between AOD risk and MHI-5 (not shown) for the set of models that added the interaction terms.

Discussion

Adolescent AOD risk is a continuing concern. The PC setting provides an optimal opportunity for querying adolescents about risk behavior, including AOD use. This study contributes new information to the literature on adolescent AOD screening by examining both AOD use and mental health status together. Another contribution of this study is its examination of a large and diverse sample of underserved adolescents to understand the extent to which AOD risk and mental health influence the care that adolescents receive. Fully 85% of the sample is from diverse racial and ethnic backgrounds and unlike earlier studies includes adolescents from the full age range (12–18 year olds) incorporating those under age 16.

We found that consistent with previous research [19, 21, 22], overall rates of screening and intervention for adolescent AOD use were low. Specifically, less than two thirds reported being screened for use, and only a third of those at risk for AOD use (yellow or red flag on the PESQ) who were screened for AOD use reported receiving some type of intervention.

We also found that the odds of being screened or receiving brief intervention for AOD use increased for adolescents who were at highest risk. This suggests that medical providers in PC are identifying and addressing those who are more dependent on substances. We did not find, however, that having both higher risk of AOD use and poorer mental health increased the odds of receiving screening and intervention. Our models that included the MHI-5 intensified the associations between AOD risk for screening and advice outcome measures but attenuated the associations for referral, counseling, or screening plus an intervention. This suggests that medical providers are identifying risky AOD use *independent* of mental health problems and that poorer mental health may also be a trigger for more screening and advice about AOD use. Given the high rates of comorbidity between AOD use and mental health among adolescents, adolescents identified as high-risk for both problems may benefit from referral to integrated models of care.

We also observed significant associations between demographic characteristics and reported care. Older adolescents were more likely to report being screened, but less likely to report being counseled which could be explained by the higher rates of use among older adolescents. Adolescents from racial/ethnic minority groups were less likely to report being screened. This suggests potential disparities in care across race/ethnicity.

This study has several strengths. It is the first to examine the likelihood of adolescents' receipt of care from a medical provider for AOD risk for varying levels of risk with a large and diverse population, as well as examining the additive effect of having poor mental health on reported care. Nevertheless, findings must be interpreted with a few caveats. The outcome measures of AOD screening and intervention are based on adolescent self-reports, which could be biased [36]. Further, we relied on a one year retrospective reporting period, which, given its length, could limit accuracy. For example, cognitive factors such as poor recall or comprehension [37] could compromise accuracy of responses and situational factors including social desirability [38], and perceived lack of confidentiality could also lead to underreporting of risky behavior. However, we designed clinic recruitment procedures for maximum confidentiality by securing private space to conduct assessments for study eligibility. Further, surveys were web-based self-reports that could be completed in private areas. We also included a fictitious drug in the survey and very few respondents reported taking it (only 10 of 1573 adolescents), which suggests that reporting was not necessarily biased [39] and estimates of AOD use in our sample match national survey norms [40]. Finally, this U.S. based study may not generalize to other areas in the U.S. or to other countries with different healthcare systems.

We also cannot determine whether the large number of adolescents who did not report receiving any form of intervention was due to a positive screening but no care or because youth were screened and deemed not to be at risk. Despite this uncertainty, we know that adolescents in the red flag group, who were current AOD users, reported not being screened for use e.g., less than 100% of those in need were screened. This suggests that PC is missing opportunities to identify adolescents at risk and intervene with them early in their lifespan to prevent future consequences of prolonged AOD use. Finally, because of the way in which the screening and intervention question was worded, we cannot separate out counseling for AOD use from counseling for mental health problems. Future research is needed to disentangle counseling for AOD use and from mental health counseling.

With continuing high prevalence of AOD use among adolescents, strategies for facilitating the opportunity to intervene and educate adolescents in primary care about AOD use may be warranted. These strategies should address some of the barriers to screening and intervention by providing organizational support and training [24] so that PC can more easily integrate screening into the adolescent's appointment and ultimately prevent or delay AOD use into adulthood when it is less risky. Such efforts, however, should acknowledge that there is inconclusive evidence for screening's effectiveness in reducing substance use among adolescents [41], and also recognize that PC providers may screen; however, competing time demands [42, 43] and/or limited training [23] may prevent them from being able to deliver effective interventions.

Although less accurate than validated interviewer-administered diagnostic instruments, single item screening questions (SISQs) are a promising approach to screening for risky health behaviors in PC settings because they are both practical and feasible [44–46]. SISQs are sufficiently brief for incorporation into busy practice settings, are less likely to be biased by social desirability, and also may facilitate conversations in a less stigmatized manner [47, 48]. Recently, a study validated the use of a self-administered SISQ for AOD use on a tablet for adult primary care patients [49]. Tablet administration decreases provider burden and may lessen stigma for patients compared with responding to provider questions directly. Such an approach could be broadly incorporated into primary care practice and may be adaptable for use with adolescents. Moreover, such a screening approach could decrease discomfort associated with discussing a sensitive topic and would also be time efficient.

However, screening alone is not enough. It must be paired with approaches for delivering brief interventions in the primary care setting. Consistent with Sterling et al. (2012) [24] implementing clinical practices and policies to address the barriers to intervention are needed. These include restructuring practice to allow for extra time needed for encounters with at-risk adolescents, such as flexible scheduling, reimbursement for longer visits with at-risk patients, or advance visit self-screening. Other facilitators to screening and intervention may include additional training for medical providers to increase comfort with addressing AOD use (e.g., de-stigmatize) [50, 51], as well as addressing concerns regarding patient confidentiality and adverse consequences of documenting AOD use in the medical record. Intervening in as little as 15 min can lead to positive behavior change [52]. Additionally, future research should examine the relative effectiveness of the screening, brief intervention, and referral to treatment model [53, 54] for risky AOD use to facilitate provider competency for delivering such care for adolescents in PC settings. Finally, given the high rates of comorbidity between AOD use and mental health issues, strategies are needed to facilitate medical providers' understanding of the importance of potential identifying the need for counseling of both AOD and mental health care for at risk youth.

Conclusion

Risky AOD use by adolescents remains a concern, particularly among adolescents with poor mental health functioning. Although there are barriers to screening [23–26], many providers are aware of the important role of screening for both of these problems so that adolescents may be referred to needed services. While screening rates were low in this large and diverse sample of adolescents, those at highest risk were significantly more likely to be screened and receive intervention. Findings highlight the continued need to decrease barriers in PC settings for screening and intervention with adolescents at risk for AOD use. Older adolescents were more likely to be screened but not to receive intervention, and were actually less likely to receive counseling. Adolescents from minority groups were significantly less likely to be screened than white adolescents but race/ethnicity was not associated with receipt of any type of intervention.

These findings underscore the importance of identifying practical, effective, and cost-effective strategies for addressing AOD risk among adolescents in PC settings. Further, to ensure that adolescents who screen positive for AOD use receive some sort of intervention and further assessment of mental health status, practice-based strategies that support the extra time needed for at-risk youth through flexible scheduling and reimbursement for expanded encounter durations are needed. Finally, strategies for facilitating PC provider competency including training about how to screen in a sensitive manner that feels comfortable and addresses issues of stigma, perceived confidentiality, and potential adverse consequences of patient disclosure are needed.

Abbreviations

AOD: Alcohol and Other Drug use; MHI-5: 5-Item Mental Health Inventory; NIAAA: National Institute on Alcohol Abuse and Alcoholism; OR: Odds Ratio; PESQ-PS: Personal Experience Screening Questionnaire-Problem Severity Scale; SAS 9.3: Statistical Analysis Software version 0.3; SISQ: Single Item Screening Questions

Acknowledgements

The authors wish to thank the clinics that participated and supported this project. We would also like to thank Kirsten Becker and Jennifer Parker for overseeing the survey administrations, Rachana Saleem for helping with statistical programming, and Rosie Velasquez for help with manuscript formatting.

Funding

Work on this article was supported by a grant from the National Institute of Alcohol Abuse and Alcoholism (R01AA021786) to Elizabeth D'Amico.

Authors' contributions

LM: Study design, data analysis, data interpretation, and manuscript preparation. BE: Data analysis, data interpretation, and manuscript preparation. BS: Study design, data interpretation, and manuscript preparation. WS: Study design, data interpretation, and manuscript preparation. SH: Data interpretation and manuscript preparation. LP: Statistical analysis, data interpretation, and manuscript preparation. ED: Study conceptualization/design; data interpretation, and manuscript preparation. All authors read and approved the final manuscript.

Consent for publication

Not applicable.

Competing interests

The authors declare that they have no competing interests.

Author details
[1]RAND Corporation, 1776 Main Street, Santa Monica, CA 90407-2138, USA. [2]VA HSR&D Center for the Study of Healthcare Innovation, Implementation, and Policy, California, Los Angeles, USA. [3]RAND Corporation, Pittsburgh, PA, USA.

References

1. Johnston LD, O'Malley PM, Miech RA, Bachman JG, Schulenberg JE. Monitoring the future national survey results on drug use, 1975–2015: overview, key findings on adolescent drug use. Ann Arbor: Institute for Social Research, The University of Michigan; 2016.
2. Adams WL. The effects of alcohol on medical illnesses and medication interactions. In: Gurnack AM, Atkinson R, Osgood NJ, editors. Treating alcohol and drug abuse in the elderly. New York: Springer Publishing Co; 2002. p. 32–49.
3. Eaton DK, Davis KS, Barrios L, Brener ND, Noonan RK. Associations of dating violence victimization with lifetime participation, co-occurrence, and early initiation of risk behaviors among U.S. high school students. J Interpers Violence. 2007;22:585–602.
4. aminer Y and Bukstein OG. Adolescent substance abuse: psychiatric comorbidity and high-risk behaviors: Taylor & Francis; 2008.
5. Martins SS, Alexandre PK. The association of ecstasy use and academic achievement among adolescents in two U.S. national surveys. Addict Behav. 2009;34:9–16.
6. Patton GC, Coffey C, Carlin JB, Degenhardt L, Lynskey M, Hall W. Cannabis use and mental health in young people: cohort study. Br Med J. 2002;325:1195–8.
7. Shrier LA, Harris SK, Kurland M, Knight JR. Substance use problems and associated psychiatric symptoms among adolescents in primary care. Pediatrics. 2003;111:e699–705.
8. Tripodi SJ, Springer DW, Corcoran K. Determinants of substance abuse among incarcerated adolescents: implications for brief treatment and crisis intervention. Brief Treatment and Crisis Intervention. 2007;7:34.
9. McCambridge J, McAlaney J, Rowe R. Adult consequences of late adolescent alcohol consumption: a systematic review of cohort studies. PLoS Med. 2011;8
10. Centers for Disease Control and Prevention. The Cost of Excessive Alcohol Use: A Drain on the U.S. Economy. CDC 24/7: Saving Lives, Protecting People: Department of Health and Human Services; 2016.
11. National Drug Intelligence Center. The economic impact of illicit drug use on American society. https://www.justice.gov/archive/ndic/pubs44/44731/44731p.pdf (2011). Accessed.
12. Bloom B, Cohen RA. Summary health statistics for U.S. children: National Health Interview Survey, 2006. Vital Health Stat 10. 2007:1–79.
13. Johnson SB, Millstein SG. Prevention opportunities in health care settings. Am Psychol. 2003;58:475–81.
14. Newacheck PW, Brindis CD, Cart CU, Marchi K, Irwin CE. Adolescent health insurance coverage: recent changes and access to care. Pediatrics. 1999;104:195–202.
15. Ozer EM, Adams SH, Orrell-Valente JK, Wibbelsman CJ, Lustig JL, Millstein SG, et al. Does delivering preventive Services in Primary Care Reduce Adolescent Risky Behavior? J Adolesc Health. 2011;49:476–82.
16. U.S. Preventive Services Task Force. Alcohol Misuse screening and behavioral counseling interventions in primary care. www.uspreventiveservicestaskforce.org/uspstf/uspsdrin.htm. 2012. Accessed 1 May 2016.
17. American Academy of Pediatrics Committee on Substance Abuse. Policy statement—alcohol use by youth and adolescents: a pediatric concern. Pediatrics. 2010;125:1078–87.
18. NIAAA. Alcohol screening and brief intervention for youth: a practioners guide. NIH publication no. 11–7805. Rockville, MD: NIAAA, DHHS and AAP; 2011.
19. Hingson RW, Heeren T, Edwards EM, Saitz R. Young adults at risk for excess alcohol consumption are often not asked or counseled about drinking alcohol. J Gen Intern Med. 2012;27:179–84.
20. Hingson RW, Zha W, Iannotti RJ, Simons-Morton B. Physician advice to adolescents about drinking and other health behaviors. Pediatrics. 2013; 131:249–57.
21. Klein DJ, Allan MJ, Elster AB, Stevens D, Cox C, Hedberg VA, et al. Improving adolescent preventive care in community health centers. Pediatrics. 2001; 107:318–27.
22. Van Hook S, Harris SK, Brooks T, Carey P, Kossack R, Kulig J, et al. The "six T's": barriers to screening teens for substance abuse in primary care. J Adolesc Health. 2007;40:456–61.
23. Ozer EM, Adams SH, Gardner LR, Mailloux DE, Wibbelsman CJ, Irwin CE. Provider self-efficacy and the screening of adolescents for risky health behaviors. J Adolesc Health. 2004;35:101–7.
24. Sterling S, Kline-Simon AH, Wibbelsman C, Wong A, Weisner C. Screening for adolescent alcohol and drug use in pediatric health-care settings: predictors and implications for practice and policy. Addict Sci Clin Pract. 2012;7:13.
25. Marcell AV, Halpern-Felsher B, Coriell M, Millstein SG. Physicians' attitudes and beliefs concerning alcohol abuse prevention in adolescents. Am J Prev Med. 2002;22:49–55.
26. Center for Mental Health Services. Mental Health Care for Youth: A National Assessment, Annual/Final Progress Report, editors. Vol. January-December 2001. Rockville, MD: Substance Use and Mental Health Services Administration; 2001.
27. SAMHSA. Results from the 2011 National Survey on drug use and health: summary of national findings. NSDUH series H-44, HHS publication no. (SMA) 12–4713. Rockville, MD: Substance Abuse and Mental Health Services Administration; 2012.
28. Turner WC, Muck RD, Muck RJ, Stephens RL, Sukumar B. Co-occurring disorders in the adolescent mental health and substance abuse treatment systems. J Psychoactive Drugs. 2004;36:455–62.
29. Burnett-Zeigler I, Walton MA, Ilgen M, Barry KL, Chermack ST, Zucker RA, et al. Prevalence and correlates of mental health problems and treatment among adolescents seen in primary care. J Adolesc Health. 2012;50:559–64.
30. D'Amico EJ, Paddock SM, Burnam A, Kung FY. Identification of and guidance for problem drinking by general medical providers: results from a national survey. Med Care. 2005;43:229–36.
31. Sturm R, Gresenz C, Sherbourne C, Minnium K, Klap R, Bhattacharya J, et al. The design of healthcare for communities: a study of health care delivery for alcohol, drug abuse, and mental health conditions. Inquiry. 1999;36:221–33.
32. Winters KC. Development of an adolescent alcohol and other drug abuse screening scale: Personal Experiences Screening Questionnaire. Addict Behav. 1992;17:479–90.
33. Berwick DM, Murphy JM, Goldman PA, Ware JE Jr, Barsky AJ, Weinstein MC. Performance of a five-item mental health screening test. Med Care. 1991;29:169–76.
34. Gelman A and Hill J. Data analysis using regression and multilevel/hierarchical models: Cambridge University press; 2006.
35. Rubin DB, Little RJA. Statistical analysis with missing data. Hoboken, NJ: J Wiley & Sons; 2002.
36. Brener ND, Billy JO, Grady WR. Assessment of factors affecting the validity of self-reported health-risk behavior among adolescents: evidence from the scientific literature. J Adolesc Health. 2003;33:436–57.
37. Eisenhower D, Mathiowetz NA, Morganstein D. Recall error: sources and bias reduction techniques. In: Biemer PP, Groves RM, Lyberg LE, et al., editors. Measurement errors in surveys. New York: John Wiley & Sons; 1991. p. 127–44.
38. DeMaio T. Social desirability and survey measurement: a review. In: Turner CF, Martin E, editors. Surveying social phenomena. New York, NY: Russell Sage Foundation; 1984. p. 257–82.
39. Poulin C, MacNeil P, Mitic W. The validity of a province-wide student drug use survey: lessons in design. Can J Public Health. 1993;84:259–64.
40. Johnston LD, O'Malley PM, Bachman JG, Schulenberg JE. Monitoring the future national survey results on drug use, 1975–2012. Volume I: secondary school students. Ann Arbor, Michigan: Institute for Social Research, The University of Michigan; 2013.
41. Patnode CD, O'Connor E, Rowland M, Burda BU, Perdue LA, Whitlock EP. Primary care behavioral interventions to prevent or reduce illicit drug use and nonmedical pharmaceutical use in children and adolescents: a systematic evidence review for the US preventive services task force. Ann Intern Med. 2014;160:612–U161.
42. Yarnall KS, Pollak KI, Ostbye T, Krause KM, Michener JL. Primary care: is there enough time for prevention? Am J Public Health. 2003;93:635–41.
43. Earls MF, Hay SS. Setting the stage for success: implementation of developmental and behavioral screening and surveillance in primary care practice - the North Carolina assuring better child health and development (ABCD) project. Pediatrics. 2006;118:E183–8.
44. Saitz R, Cheng DM, Allensworth-Davies D, Winter MR, Smith PC. The ability of single screening questions for unhealthy alcohol and other drug use to

identify substance dependence in primary care. Journal of studies on alcohol and drugs. 2014;75:153–7.

45. Smith PC, Schmidt SM, Allensworth-Davies D, Saitz RA. Single-question screening test for drug use in primary care. Arch Intern Med. 2010;170: 1155–60.
46. Smith PC, Schmidt SM, Allensworth-Davies D, Saitz R. Primary care validation of a single-question alcohol screening test. J Gen Intern Med. 2009;24:783–8.
47. McCormick KA, Cochran NE, Back AL, Merrill JO, Williams EC, Bradley KA. How primary care providers talk to patients about alcohol: a qualitative study. J Gen Intern Med. 2006;21:966–72.
48. Stockwell T, Donath S, Cooper-Stanbury M, Chikritzhs T, Catalano P, Mateo C. Under-reporting of alcohol consumption in household surveys: a comparison of quantity-frequency, graduated-frequency and recent recall. Addiction. 2004;99:1024–33.
49. McNeely J, Cleland CM, Strauss SM, Palamar JJ, Rotrosen J, Saitz R. Validation of self-administered single-item screening questions (SISQs) for unhealthy alcohol and drug use in primary care patients. J Gen Intern Med. 2015;30:1757–64.
50. Buckelew SM, Adams SH, Irwin CE Jr, Gee S, Ozer EM. Increasing clinician self-efficacy for screening and counseling adolescents for risky health behaviors: results of an intervention. J Adolesc Health. 2008;43:198–200.
51. Ozer EM, Adams SH, Lustig JL, Gee S, Garber AK, Gardner LR, et al. Increasing the screening and counseling of adolescents for risky health behaviors: a primary care intervention. Pediatrics. 2005;115:960–8.
52. D'Amico EJ, Miles JN, Stern SA, Meredith LS. Brief motivational interviewing for teens at risk of substance use consequences: a randomized pilot study in a primary care clinic. J Subst Abus Treat. 2008;35:53–61.
53. Ambresin AE, Otjes CP, Patton GC, Sawyer SM, Thuraisingam S, English DR, et al. Training general practitioners to detect probable mental disorders in young people during health risk screening. J Adolesc Health. 2017;
54. Ozechowski TJ, Becker SJ, Hogue A. SBIRT-A: adapting SBIRT to maximize developmental fit for adolescents in primary care. J Subst Abus Treat. 2016;62:28–37.

10

An overview of systematic reviews on the collaboration between physicians and nurses and the impact on patient outcomes

Evi Matthys*, Roy Remmen and Peter Van Bogaert

Abstract

Background: Primary care needs to be strengthened in order to address the many societal challenges. Group practices in primary care foster collaboration with other health care providers, which encourages care co-ordination and leads to a higher quality of primary care. Nursing roles and responsibilities expanded over time and nurses have been found to often provide equal high-quality chronic patient care compared to physicians, even with higher patient satisfaction. Inter-professional collaboration between primary care physicians and nurses is a possible strategy to achieve the desired quality outcomes in a strengthened primary care system. The objective of this research is to synthesize the evidence presented in literature on the impact of collaboration between physicians and nurses on patient outcomes in primary care or in comparable care settings.

Methods: A systematic review of peer-reviewed reviews was performed in four databases: COCHRANE, MEDLINE, EMBASE and CINAHL. All studies from 1970 until May 22 2016 were included in the search strategy. Titles, abstracts and full texts were respectively reviewed. At least two of the three authors independently reviewed each of the 277 abstracts and 58 full texts retrieved in the searches to identify those which contained all the inclusion criteria. Two authors independently appraised the methodological quality of the reviews, using the AMSTAR quality appraisal tool.

Results: A total of eleven systematic reviews met all the inclusion criteria and almost fifty different patient outcomes were described. In most reviews, it was concluded that nurses do have added value. Blood pressure, patient satisfaction and hospitalization are patient outcomes where three or more systematic reviews concluded better results when physicians and nurses collaborated, compared to usual care. Colorectal screening, hospital length of stay and health-related quality of life are outcomes where collaboration appeared not to be effective.

Conclusions: Collaboration between physicians and nurses may have a positive impact on a number of patient outcomes and on a variety of pathologies. To address future challenges of primary care, there is a need for more integrated inter-professional collaboration care models with sufficiently educated nurses.

Keywords: Nurse, Physician, Primary care, Collaboration, Inter-professional, Patient outcome, Education

* Correspondence: Evi.Matthys@uantwerp.be
University of Antwerp, Campus Drie Eiken DR334, Universiteitsplein 1, 2610 Wilrijk, Belgium

Background

Populations around the world are rapidly ageing. It is estimated that between 2015 and 2050, the world's population of over 60 year olds' will nearly double from 12 to 22% [1]. As people age, they are more likely to experience several health conditions at the same time. The demand for health care is evolving rapidly in the context of an ageing population and the growing number of people living with one or more chronic conditions [2]. In Europe, patients are more demanding and expect health care to be accessible and high qualitative at the same time [2, 3]. Professional caregivers, on the other hand, experience a high workload and demand a better work-life balance [4, 5]. At the same time, financial resources in health care are decreasing, while the demand for financial support is increasing [6–8]. In an attempt to address these challenges, the following four aims have the potential to guide innovations in health care delivery: improving the health of populations, improving the experience of care, reducing per capita costs of health care, and diminishing the workload for professional caregivers so they can rediscover meaning and joy in their work [7, 9, 10].

Reforms are shifting care from hospitals to community, partly due to a growing prevalence of chronic diseases [11, 12]. In addition, countries in the European Union show many potentially avoidable hospital admissions for several chronic conditions including diabetes mellitus, chronic heart failure, chronic obstructive pulmonary disease and asthma. Potentially avoidable hospitalizations for these conditions are commonly used to measure access and quality of primary care systems [13, 14]. In order to address the needs of ageing populations and to reduce the unnecessary use of hospital care, primary care systems should be strengthened [2].

It was suggested that group practices in primary care foster collaboration with other health care providers, which encourages care co-ordination and leads to a higher quality of primary care [8]. Primarily, nurses were introduced in primary care practices to meet a perceived shortage of primary care physicians [15]. Over time, nursing roles and responsibilities expanded. Practice nurses were able to provide holistic care for patients that was not limited to traditional nursing boundaries [16]. Nurses have been found to often provide cost effective patient care and equal high-quality chronic patient care compared to primary care physicians, even with higher patient satisfaction [2, 12, 16, 17]. By expanding the roles and responsibilities of nurses, primary care systems can be strengthened.

Improved inter-professional collaboration is important and diversity of disciplines is needed in a time when the provision of primary health care becomes more complex and one health professional can no longer meet all patient needs [18, 19]. As the largest health care workforce group, and because of their specific skills and competencies, nurses are in an ideal position to collaborate with other team members in the delivery of more accessible and effective chronic disease management in primary care. Inter-professional collaboration between primary care physicians and nurses is a possible strategy to achieve the desired quality outcomes in an effective and efficient manner in an integrated health system. Therefore, there's a need to explore to what extent an integration of physician and nurse competencies impacts patient outcome.

The objective of this research is to synthesize the evidence presented in literature on the impact of collaboration between physicians and nurses on patient outcomes in primary care or in comparable care settings.

Methods

Data sources

We searched for reviews of the literature containing synthesized evidence relating to collaboration between physicians and nurses, and the impact of their collaboration on patient outcomes.

Searches were performed in four literature databases: COCHRANE, MEDLINE, EMBASE and CINAHL. All databases were searched from 1970 (or from their inception if this was later than 1970) until May 2016. In addition, reference lists of the selected reviews were reviewed to identify other eligible reviews, but no additional review articles were identified.

All detailed search strategies can be found in Additional file 1.

The retrieved references were entered into Endnote© and duplicates were removed.

Study selection

The included studies had to fulfil a number of criteria in order to be included. First, the manuscript had to be a systematic review of the literature. A review was considered a systematic review if two of the following criteria were met: a search strategy was reported, a search was performed in Medline(PubMed) at least, and the included studies were subjected to a methodological assessment. There were no inclusion criteria based upon the research design of the primary research articles included in the systematic reviews.

Second, the manuscript needed to concern 'collaboration between physicians and nurses' in a primary care setting or in a hospital setting. Since there is no generally accepted definition of what inter-professional collaboration means, the intervention was defined as collaboration by the researchers if at least one physician provided care along with at least one nurse.

Third, the outcomes in the reviews needed to concern clinical patient outcomes and/or patient satisfaction outcomes. The review also needed sufficient methodological quality according to the AMSTAR quality appraisal tool (studies with a score ≥ 11 were included) [15–17]. And finally, none of the exclusion criteria listed below were met.

Research publications were excluded when they were primary research studies, when they were written in a language other than English or Dutch, or when the setting was considered 'inappropriate'. Settings were defined as inappropriate when the presented patient population was dissimilar or incomparable to the primary care population. Inappropriate settings were determined as; an intensive care unit (ICU), radiology, neonatology intensive care unit (NICU), obstetrics and gynecology. Studies were also excluded when the outcomes merely concerned nurse/physician outcomes.

A four-stage inclusion process was applied. Initially, titles and abstracts of research articles identified from the search strategies were screened, in order to determine their relevance and whether they met the inclusion criteria. No further analysis was done on the subsequent criteria as soon as one criterion was not met. In the first stage, one reviewer screened all references. When the title provided insufficient information to determine inclusion or exclusion, the research article proceeded to the second stage.

In the second stage, two reviewers independently examined all abstracts of the articles selected in the first stage, in order to determine whether they met the inclusion criteria. Any disagreements were resolved by discussion between the two reviewers.

In the third stage, two reviewers independently examined all full texts of the articles selected in the second stage. Any disagreements were resolved by discussion between the two reviewers. If no agreement could be reached, a third reviewer decided.

The final stage of inclusion related to the methodological assessment of the reviews. All reviews remaining after the third stage, were assessed with the AMSTAR quality appraisal tool [15, 17]. This assessment tool was formed by combining the enhanced Overview Quality Assessment Questionnaire (OQAQ), a checklist created by Sacks, and three additional items judged to be of methodological importance. 11 different components were identified [15]. The eleven criteria were scored as followed: 2 points were given when the criterion was fully met, 1 point when it was partly met and zero points when it was not met. Therefore, a maximum of 22 points on methodological quality could be achieved (see Table 2). Two reviewers independently examined the methodological quality of the reviews, using the AMSTAR quality appraisal tool [18]. The mean of the scores of the two reviewers was computed and classified as the final quality score [17]. In case the scores of the reviewers differed more than two points, reviewers reached consensus by discussion. Only moderate and high quality reviews (mean scores ≥11) were used for data extraction.

Data-analysis and synthesis

Data were extracted about the search strategies, time frame of the searches, studied interventions, selected outcomes, selected patient populations, selected study setting, the collaboration between physician(s) and nurse(s) and the different nursing roles within the collaboration.

Data-analysis was done primarily by description of the characteristics, interventions and outcomes. Meta-analyses and quantitative assessments from the included reviews were described. No quantitative pooling was performed across the reviews.

Results

Search and inclusion results

After duplicates were removed, the searches in the different databases resulted in one unique database, encompassing 4004 studies. Titles, abstracts and full texts were respectively reviewed and subsequently 277 studies and 58 studies were identified as potentially meeting the inclusion criteria (See Fig. 1). A total of 36 systematic reviews met all the inclusion criteria. Two reviewers independently assessed the remaining 36 reviews on their methodological quality, using the AMSTAR quality appraisal tool. A mean of the two scores was computed and classified as the final quality judgement. Eleven systematic reviews had a mean quality score higher than 11 and were included for data-extraction and analysis.

The flow diagram of the inclusion process is shown in Fig. 1.

Characteristics of the 11 included systematic reviews.

Search periods for each systematic review are shown in Table 1.

A narrative overview of the included review articles is described in Table 2. The eleven reviews only included quantitative studies. Four reviews [19–22] were limited to randomized controlled trials only, while the other seven reviews also included other comparative designs such as controlled before and after studies, interrupted time series and intervention studies. Three reviews included observational studies [23–25]. One review author additionally included other systematic reviews [26].

Four systematic reviews performed a meta-analysis [21, 26–28]. The methodological quality of the included review articles varies from moderate [20, 24] to high [21, 28, 29]. Nine review articles included

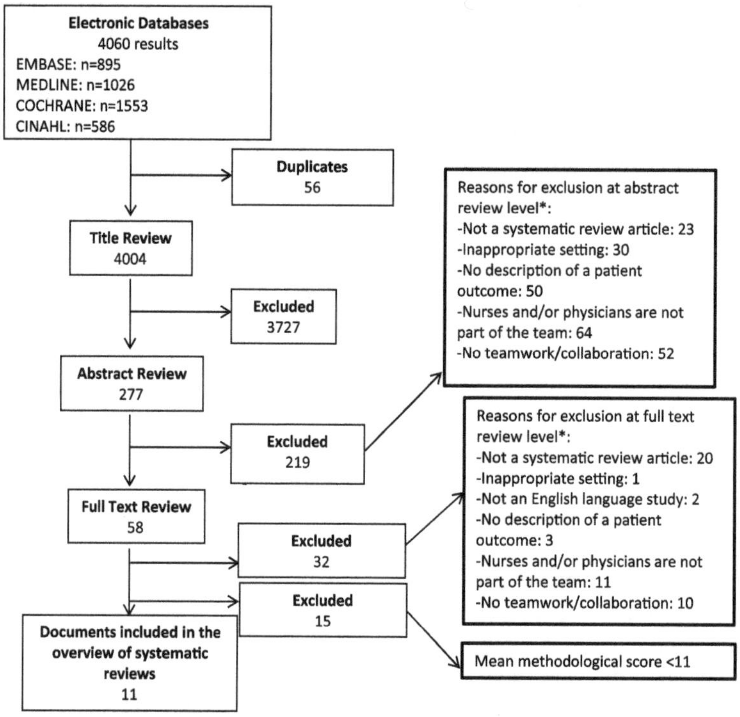

Fig. 1 Search strategy. Presents the search strategy of this overview of systematic reviews. The reasons for exclusion after reviewing the abstracts and full texts are presented on the right. *Reasons for study exclusion can be attributable to more than one category

studies that were conducted in both a primary care setting and a hospital setting [19–24, 26, 28, 29]. Two review articles included studies that were exclusively conducted in a hospital setting [25, 27].

The eleven systematic reviews included a total of 285 different primary studies, the number of primary studies included in the review articles varies from 6 to 69. Most of the primary studies were included only once in a review, with the exception of 12 papers that were included in two reviews. Additional file 2 presents a list of all primary studies included in at least one of the reviews.

Table 1 Search periods in included review articles

Review article	Search period
Allen et al. 2014	1990–2013
Aubin et al. 2012	1947–2009
Health Quality Ontario. 2013	Inception-2012
Health Quality Ontario. 2014	2000–2013
Martin et al. 2010	1999–2009
Newhouse et al. 2011	1990–2008
Renders et al. 2000	1966–1999
Shaw et al. 2014	1980–2014
Smith et al. 2014	1990–2011
Snaterse et al. 2016	1990–2015
Stalpers et al. 2015	2004–2012

Table 3 presents the main findings of the meta-analyses. Four different review articles are presented. The table includes: intervention, control group and the different outcomes. The number of studies within the systematic review and the total number of patients are presented, followed by the (weighted median) effect size, a measure of heterogeneity and an appraisal of the quality of evidence/risk of bias (if available). The included systematic reviews provided no information on the performance of a statistical process for small-study effects. The table shows that interdisciplinary teams targeting either informational or management continuity had a positive impact, with a weighted median effect size (95% confidence interval) of respectively 2.0% (−0.03, 3.20) and 2.0% (−1.90, 3.20), on the quality of life of patients diagnosed with cancer. A measure of heterogeneity was not available. The quality of evidence of the included research articles, according to GRADE, was rated very low. Team based models of end-of-life care (home and comprehensive) caused a decrease in the number of people admitted to hospital and an increase of the number of people dying at home. Nurse-coordinated care as well as nurse-managed protocols had a positive effect on patients' blood pressure and caused a decrease in patients' low-density lipoprotein cholesterol levels.

Table 2 Characteristics of the systematic reviews ($n = 11$)

Author, country, year	Objectives	Design	Patient population + setting	(Patient) Outcomes	Results/Conclusions	Quality assessment
1. Allen et al., Australia, 2014	To locate and synthesise research using randomized control trial designs on quality of outcomes following transitional care interventions compared with standard hospital discharge for older people with chronic illnesses. To make recommendations for research and practice.	Systematic review. 12 quantitative studies included: - 12 randomized controlled trials	- Older patients diagnosed with chronic illnesses - Transition from acute hospital care to (nursing) home	- Length of hospital stay - Length of time till re-hospitalization - Length of re-hospitalization - Costs - Functional status - Depression - Patient satisfaction - Quality of life - General practitioner (GP) satisfaction	Collaboration between nurses and physicians in the 'Discharge protocol and advanced practice nurse' intervention: - Delay in re- hospitalization. - Fewer days of re- hospitalization. - Fewer days of hospitalization. - Lower costs. - No significant difference in functional status, depression or patient satisfaction. Collaboration between nurses and physicians in the 'General practitioner and primary care nurse models' intervention: - Mixed results for (re-)hospitalization. - Higher patient satisfaction. - Improved referral to community services. - Higher GP satisfaction. - Faster discharge communication to GPs. General practitioner and practice nurse interventions were not effective in the reduction of hospitalization rates or length of stay. Low response rate of general practitioners makes interpretation of the results difficult.	19
2. Aubin et al., Canada, 2012	To describe and classify the various interventions studied in the literature to improve continuity of care in the follow- up of patients with cancer. To determine the effectiveness of interventions aiming to improve continuity of cancer care, on patient, healthcare provider and process outcomes.	Systematic review and meta- analysis. 51 quantitative studies included: - 49 randomized controlled trials - 2 controlled clinical trials (5 studies had a multi-disciplinary approach as intervention)	- Patients (65 years and older) with a cancer diagnosis - Patients admitted to the hospital with a terminal prognosis of 2 weeks to 6 months - Patients diagnosed with cancer and receiving Medical oncology outpatient clinic - Hospital setting	Patient outcomes: - Quality of life - Functional status - Physical performance - Pain - Depression - Anxiety - Satisfaction - Survival - Emotional adjustment - Cognitive functioning Informal caregiver outcomes Process outcomes	Three out of the five studies assessing interdisciplinary team models of care reported significant improvements in one or more classes of patient health- related outcomes during the study follow- up period. Patients supported by the multidisciplinary specialist Palliative Care Team had: - Significant improvements in scores of symptom severity. - A significantly better mood and were less bothered by emotional problems. - Significantly better quality of life scores at one and four weeks of follow- up, compared to patients assigned to the control group. Based on the median effect size estimates and the 95% CI, no significant difference in patient health measures was found.	20

Table 2 Characteristics of the systematic reviews ($n = 11$) *(Continued)*

Author, country, year	Objectives	Design	Patient population + setting	(Patient) Outcomes	Results/Conclusions	Quality assessment
					According to the descriptive analysis of single interventions on the improvement of patient health- related outcomes, case management and interdisciplinary teams seemed to be the most favourable models of care to improve one or more classes of patient outcomes.	
3. Health Quality Ontario, Ontario, 2013	To determine the effectiveness of specialized nurses who have a clinical role in patient care in optimizing chronic disease management among adults in the primary health care setting.	An evidence based analysis. 6 quantitative studies included: - 6 randomized controlled trials (8 papers)	- Patients with a chronic disease(s)/type 2 diabetes/ asthma/hypertension/ dementia/chronic obstructive pulmonary disease (COPD)/cancer/ coronary artery disease (CAD)/congestive heart failure (CHF) - Primary health care setting - General internal medicine clinic	- Hospitalizations - Length of stay - Mortality - Emergency department visits - Specialist visits - Health- related quality of life (HRQOL) - Patient satisfaction - Disease- specific measures - Process measures - Examination or medication prescribing - Health- system efficiencies - Number and length of primary health care visits - Physician workload	Specialized nurses working with physicians showed a general increase in process measures related to clinical examinations and medication management based on guidelines. - Significant reduction in HbA1c among diabetes patients. - Significant increase in the proportion of CAD patients with controlled BP and total cholesterol. - Significant reduction in hospitalization after 1 year for CAD patients receiving secondary prevention. - More patient satisfaction with care provided by the nurse plus physician intervention. - Inconsistency regarding outcomes related to HRQOL. No outcomes indicated specialized nursing interventions to be more harmful than physicians alone. Unclear role of the specialized nurse, making it difficult to determine the impact on efficiency. More research is needed to better understand the impact of specialized nurses on primary health care efficiency.	15
4. Health Quality Ontario, Ontario, 2014	To systematically review team- based models of care for end- of- life service delivery, to determine whether an optimal model exists.	Systematic review and meta- analysis. 12 quantitative studies included: - 2 systematic reviews - 10 randomized controlled trials	- Patients (adults) with advanced diseases (cancer, dementia, organ failure, stroke, chronic heart failure) receiving end of life care. - Home care - Hospital care	- Patient quality of life - Symptom management - Patient satisfaction - Informal caregiver satisfaction - Health care provider satisfaction - (Nursing) home death - Advance care planning - Emergency department visits - Hospital/ intensive care admission	The review considered the core model components of team membership, services offered, mode of patient contact, and setting. Team membership includes at minimum a physician and nurse, one of who is specialized in end- of- life health care. Team services included: symptom management, psychosocial care, and development of patient care	16

Table 2 Characteristics of the systematic reviews ($n = 11$) *(Continued)*

Author, country, year	Objectives	Design	Patient population + setting	(Patient) Outcomes	Results/Conclusions	Quality assessment
				- Hospital length of stay	plans, end- of- life care planning, and coordination of care. Comprehensive team- based model: moderate- quality evidence that a comprehensive team- based model with direct patient contact significantly: - Improves patient QOL, symptom management and patient and informal caregiver satisfaction. - Increases the patient's likelihood of dying at home. - Decreases the patient's likelihood of dying in a nursing home. - Has no impact on hospital admissions or hospital length of stay. Hospital team- based model: no impact on length of hospital stay, significant reduction of ICU admissions. Home team- based model: significantly increases patient satisfaction, increases the patient's likelihood of dying at home and significantly decreases emergency department visits and hospital admissions. Findings are applicable to deliver care to people with an estimated survival of up to 24 months.	
5. Martin et al., Switzerland, 2010	To provide an overview of the evidence base for inter- professional collaboration and new models of care in relation to patient outcomes.	A qualitative synthesis. 14 quantitative studies included: - 14 randomized controlled trials	Elderly with: - acute/ chronic diseases - risk factors - Patients after stroke - Patients with hip fracture/ type 2 diabetes/Alzheimer disease/ chronic heart failure/ multi- morbidity/problems in cognition, activities of daily living (ADL) - Children with asthma - Patients with bipolar disease/depression - Primary care - Hospital setting - Outpatient clinic	- Mortality - Clinical outcomes - Functional outcomes - Social outcomes - Utilisation of medical services - Patient- reported outcomes: QOL, ADL and satisfaction with care.	Mixed results were reported regarding: - Mortality. - Physical, emotional and social functioning. - Utilisation of medical services. - Hospitalization rates and length of hospital stay. Patient reported outcomes: significantly higher score of self- perceived health and life satisfaction. Mixed results regarding activities of daily living. Four studies showed that participants who experienced collaborative care management models were significantly more satisfied with their care than usual- care recipients. The evidence base of inter- professional collaboration shows promising results in relation to patient outcomes.	13.5

Table 2 Characteristics of the systematic reviews ($n = 11$) *(Continued)*

Author, country, year	Objectives	Design	Patient population + setting	(Patient) Outcomes	Results/Conclusions	Quality assessment
6. Newhouse et al., USA, 2011	Compared to other providers (physicians or teams without advanced practice registered nurses (APRN)), are APRN patient outcomes of care similar?	Systematic review. 69 quantitative studies included: - 20 randomized controlled trials (RCTs) - 49 observational studies	- Pregnant women - Neonates - New- borns - Children - Adults - Elderly - Community - Primary care - Inpatient - Nursing home - Ambulatory - Surgery - Prenatal- inpatient - Hospital	- Patient satisfaction - Self- reported perceived health - Functional status - Glucose control - Lipid control - Blood pressure (BP) - Emergency department/ urgent care visits - Hospitalization - Duration of mechanical ventilation - Length of stay - Mortality - Cost - Complication	37 studies examined patient outcomes of care by nurse practitioners (NP care group) compared with care management exclusively by physicians. - High level of evidence to support equivalent levels of patient satisfaction, self- reported perceived health, functional status outcomes, glucose control and BP control. - High level of evidence to support equivalent rates of emergency department visits, hospitalization and mortality. - High level of evidence to support better serum lipid levels. - Moderate level of evidence to support equivalent length of stay. 11 studies examined clinical nurse specialist (CNS) outcomes. - High level of evidence to support equivalent patient satisfaction scores. - High level of evidence to support equivalent or lower length of stay for patients cared for in the CNS group. - High level of evidence to support the CNS group has a lower cost of care High level of evidence that APRNs provide safe, effective quality care to a number of specific populations in a variety of settings. APRNs have a significant role in the promotion of health in partnership with physicians and other providers,	17.5
7. Renders et al., Amsterdam, 2000	To determine the effectiveness of different interventions, targeted at health care professionals or the structure in which health care professionals deliver their care, to improve the care for patients with diabetes in primary care, outpatient and community settings.	Systematic review. 41 quantitative studies included: - 27 randomized controlled trials - 12 controlled before and after studies - 2 interrupted time series	- Non- hospitalised patients with Type 1 or Type 2 diabetes mellitus. - A primary care setting - Outpatient (ambulatory care) setting - Community setting (managed care organisations, general medical clinics)	- Glycaemic control - Micro- or macro- vascular complications - Cardiovascular risk factors - Hospital admissions - Mortality - Well- being - Perceived health - Quality of life - Functional status - Patient satisfaction	The addition of patient education or a more enhanced role of a nurse to a complex intervention strategy seems to be important to improve patient outcomes besides process outcomes. Nurses can play an important role in facilitating compliance or giving patient education. They can even replace physicians in delivering many aspects of diabetes care, if detailed management protocols are available, or if they receive training. The seven studies in which nurses replaced (partly) physicians in providing diabetes care generally	21

Table 2 Characteristics of the systematic reviews ($n = 11$) *(Continued)*

Author, country, year	Objectives	Design	Patient population + setting	(Patient) Outcomes	Results/Conclusions	Quality assessment
					demonstrated a positive impact on glycaemic control. The effectiveness of the implementation of revision of professional roles as a single intervention remains unclear.	
8. Shaw et al., USA, 2014	To synthesize the current literature describing the effects of nurse- managed protocols, including medication adjustment, for the outpatient management of adults with common chronic conditions, namely diabetes, hypertension and hyperlipidaemia.	Systematic review and meta- analysis. 18 quantitative studies included: - 16 randomized controlled trials - 2 controlled before- and- after studies. (2 companion articles-methods or follow- up)	- Adults with elevated cardiovascular risk - General medical hospital - Specialty hospital - Primary care clinic - Telephone delivered care	- Haemoglobin A1c level - BP - Cholesterol level - Performance measure - Behavioural adherence (medication) - Protocol adherence	The 'medical home' is a team approach which may involve nurse- managed protocols. Nurse- managed protocols were associated with: - A highly variable mean decrease in HbA1c level. - A mean decrease in systolic and diastolic BP. - A mean decrease in total and low-density lipoprotein (LDL) cholesterol levels. Nurse- managed protocols were statistically significantly more likely to achieve target total cholesterol levels than control protocols. Effects of lifestyle changes and medication adherence showed an overall pattern of small positive effects associated with nurse-managed protocols. Adherence to protocol: pharmacologic therapy was started or doses were increased by nurses following treatment protocols more often than in usual care groups. Team approaches using nurse-managed protocols help improve health outcomes among patients with moderately severe diabetes, hypertension and hyperlipidemia.	22
9. Smith et al., England, 2014	To review the current literature on the participation and roles of APRNs/ Physician assistants (PAs) in providing cancer screening and prevention recommendations in primary care settings in the USA.	Systematic review. 15 quantitative studies included: - 3 intervention studies - 12 observational studies	- Adults (Smoking) - Pregnant women - Primary care settings - Private practices - Primary care health centres - Study hospitals - Obstetric clinic - Hospital ambulatory settings	7 studies reported outcomes on screening for - Cervical cancer (Pap test) - Breast cancer (Mammogram) - Colorectal cancer 10 studies reported outcomes on cancer prevention recommendations for - smoking cessation - diet - physical activity	Cervical cancer screening: - Physicians who work in teams that include NPs and PAs are more supportive of NPs and PAs performing Pap tests than physicians who do not practice in provider teams that include NPs and PAs. - The annual rate of women screened for cervical cancer by a NP increased significantly at the intervention location. Breast cancer screening:	13

Table 2 Characteristics of the systematic reviews ($n = 11$) *(Continued)*

Author, country, year	Objectives	Design	Patient population + setting	(Patient) Outcomes	Results/Conclusions	Quality assessment
					- 69- 91% of the patients who see NPs receive mammograms. - NPs recommend a similar number of mammograms as physicians. - The annual rate of mammography screening increased more among women seen at the NP screening recommendation site. Colorectal cancer screening: - Findings about APRN/PAs involvement in colorectal screening are mixed. - 2 studies showed physicians reporting more colorectal cancer screening than APRN/PAs. Smoking cessation recommendations: - Both physicians and APRN/PAs report frequently providing smoking cessation recommendations. - Patients are more likely to receive recommendations for smoking cessation during visits with NPs than during visits without NPs. Diet and physical activity recommendations: APRN/PAs do not frequently provide recommendations on diet and physical activity (12–52%), they do provide more recommendations than their physician counterparts (3–15%).	
10. Snaterse et al., The Netherlands, 2016	To systematically review the available evidence on the efficacy of nurse- coordinated care (NCC) in secondary prevention of coronary heart diseases.	Systematic review and meta- analysis. 18 quantitative studies included: - 18 randomized controlled trials	- Patients with coronary heart diseases (adults) - Hospital setting - Outpatient clinics - Community health clinic - Secondary prevention unit - General practices	30 NCC outcomes were measured. Observed outcomes were grouped into four categories: - Risk factor levels - Clinical events - Patient perceived health - Guideline adherence	NCC programs were grouped into three strategies: - Risk factor management: education, lipid/BP control, advice on healthy diet and encouraging physical activity, prescription and or titration of drug therapy, enhancing adherence and smoking cessation counselling. - Multidisciplinary consultation: involvement of multidisciplinary team (>2 disciplines), consultation with general practitioner, referral to specialized disciplines. - Shared decision- making: personalized action plan, goal setting for cardiac risk factor control and family support. Effective components regarding behavioural interventions were goal	21

Table 2 Characteristics of the systematic reviews ($n = 11$) *(Continued)*

Author, country, year	Objectives	Design	Patient population + setting	(Patient) Outcomes	Results/Conclusions	Quality assessment
					setting for cardiac risk factor control plus identification of barriers. 8 Trials found positive outcomes for NCC compared with usual care: - Risk factor levels: total cholesterol, LDL cholesterol, triglyceride, pharmacological treatment, BP, diet, SCORE (a comprehensive cardiovascular risk algorithm designed for the primary prevention setting) and smoking cessation. - Clinical events: all- cause and cardiovascular readmission (days). - Guideline adherence.	
11. Stalpers et al., The Netherlands, 2015	To systematically review the literature and to provide an overview of associations between characteristics of the nurse work environment (e.g., nurse staffing, nurse- physician collaboration) and five nurse-sensitive patient outcomes (i.e., delirium, malnutrition, pain, patient falls and pressure ulcers).	Systematic review. 29 quantitative studies included: - 1 randomized controlled trial - 28 observational studies	- Hospitalized patients - Hospital setting: surgical/general/ emergency/intensive care/obstetric/cardiology/ cardiothoracic surgery/ respiratory units.	Nurse- sensitive outcomes: - 12 studies examined pressure ulcers. - 11 studies examined patient falls. - 6 studies analysed both pressure ulcers and patient falls among which one also elaborated on pain management.	Patient falls: - Collaborative nurse- physician relationships: 2/3 studies reported significant associations. Specifically, positively appreciated communication was associated with fewer adverse events and lower number of patient falls. Pressure ulcers: - Collaborative nurse- physician relationships: positively appreciated communication was associated with a lower number of pressure ulcers. Another study did not find significant associations.	15

Table 3 Meta-analyses ($n = 4$)

Aubin et al., 2012

Intervention	Control	Outcome	Number of studies	Number of patients	Median effect size[a] % (95% BCI)[b]	Hetero-geneity	Quality of evidence: GRADE
Interdisciplinary teams (targeting informational continuity)	Usual care	Functional status	11	3057	0 (−3.40, 2.70)	NAV	Very low
		Physical status	16	3589	0 (−0.50, 0.50)	NAV	Very low
		Psychological status	13	3228	−0.24 (−3.00, 0.02)	NAV	Very low
		Social status	4	589	−0.01 (−10.70, 0.30)	NAV	Very low
		Global quality of life	**9**	**2472**	**2.0 (−0.03, 3.20)**	**NAV**	**Very low**
Interdisciplinary teams (targeting management continuity)	Usual care	Functional status	11	2612	0 (−3.40, 2.00)	NAV	Very low
		Physical status	18	3439	0 (−0.50, 0.03)	NAV	Very low
		Psychological status	15	3687	−1.1 (−6.30, 0.00)	NAV	Very low
		Social status	4	528	−0.7 (−7.00, 0.30)	NAV	Very low
		Global quality of life	**7**	**1717**	**2.0 (−1.90, 3.20)**	**NAV**	**Very low**

Health Quality Ontario, 2014

Intervention	Control	Outcome	Number of studies	Number of patients	Effect size (95% CI)	Hetero-geneity	Quality of evidence: GRADE
Home team-based model of care	Medicare guidelines for home health care	**Home death (number of people)**	**1**	**310**	**Odds ratio 2.20 (1.30, 3.72)**	**NA**	Low
		Hospital admission (number of people admitted to hospital)	**1**	**310**	**Odds ratio 0.39 (0.24, 0.62)**	**NA**	Low
Home (indirect) team-based model of care	Usual care by a management care organization	**Advanced care planning (number of people)**	**1**	**190**	**Odds ratio 1.30 (0.58, 2.90)**	**NA**	Very low
Hospital team-based model of care	Hospital care/ primary care team only	**Advanced care planning**	**2**	**616**	**Odds ratio 2.77 (0.48, 16.11)**	**I-square 48%**	Very low
Comprehensive team-based model of care	Usual care	**Home death (number of people)**	**1**	**434**	**Odds ratio 1.89 (1.13, 3.16)**	**NA**	Moderate
		Nursing home death (number of people)	**1**	**434**	**Odds ratio 0.37 (0.20, 0.67)**	**NA**	Moderate
		Hospital admission	**1**	**434**	**Odds ratio 0.90 (0.42, 1.89)**	**NA**	Moderate
Comprehensive, early start, team-based model of care	Routine oncologic care	**Hospital admission**	**1**	**151**	**Odds ratio 0.84 (0.34, 2.03)**	**NA**	Low

Table 3 Meta-analyses ($n = 4$) *(Continued)*

Shaw et al., 2014

Intervention	Control	Outcome	Number of studies	Number of patients	Effect size (95% CI)	Hetero-geneity	Quality of evidence- risk of bias
Nurse-managed protocols	Usual care	**Systolic blood pressure (difference in mmHg)**	**12**	**Intervention:5244 Control:4980**	**Weighted mean difference – 3.68 (−6.31, −1.05)**	**I-square 75.1%**	According to the approach recommended by the Agency for Healthcare Research and Quality: 4 articles: Low risk of bias/good quality 12 articles: Moderate risk of bias/fair quality 2 articles: High risk of bias/poor quality
	Usual care	**Diastolic blood pressure (difference in mmHg)**	**12**	**Intervention:5244 Control:4980**	**Weighted mean difference – 1.56 (−2.76, −0.36)**	**I-square 75.1%**	
	Usual care	**Total cholesterol (difference in mg/dL)**	**9**	**Intervention:1879 Control:1615**	**Weighted mean difference – 9.37 (−20.77, 2.02)**	**I-square 90.8%**	
	Usual care	**Low-density lipoprotein cholesterol (difference in mg/dL)**	**6**	**Intervention:564 Control:555**	**Weighted mean difference – 12.07 (−28.27, 4.13)**	**I-square 89.1%**	
	Usual care	**Hemoglobin A1c level**	**8**	**Intervention:1444 Control: 1189**	**Weighted mean difference – 0.40 (−0.70, −0.10)%**	**I-square 69.8%**	

Snaterse et al., 2016

Intervention	Control	Outcome	Number of studies	Number of patients	Effect size (95% CI)	Hetero-geneity	Quality of evidence– risk of bias
Nurse-coordinated care	Usual care	**Blood pressure (difference in mmHg)**	**7**	**3514**	**Weighted mean difference −2.96 (−4.40, −1.53)**	**I-square 37.1% $p = 0.146$**	Cochrane Collaboration's risk of bias tool: low/unclear risk of bias.
	Usual care	**Low-density lipoprotein cholesterol (difference in mmol/L)**	**8**	**3441**	**Weighted mean difference −0.23 (−0.36, −0.10)**	**I-square 74.3% $p = 0.000$**	
	Usual care	**Smoking cessation rates (Relative risk of quitting)**	**8**	**3265**	**Relative risk 1.25 (1.09, 1.43)%**	**I-square 0.0% $p = 0.459$**	

Table 3 presents the results of the meta-analyses of four of the included systematic reviews. The different 'collaboration interventions' are presented, followed by the control group, patient outcomes, number of studies, number of patients, effect size, a measure of heterogeneity (if available) and a measure of quality of evidence/risk of bias (if available). The improved patient outcomes are written in bold

NA 'not applicable', *NAV* 'not available'

[a]To handle the diverse set of outcomes within each individual study, the median value was computed of all the measured effects across all the outcomes of the same class. To pool the results from multiple studies, the median effect size was calculated for each class of outcome, by computing the median from all the median effects in outcomes obtained from individual studies. The researchers chose this pooling strategy to be consistent with the median approach used in other reviews [45–47]

[b]non-parametric bootstrap confidence intervals

Table 4 presents an overview of the systematic reviews that did not provide a meta-analysis. Seven different review articles are presented. The table includes: intervention, control group and the different outcomes. The number of studies within the systematic review and the total number of patients are presented, followed by a statement on heterogeneity (if available) and an appraisal of the quality of evidence/risk of bias (if available).

All eleven articles describe the impact of collaboration between physicians and nurses on patient outcomes. Table 5 presents an overview of the different outcomes described in the review articles. Table 5 provides an overview of the improved patient outcomes (collaboration between physicians and nurses led to better results for these outcomes), Table 6 shows an overview of the equivalent patient outcomes (collaboration between physicians and nurses led to equal results for these outcomes) and Table 7 presents an overview of the mixed patient outcomes (collaboration between physicians and nurses led to better and/or equal and/or worse results for these outcomes). Blood pressure, patient satisfaction and hospitalization are the outcomes where three or more systematic reviews concluded better results when physicians and nurses collaborated, compared to usual care. Systematic reviews often described a combination of improved and equivalent patient outcomes when the included articles showed mixed results.

Table 8 describes the collaboration between physicians and nurses in the different review articles. Collaboration was described as a 'multidisciplinary', 'inter-disciplinary' or 'inter-professional'. Other health care providers are often part of the team [20, 21, 26, 27].

Figure 2 presents the nursing roles/tasks in the collaboration with physicians in the included systematic reviews. The most frequently represented tasks are: specific nursing tasks (e.g. blood pressure control), communication/consultation tasks (e.g. communication with the multidisciplinary team), patient education tasks (e.g. lifestyle counseling) and coordination/organization/referral tasks (e.g. coordination of care, conducting a discharge planning). Two review articles did not clearly describe the tasks performed by the nurses.

Discussion

Eleven systematic reviews describing the impact of collaboration between physicians and nurses on patient outcome were included in this overview of systematic reviews. Collaboration between physicians and nurses may have a positive impact on a number of patient outcomes and on a variety of pathologies.

Almost fifty different patient outcomes were described (Table 3). In most reviews, it was concluded that nurses do have added value. Maybe we observe some publication bias here since most of the author groups included nurses [30]. We also obtained mixed results in the other reviews. Blood pressure was the only patient outcome exclusively reported as improved in three different systematic reviews [19, 21, 28]. Two of them even performed a meta-analysis [21, 28]. Patient satisfaction is an improved patient outcome as well. No less than five different systematic reviews confirmed this [19, 20, 22, 26, 27]. However, two systematic reviews reported an equivalent patient satisfaction when physicians and nurses collaborated [22, 23]. Number of hospitalization is another improved patient outcome, confirmed by four different systematic reviews [19, 20, 22, 26]. However, three systematic reviews [20, 23, 26] also reported an equivalent number of hospitalizations and one [22] even reported an increase of hospitalizations when physicians and nurses collaborated. These mixed results make it difficult to make an accurate interpretation and conclusion towards the different patient outcomes.

Colorectal screening, hospital length of stay and health-related quality of life are three patient outcomes that also improved when physicians and nurses did not collaborate. However, only colorectal screening and health-related quality of life were merely categorized as negative outcomes. Allen et al. reported the length of hospital stay as a negative outcome. But the same review article also reported improvement in length of hospital stay, as well as two other review articles [20, 23]. Quality of life in general was reported as an improved outcome when physicians and nurses collaborated in two different review articles [26, 27].

The included systematic reviews often combined different interventions such as patient education [22, 29], medication adjustment [28], discharge planning protocol and shared decision making [21, 22] while measuring patient outcomes. Adding one or more interventions, besides collaboration between physicians and nurses, also makes it more difficult to determine which effect can be attributed to which intervention.

The evidence of collaboration between physicians and nurses on patient outcome can be applied to the primary care setting for almost all the measured patient outcomes. Only two systematic reviews included articles conducted in a hospital setting [25, 27]. Therefore, the improvement of global quality of life, and the decline of patient falls and pressure ulcers cannot be allotted to collaboration between physicians and nurses in the primary care setting.

Collaboration

The different systematic reviews used a variety of terms describing the collaboration between health care providers including inter-professional collaboration, multidisciplinary collaboration, coordination, communication, teamwork and shared care. A clear definition and subsequent

Table 4 Overview systematic reviews without meta- analysis ($n = 7$)

Intervention	Control	Outcome	Number of studies	Number of patients	Heterogeneity	Quality of evidence- risk of bias
Allen et al., 2014						
Discharge protocol and advanced practice nurse	Usual care	- Length of hospital stay - Length of time till re-hospitalization - Costs - Functional status - Depression - Patient satisfaction - Quality of life - GP satisfaction	5 (RCT)	918	Due to heterogeneity in the transitional care interventions and outcomes, data were not pooled.	Cochrane Collaboration's tool – high risk of performance bias in the included research articles
General practitioner and primary care nurse models	Usual care		3 (RCT)	1949		
Health Quality Ontario, 2013						
Nurse and physician care	Physician care	- Hospitalizations - Length of stay - Mortality - ED visits - Specialist visits - Health- related quality of life - Patient satisfaction - Disease specific measures - Examination or medication prescribing - Health- system efficiencies - Number and length of primary health care visits - Physician workload	6 (RCT)	Intervention: 1403 Control:1538	Due to clinical heterogeneity in the study populations evaluated, and differences in provider roles and characteristics, the pooling of outcomes was thought to be inappropriate and a meta- analysis was not conducted.	Quality of evidence: GRADE Low- Moderate quality
Martin et al., 2010						
Inter- professional collaboration – new models of care	Usual care	- Mortality - Clinical outcomes - Functional outcomes - Social outcomes - Utilization of medical services - Patient- reported outcomes: quality of life, activities of daily living	14 (RCT)	Intervention: 2788 Control: 2563	NAV	NAV
Newhouse et al., 2011						
Nurse practitioner/clinical nurse specialist care groups	Care management exclusively by physicians	- Patient satisfaction - Self- reported perceived health - Functional status - Glucose control - Lipid control - Blood pressure - ED visits - Hospitalizations - Duration of mechanical ventilation	69: 20 (RCT) + 49 (obser- vational)	NAV	Effect sizes were not calculated for the multiple outcomes. Because of the widely varying populations, definitions, time periods, and study designs. Also, the publications did not consistently include the necessary data to calculate effect size.	Quality assessment by the Jadad scale 46 articles: High quality 12 articles: Low quality

Table 4 Overview systematic reviews without meta- analysis ($n = 7$) *(Continued)*

Intervention	Control	Outcome	Number of studies	Number of patients	Heterogeneity	Quality of evidence- risk of bias
		- Length of stay - Mortality - Cost - Complications				
Renders et al., 2000						
Interventions targeted at health care professionals or the structure in which health care professionals deliver their care. A more enhanced nursing role.	Usual care	- Glycemic control - Micro- or macro- vascular complications - Cardiovascular risk factors - Hospital admissions - Mortality - Well- being - Perceived health - Quality of life - Functional status - Patient satisfaction	41: 27 (RCT) + 12 (CBA) + 2 (ITS)	48,598	Given the likely heterogeneity of interventions, there is decided a priori not to use meta- analysis to pool the results of studies. Differences in guidelines and also in methods and reference values to assess glycated hemoglobin meant that a uniform effect size could not be valued and presented, thereby hindering between-study comparisons.	The quality criteria applied to RCT's, CBAs and ITS are described in detail in the EPOC module of the Cochrane library. Allocation concealment: 17 articles clearly concealed Blind outcome assessment: 20 articles adequate 16 articles partly adequate Reliable outcome assessment: 22 articles adequate
Smith et al., 2014						
Participation of APRNs/PAs in providing cancer screening and prevention recommendations in primary care settings	Cancer screening and prevention provider teams with physicians that do not include APRNs/PAs	- Cervical cancer (Pap test) - Breast cancer (Mammogram) - Colorectal cancer - Smoking cessation - Diet - Physical activity	15: 3 intervention studies +12 observational studies	NAV	NAV	NAV
Stalpers et al., 2015						
Nurse- physician collaboration	Usual care	- Pressure ulcers - Patient falls - Pain management	29: 1 RCT + 28 observational studies	NAV	Fundamental problems with assessing and comparing data from primary studies prevents conducting an adequate quantitative meta- analysis of the literature.	Dutch version of Cochrane's critical appraisal instrument: validity: moderate reliability: moderate applicability: moderate

NAV 'not available', *RCT* 'randomized controlled trial', *CBA* 'controlled before and after study', *ITS* 'interrupted time series'

Table 4 presents the 'collaboration intervention', control, patient outcome, number of studies, number of patients (if available), a statement on heterogeneity (if available) and a measure of quality of evidence/risk of bias (if available) of seven included systematic reviews that did not conduct a meta- analysis

Table 5 Overview improved patient outcomes

Serum lipid levels	Newhouse et al., Snaterse et al.
Cervical and breast cancer screening	Smith et al.
Lower cost of care	Newhouse et al., Allen et al.
Patient falls	Stalpers et al.
Pressure ulcers	Stalpers et al.
Guideline adherence	Snaterse et al.
Total cholesterol	Health Quality Ontario 2013, Snaterse et al.
Low density lipoprotein cholesterol	Shaw et al., Snaterse et al.
Triglyceride	Snaterse et al.
Pharmacological treatment	Snaterse et al.
Blood pressure	Health Quality Ontario 2013, Shaw et al., Snaterse et al.
SCORE[a]	Snaterse et al.
All-cause and cardiovascular readmission days	Snaterse et al.
Reduction in HbA1c levels	Heath Quality Ontario 2013, Shaw et al.
Self-perceived health	Martin et al.
Life satisfaction	Aubin et al., Martin et al.
Symptom severity	Aubin et al., Health Quality Ontario 2014.
Quality of life	Aubin et al., Health Quality Ontario 2014.
Delay in re-hospitalization	Allen et al.
Improved referral to community services	Allen et al.
General practitioner satisfaction	Allen et al.
Discharge communication to general practitioners	Allen et al.
Informal caregiver satisfaction	Health Quality Ontario 2014.
Increase likelihood of dying at home (end-of-life care)	Health Quality Ontario 2014.
Decrease likelihood of dying in a nursing home (end-of-life care)	Health Quality Ontario 2014.
Reduction of intensive care unit admission	Health Quality Ontario 2014.
Number of clinical examinations for blood pressure, BMI[b] and smoking status	Health Quality Ontario 2013.
Number of foot examinations (diabetes)	Health Quality Ontario 2013
Patient outcomes also presented in Tables 6 or 7	
Smoking cessation recommendations	Smith et al., Snaterse et al.
Hospital length of stay	Allen et al., Martin et al., Newhouse et al.
Diet	Snaterse et al.
Patient satisfaction	Aubin et al., Allen et al., Health Quality Ontario 2013, Health Quality Ontario 2014., Martin et al.
Hospitalization rates	Allen et al., Health Quality Ontario 2013, Health Quality Ontario 2014., Martin et al.
Emergency department visits	Health Quality Ontario 2014., Martin et al.
Glycaemic control	Renders et al.
Mortality	Martin et al.
Physical, emotional and social functioning	Martin et al.

Table 5 presents the patient outcomes that were found to be improved (by one or more systematic reviews) when physicians and nurses collaborate, compared to no collaboration

[a]*SCORE* Systematic Coronary Risk Evaluation. It's a comprehensive cardiovascular risk algorithm designed for the primary prevention setting

[b]*BMI* Body Mass index

elaboration of the nature of the collaboration was lacking in most of the reviews. This is consistent with findings in the existing literature, where there seems to be no agreement on the use of terms to describe collaboration between health professionals [31]. This also makes it difficult to know how the collaboration translates itself in daily

Table 6 Overview equivalent patient outcomes

Patient satisfaction	Allen et al., Newhouse et al.
Self-reported perceived health	Newhouse et al.
Functional status outcomes	Allen et al., Newhouse et al.
Glycaemic control	Newhouse et al.
Blood pressure control	Newhouse et al.
Emergency department visits	Newhouse et al.
Hospitalization rates	Health Quality Ontario 2014., Martin et al., Newhouse et al.
Mortality	Martin et al., Newhouse et al.
Hospital length of stay	Health Quality Ontario 2014., Martin et al., Newhouse et al.
Recommendation of mammograms	Smith et al.
Smoking cessation recommendations	Smith et al.
Diet and physical therapy recommendations	Smith et al.
Depression	Allen et al.
Number of clinical examination of cholesterol	Health Quality Ontario 2013.
Utilisation of medical services	Martin et al.
Number of transfers	Martin et al.
Physical, emotional and social functioning	Martin et al.
Activities of daily living (ADL)	Martin et al.

Table 6 presents the patient outcomes that were found to be equal (by one or more systematic reviews) when physicians and nurses collaborate, compared to no collaboration

practice: were the studied collaborations between physicians and nurses merely focused on nurses performing dedicated tasks, based on physicians orders (a rather more instrumental collaboration)? Or were the studied collaborations focused on nurses' competences and tasks with autonomous decision-making capacity, based on structured agreements between nurses and physicians (a rather more integrated collaboration)?

A total of 173 RCTs were finally included in this overview of systematic reviews. Although RCTs are the gold standard in establishing a firm evidence base in quantitative research, complex practice settings like health service settings, often require a more diverse methodology [32]. The relationship between teamwork and patient outcomes seems to be difficult to investigate with RCTs. A Cochrane review on interventions to promote collaboration between nurses and physicians concluded that rigorous evaluations are difficult to conduct. This is because the interventions are complex and the intermediate processes are difficult to assess [33]. Researchers in the United Kingdom increasingly use qualitative research methods alongside RCTs to gain a more comprehensive understanding of the impact of health service delivery [32]. Direct observation of collaborative practice in primary care settings holds promise as a method to better understand and articulate the complex phenomena of inter-professional collaboration. Despite methodological challenges, observation data may contribute in a unique way to the teamwork discourse by identifying elements of inter-professional collaboration that are not so obvious to caregivers when asked to self-report [34].

Table 7 Overview mixed patient outcomes

Colorectal screening	Smith et al.
hospitalization rates	Allen et al.
Hospital length of stay	Allen et al.

Table 7 presents the patient outcomes that were found to be improved and/or equivalent and/or declined

Open communication between physicians and nurses is an important element of collaboration that appeared to be appreciated [25]. More often, researchers reported that deficiencies in collaboration and communication between healthcare professionals have a negative impact on the provision of health care and patient outcomes [35–37]. In addition to open communication, trust, respect, shared leadership, recognition of unique contribution and collegiality are mentioned by researchers as enabling factors for good inter-professional relationships [38]. On the other hand, barriers to good inter-professional collaboration reported by researchers are time pressure, lack of explicit descriptions of each other's roles and tasks (and therefore unawareness of one another's roles and competencies), poor organizational support, absence of clear leadership, different standards and professional values, different aims and priorities, and

Table 8 Collaboration between physicians and nurses

Authors	Collaboration
1. Allen et al.	Collaboration between a general practitioner and a primary care nurse in transitional care. Collaboration between an advanced practice nurse and a physician during the discharge plan.
2. Aubin et al.	Interdisciplinary team models of care for patients with cancer. These interventions used organizational strategies such as staff organization and the creation of teams of healthcare professionals working together to care for patients. These interventions also used local consensus processes, formal integration of services, arrangement for follow- up, coordination of assessment and treatment, and implementation of follow- up care plans. The interdisciplinary treatment team included: medical oncology, social work, occupational therapy, nursing, nutrition and dietetics and pastoral care.
3. Health Quality Ontario 2013.	Nurses/nurse practitioners/registered nurses and physicians working in a partnership. Nurses who worked in this collaboration could have been substituting or supplementing aspects of physician care.
4. Health Quality Ontario 2014.	An end- of- life care team contained at least a medical doctor and a registered nurse. Other possible team members: - social worker - spiritual advisor - nutritionist - geriatrician - pharmacist - dietician Team services included: - symptom management - psychosocial care - development of patient care plans - end- of- life care planning - coordination of care
5. Martin et al.	Inter- professional collaboration in the care for elderly with (chronic) diseases. Collaboration between at least (advanced practice) nurses and (primary care) physicians. Other care providers: - social worker - physio- occupational therapist - pharmacist - psychiatrist - ...
6. Newhouse et al.	Advanced practice registered nurses (APRN)/ clinical nurse specialists delivered care in collaboration with physicians.
7. Renders et al.	The multidisciplinary team was led by a nurse educator. There was a joint general practitioner- nurse review system in combination with arrangements for follow up.
8. Shaw et al.	Collaboration according to nurse- managed protocols in the care for adults with elevated cardiovascular risk.
9. Smith et al.	APRN and Practice Assistants (PAs) provided cancer screening and prevention recommendations in collaboration with physicians.
10. Snaterse et al.	Multidisciplinary consultation for patients with coronary heart diseases. Collaboration between nurses and general practitioners or cardiologists. The following strategies were used: - Risk factor management. - Multidisciplinary consultation. - Shared decision- making.
11. Stalpers et al.	Collaborative nurse- physician relationships in the care for hospitalized patients.

Table 8 presents an overview of the interpretation of collaboration between physicians and nurses (and other health care providers) within the eleven included systematic reviews

vertical management structures with discriminatory power structures [39–41].

Nursing roles

Although the review articles often lacked a comprehensive description of the nursing roles in collaboration with physicians, we identified seven different categories of nursing roles in the systematic reviews in our review. 'Nursing tasks' and 'drug prescription' may be more distinct instrumental roles or nursing tasks, and are probably based on physicians' orders. 'Communication/consultation' and 'coordination/organization/referral' may be rather more related to integrated nursing roles with nurses' autonomous decision-making capacity based on structured agreements between nurses and physicians. Existing literature confirms the nursing skill mix, and the shift from task delegation to team care with shared responsibilities [42, 43]. Two systematic

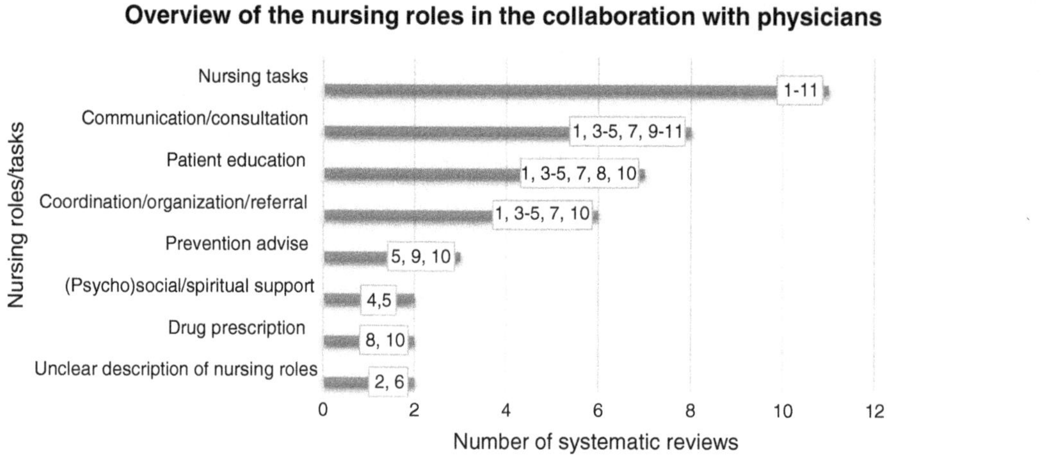

Fig. 2 Overview of the nursing roles in the collaboration with physicians. Presents an overview of the 7 different nursing roles in collaboration with physicians within the eleven included systematic reviews. 2 systematic reviews failed to give a clear description of the nursing roles. The numbers within the graph represent the eleven included systematic reviews

reviews failed to describe the nature of the nursing roles and their responsibilities [23, 27]. Furthermore, nursing titles differed across the included systematic review articles and ranged from 'advanced practice (registered) nurses', 'nurse practitioners', 'registered nurses', 'primary care nurses', 'clinical nurses specialists' and 'practice assistants'. The literature confirms the increasing diversity of the primary care workforce. A wider range of health professionals is included, such as those mentioned above [43]. The difference in professional titles might be attributed to a difference in education, which points out the importance of (post-graduate) education of nurses, especially in collaboration with physicians [29]. Expanding the role of primary care nurses is possible with appropriate training and on-going support from primary care physicians [44]. Improving care quality requires investing in a distinct primary care workforce that has followed a defined program of post-graduate training in primary care [2].

Strengths and limitations

A comprehensive research was performed and the methodological quality of the included review articles was carefully assessed. Overall, the quality of available systematic reviews on this research topic appeared to be limited. 15 potentially useful systematic reviews were excluded based upon an inadequate methodological quality. The included systematic review articles were heterogeneous in terms of patient populations, setting, type of nurse and geographic region. Limited descriptions of the collaboration, and the different nursing and physician roles in the included systematic reviews are limitations of this overview of systematic reviews. The included systematic reviews often lacked a detailed description of the evidence of the different primary studies, therefore it is difficult to make conclusions about the strength of the evidence of the results. For future systematic reviews concerning this research topic we suggest to define more precisely the nature of the collaboration between the two professions and to provide a clear description of the concept of inter-professional collaboration.

Primary research articles concerning this research topic within the primary care setting are often limited to one pathology or diagnosis. However, the patient population in primary care presents itself with a wide range of pathologies. This overview of systematic reviews provides a more comprehensive view on the impact of collaboration between physicians and nurses in primary care on a wide variety of patient outcomes, for a wide range of patients.

Future research is necessary to define 'integrated inter-professional collaboration' in primary care more clearly, and to explore the impact of this collaboration on relevant patient and health care provider outcomes. These include hospital (re)admissions of patients with chronic conditions, patient satisfaction and primary health care provider satisfaction. We suggest using complementary methods to find a more robust evidence base for the collaboration of nurses and general practitioners in primary care.

Implications for practice

This overview of systematic reviews provides a firm evidence base to engage practice nurses in general practices. Moreover, current and future challenges in primary care require a more integrated inter-professional collaboration instead of a task shift between general practitioners and nurses. Therefore, we recommend that collaboration between health care providers should be well described and discussed concerning roles, tasks and responsibilities of individual caretakers. A clear description is important in order to address the needs of the patient populations, and in order to address the individual patient needs.

Conclusion

This overview of systematic reviews shows that collaboration between physicians and nurses may have a positive impact on a number of patient outcomes and on a variety of pathologies. To address future challenges of primary care, there is a need for more integrated inter-professional collaboration and sufficiently educated nurses.

Abbreviations

(HR)QOL: Health related quality of life; ADL: Activities of daily living; APRN: Advanced practice registered nurse; BCI: Bootstrap confidence interval; BMI: Body mass index; BP: Blood pressure; CAD: Coronary artery disease; CBA: Controlled before and after study; CHF: Chronic heart failure; CI: Confidence interval; CNS: Clinical nurse specialist; COPD: Chronic obstructive pulmonary disease; GP: General practitioner; ICU: Intensive care unit; ITS: Interrupted time series; LDL: Low density lipoprotein; NA: Not applicable; NAV: Not available; NCC: Nurse coordinated care; NICU: Neonatal intensive care unit; NP: Nurse practitioner; PA: Physician assistant; RCT: Randomized controlled trial; SCORE: Systematic coronary risk evaluation

Acknowledgements

We thank native speaker mrs Jude Murison for providing feedback on the manuscript.

Funding

The first author, Evi Matthys, received a scholarship from the home care organization 'Wit-Gele Kruis van Antwerpen VZW', to perform a part time PhD. Prof. Dr. Peter Van Bogaert and Prof. Dr. Roy Remmen are full-time academics. All authors declare no conflict of interest. 'Wit-Gele Kruis van Antwerpen VZW' has no role in the design of the study and collection, analysis, and interpretation of data in writing the manuscript.

Authors' contributions

EM searched the databases, reviewed titles, abstracts and full texts, and drafted the manuscript. RR reviewed titles, abstracts and full texts, and drafted the manuscript. PVB reviewed titles, abstracts and full texts, and drafted the manuscript. All authors read and approved the final manuscript.

Consent for publication

Not applicable.

Competing interests

The authors declare that they have no competing interests.

References

1. World Health Organization. Global strategy and action plan on ageing and health (2016–2020). 2016. http://www.who.int/ageing/global-strategy/en/. Accessed 20 May 2017.
2. OECD. Health at a Glance: Europe 2016. State of Health in the EU Cycle. 4th edition. OECD publishing; 2016. p. 204.
3. Ogden J, et al. I want more time with my doctor: a quantitative study of time and the consultation. Fam Pract. 2004;21(5):479–83.
4. Kacenelenbogen N, Offermans AM, Roland M. Burnout of general practitioners in Belgium: societal consequences and paths to solutions. Rev Med Brux. 2011;32(4):413–23.
5. Goetz K, et al. The influence of workload and health behavior on job satisfaction of general practitioners. Fam Med. 2013;45(2):95–101.
6. Gerkens SM, Belgium S. Health System Review. Health Systems in Transition. 2010;12(5):1–266.
7. Berwick DM, Nolan TW, Whittington J. The triple aim: care, health, and cost. Health Aff (Millwood). 2008;27(3):759–69.
8. Kringos DSB, Hutchinson A WGW, Saltman RB. Building Primary Care in a Changing Europe: Case Studies. European Observatory on Health Systems and Policies. 2015;38:172.
9. Hildebrandt H, et al. Pursuing the triple aim: evaluation of the integrated care system Gesundes Kinzigtal: population health, patient experience and cost-effectiveness. Bundesgesundheitsblatt Gesundheitsforschung Gesundheitsschutz. 2015;58(4–5):383–92.
10. Sikka R, Morath JM, Leape L. The quadruple aim: care, health, cost and meaning in work. BMJ Qual Saf. 2015;24(10):608–10.
11. van Uden CJ, Crebolder HF. Does setting up out of hours primary care cooperatives outside a hospital reduce demand for emergency care? Emerg Med J. 2004;21(6):722–3.
12. Laurant M, et al. Substitution of doctors by nurses in primary care. Cochrane Database Syst Rev. 2005. doi:10.1002/14651858.CD001271.pub2.
13. van Loenen T, et al. Organizational aspects of primary care related to avoidable hospitalization: a systematic review. Fam Pract. 2014;31(5):502–16.
14. Longman JM, et al. Admissions for chronic ambulatory care sensitive conditions - a useful measure of potentially preventable admission? BMC Health Serv Res. 2015;15:472.
15. Shea BJ, et al. Development of AMSTAR: a measurement tool to assess the methodological quality of systematic reviews. BMC Med Res Methodol. 2007;7:10.
16. Shea BJ, et al. AMSTAR is a reliable and valid measurement tool to assess the methodological quality of systematic reviews. J Clin Epidemiol. 2009; 62(10):1013–20.
17. Pollock M, Fernandes RM, Hartling L. Evaluation of AMSTAR to assess the methodological quality of systematic reviews in overviews of reviews of healthcare interventions. BMC Med Res Methodol. 2017;17(1):48.
18. Shea BJ, et al. External validation of a measurement tool to assess systematic reviews (AMSTAR). PLoS One. 2007;2(12):e1350.
19. Specialized nursing practice for chronic disease management in the primary care setting: an evidence-based analysis. Ont Health Technol Assess Ser. 2013;13(10):1–66.
20. Martin, J.S., et al., Interprofessional collaboration among nurses and physicians: Making a difference in patient outcome. Swiss Med. Wkly, 2010. 140(SEPTEMBER).
21. Snaterse M, et al. Effective components of nurse-coordinated care to prevent recurrent coronary events: a systematic review and meta-analysis. Heart. 2016;102(1):50–6.
22. Allen J, et al. Quality care outcomes following transitional care interventions for older people from hospital to home: a systematic review. BMC Health Serv Res. 2014;14:346.
23. Newhouse, R.P., et al., Advanced practice nurse outcomes 1990-2008: a systematic review. Nurs Econ, 2011. 29(5): p. 230–250; quiz 251.
24. Smith AA, Kepka D, Yabroff KR. Advanced practice registered nurses, physician assistants and cancer prevention and screening: a systematic review. BMC Health Serv Res. 2014;14:68.
25. Stalpers D, et al. Associations between characteristics of the nurse work environment and five nurse-sensitive patient outcomes in hospitals: a systematic review of literature. Int J Nurs Stud. 2015;52(4):817–35.
26. Team-Based Models for End-of-Life Care: An Evidence-Based Analysis. Ont Health Technol Assess Ser. 2014;14(20):1–49.
27. Aubin M, et al. Interventions to improve continuity of care in the follow-up of patients with cancer. Cochrane Database Syst Rev. 2012. doi:10.1002/14651858.CD007672.pub2.
28. Shaw RJ, et al. Effects of nurse-managed protocols in the outpatient management of adults with chronic conditions: a systematic review and meta-analysis. Ann Intern Med. 2014;161(2):113–21.
29. Renders Carry M, et al. Interventions to improve the management of diabetes mellitus in primary care, outpatient and community settings. Cochrane Database Syst Rev. 2000. doi:10.1002/14651858.CD001481..
30. Dwan K, et al. Systematic review of the empirical evidence of study publication bias and outcome reporting bias - an updated review. PLoS

One. 2013;8(7):e66844.
31. Mahler C, et al. Terminology for interprofessional collaboration: definition and current practice. GMS Z Med Ausbild. 2014;31(4):Doc40.
32. O'Cathain A, Murphy E, Nicholl J. Why, and how, mixed methods research is undertaken in health services research in England: a mixed methods study. BMC Health Serv Res. 2007;7:85.
33. Zwarenstein M, Bryant W. Interventions to promote collaboration between nurses and doctors. Cochrane Database Syst Rev. 2000;2:CD000072.
34. Morgan S, Pullon S, McKinlay E. Observation of interprofessional collaborative practice in primary care teams: an integrative literature review. Int J Nurs Stud. 2015;52(7):1217–30.
35. Rosenstein, A.H. and M. O'Daniel, Disruptive behavior and clinical outcomes: perceptions of nurses and physicians. Am J Nurs, 2005. 105(1): p. 54–64; quiz 64-5.
36. Manojlovich M, DeCicco B. Healthy work environments, nurse-physician communication, and patients' outcomes. Am J Crit Care. 2007;16(6):536–43.
37. Zwarenstein M, et al. Structuring communication relationships for Interprofessional teamwork (SCRIPT): a cluster randomized controlled trial. Trials. 2007;8:23.
38. Schmalenberg C, et al. Excellence through evidence: securing collegial/collaborative nurse-physician relationships, part 1. J Nurs Adm. 2005;35(10): 450–8.
39. Xyrichis A, Lowton K. What fosters or prevents interprofessional teamworking in primary and community care? A literature review. Int J Nurs Stud. 2008;45(1): 140–53.
40. Supper I, et al. Interprofessional collaboration in primary health care: a review of facilitators and barriers perceived by involved actors. J Public Health (Oxf). 2015;37(4):716–27.
41. Davies C. Getting health professionals to work together. BMJ. 2000; 320(7241):1021–2.
42. Walker L, Clendon J, Nelson K. Nursing roles and responsibilities in general practice: three case studies. J Prim Health Care. 2015;7(3):236–43.
43. Freund T, et al. Skill mix, roles and remuneration in the primary care workforce: who are the healthcare professionals in the primary care teams across the world? Int J Nurs Stud. 2015;52(3):727–43.
44. Maier, C.E.A., Nurses in Advanced Roles in Primary Care: Policy Levers for Implementation OECD Health Working Papers. Paris: OECD Publishing.
45. Steinman MA, et al. Improving antibiotic selection: a systematic review and quantitative analysis of quality improvement strategies. Med Care. 2006; 44(7):617–28.
46. Walsh JM, et al. Quality improvement strategies for hypertension management: a systematic review. Med Care. 2006;44(7):646–57.
47. Shojania KG, et al. The effects of on-screen, point of care computer reminders on processes and outcomes of care. Cochrane Database Syst Rev. 2009;3:Cd001096.

11

Support needs of patients with obesity in primary care: a practice-list survey

Elizabeth H. Evans[1*†], Kirby Sainsbury[1†], Dominika Kwasnicka[2], Alex Bolster[1], Vera Araujo-Soares[1] and Falko F. Sniehotta[1]

Abstract

Background: UK guidelines recommend that patients with obesity in primary care receive opportunistic weight loss advice from health care professionals, but there is a lack of research into the characteristics and existing weight management practices of these patients. The aim of this study was to characterise primary care patients with obesity in England, to inform the screening, support, and referral options appropriate to this group.

Methods: We surveyed 1309 patients registered at 15 GP practices in North East England, aged ≥18 years and with objectively recorded obesity (BMI ≥ 30 kg/m^2). Study participants reported their weight history, health status, past and current weight loss activities, motivating factors, weight loss strategies used, professional support received, and perceived barriers to weight loss.

Results: 62% of participants were actively trying to lose weight, and a further 15% had attempted and discontinued weight loss in the last 12 months. Only 20% of the sample had sought GP support for weight loss in the last 12 months; instead, most efforts to lose weight were self-guided and did not use evidence-based strategies. Those who sought GP weight loss support were likely to use it and find it motivating. Participants had attempted weight loss on multiple previous occasions and overall felt less confident and successful at maintaining weight loss than losing it. Participants at greatest clinical risk (higher BMI and more health conditions) reported particularly low confidence and multiple barriers to weight loss, but were nevertheless highly motivated to lose weight and keep it off.

Conclusions: We identified the need for informational, structural, and weight loss maintenance-specific support for GP patients with objectively-recorded obesity. Study participants were motivated to lose weight and keep it off, but lacked the confidence and understanding of effective strategies required to do this. GP weight loss support was acceptable and useful but underutilised, indicating that screening and brief referral interventions to structured programmes may augment patients' current weight management activities and meet key support needs whilst optimising limited primary care resources.

Keywords: Obesity, Overweight, Primary health care

Background

A quarter of UK adults have a body weight that places them in the range for obesity (≥30 kg/m^2) [1], and consequently at elevated risk for weight-related morbidity [2] and mortality [3]. Sustained weight loss of 5–10% is effective in reducing medical risk for these individuals [4]. UK guidelines therefore recommend that primary care staff screen for obesity in the office setting, and opportunistically encourage affected individuals to lose weight by offering advice and signposting to available lifestyle management services [5–7]. Despite recent evidence that brief referral interventions initiated in GP settings are effective [8, 9], concerns about the acceptability of providing weight loss advice [10] have meant that advice and referral are seldom done in practice [11].

Little is known about the potential recipients of weight loss advice: the characteristics, needs and weight management experiences of patients classified as obese presenting in primary care. Most previous research into weight loss attempts in the UK has focused upon the

* Correspondence: elizabeth.evans@newcastle.ac.uk
†Equal contributors
[1]Institute of Health & Society, Newcastle University, Newcastle upon Tyne NE2 4AX, UK
Full list of author information is available at the end of the article

general population, notably via the Health Survey for England (HSE) [12, 13]. HSE participants with a BMI ≥30 kg/m^2 were more likely to report an ongoing weight loss attempt than those with a BMI in the healthy range (76 vs. 30%), and this likelihood was higher still if weight loss had been advised by a health care professional [14]. It is not known whether weight loss attempts in the general practice population with obesity are equally prevalent. Overall, information is needed about the broader weight-related context of patients with obesity in primary care, particularly given the higher intensity of primary healthcare usage in this group [15]. Individuals with obesity are frequently subject to stigmatisation and discrimination [16, 17], and it is vital that weight management offered in primary care is non-judgemental, supportive and both informed by and sensitive to patients' previous experiences.

In the current study, we therefore examined the weight management activities, experiences, needs and attitudes of individuals with obesity in a primary care population, using a postal survey distributed via GP surgeries. We asked participants about their weight history, the importance they placed on weight loss and weight loss maintenance, confidence, past success, motivating factors, use of weight loss strategies, the impact of health conditions on weight control, and other perceived barriers. The aim of this study was to characterise primary care patients with obesity in England, with a view to informing recommendations for the screening, support, and referral options appropriate to this previously undescribed group.

Method

Participants and recruitment procedure

Practice administrative staff identified potential participants at 15 General Practices in North East England (Northumberland and Tyne & Wear) by screening medical record databases in July and August 2015. Patients were eligible if they were aged ≥18 years and had a read code for BMI ≥30 kg/m^2 or for obesity (any type of obesity coded within EMIS/SystmOne) recorded in their notes within the past 12 months. The practice sent a study pack to eligible patients consisting of a personalised letter from the practice, an information sheet and consent form, the study survey, and a postage-paid return envelope addressed to the University. As a gesture of thanks, participants were invited to enter a prize draw to win one of three £100 shopping vouchers by completing an entry form and returning it with the survey in the envelope. The North East and Cumbria Clinical Research Network facilitated recruitment of practices to the study and survey distribution. Ethics approval was obtained on 6 February 2014 from the East Midlands-Derby National Research Ethics Service (REC: 14/EM/0069).

Materials

The survey was designed to obtain the following information from participants:

1. Demographic details, self-rated health (rated from 1 to 5, excellent to poor), and details of current health conditions;
2. Current height and weight, highest and lowest adult weights (excluding pregnancy), number of previous weight loss attempts (lifetime), whether a weight loss attempt was ongoing and, if not, the length of time since last trying to lose weight;
3. In reference to participants' previous weight management efforts *overall*, confidence to lose weight and maintain weight loss, the perceived importance of weight loss and weight loss maintenance, and previous weight loss and weight loss maintenance success (all rated from 1 to 6, very low to very high);
4. Motivating factors for weight loss in participants' most recent weight management efforts (participants selected from a list of 13 common motivating factors and/or specified any other factor(s));
5. Use of weight loss methods within the last 12 months (participants selected from a list of 21 common weight loss strategies and/or specified 'any other strategy/ies), use and source of professional weight loss support within this timeframe, usual frequency of self-weighing, and current levels of physical activity (vigorous, moderate and walking), using the International Physical Activity Questionnaire - Short Form (IPAQ-SF) [18];
6. Perceived barriers to weight loss in participants' most recent weight management efforts (participants selected from a list of 9 common barriers to weight loss and/or specified any other barrier(s)).
7. Any other information participants wished to provide, in a free-text box.

The complete set of questions is provided as an additional file (Additional file 1).

Data analysis

Data were manually entered and analysed using SPSS version 21 [19]; a subset were second-entered to check for accuracy. Ratio and interval-level data were examined for the assumptions of parametric analysis through visual inspection of histograms and Kolmogorov-Smirnov calculations. BMI was computed from self-reported height and weight data using the following formula: BMI = weight (kg) / height^2 (m). The p value threshold was set a priori at $p < 0.001$ to avoid type 1 errors as a result of multiple comparisons. Missing data were dealt with using pairwise deletion as appropriate, and non-plausible height and weight data were excluded from analyses. Pearson's correlation coefficient was used to express associations between variables, and between-group differences were examined using independent-samples t-tests and Pearson chi-squared tests. Free-text data provided in the comments box were analysed using a content-analytic approach [20], in which a coding frame was developed to describe the thematic content and codes assigned to comments by two independent coders.

Results

Sample characteristics

Participants returned 1309 completed surveys out of 5800 sent (response rate = 23%). The sample had a mean age of 59 ± 14 years (range = 18–97) and 54% were women. The majority (90%) self-identified as white British, whilst the remainder self-identified as belonging to other categories (e.g., White European: 1%; mixed race: 1%) or preferred not to say (8%). Roughly a third of the sample was married or cohabitating (61% and 7% respectively); the remainder was single (11%), separated or divorced (10%), or widowed (8%). Just over half the sample had completed education beyond sixth form (degree: 18%; vocational: 35%); the other half had completed A-levels (6%); GCSEs (14%); other (1%); or had education below high school level (20%; prefer not to say/ missing: 6%).

Health status and health conditions

Most participants (83%) reported at least one current health condition, including hypertension (45%), chronic pain (42%), mobility problems (34%), diabetes (27%), and depression and/or anxiety (25%). Respondents who reported at least one health condition were older ($r = 0.29$, $p < 0.001$) and had a significantly higher BMI ($r = 0.13$, $p < 0.001$) than those without. Participants described their overall health as poor (12%), fair (35%), good (38%), very good (13%), or excellent (1%). Participants with higher BMIs reported poorer health ($r = -0.17$, $p < 0.001$); self-rated health did not vary with age ($r = -0.05$, $p = 0.11$) or gender ($r = 0.01$, $p = 0.85$).

Weight and weight loss history

Table 1 summarises participants' weight, weight history, and BMI by gender. According to current self-reported weight, 83% of the sample fell into the obese category (BMI ≥30 kg/m^2), whilst 17% was classified as overweight (BMI 25–29.9 kg/m^2). A BMI in the healthy range was reported by 7 participants (0.5%). Women had significantly higher current ($t_{(1243)} = -7.5$, $p < 0.001$) and lifetime highest ($t_{(1238)} = -7.5$, $p < 0.001$) BMIs compared to men, but lower lifetime lowest BMIs than men

Table 1 Current and lifetime highest/lowest weights and corresponding BMIs by gender

	Women ($n = 703$)				Men ($n = 583$)			
	N	Mean	SD	Min-max	*N*	Mean	SD	Min-max
Current weight (kg)	684	94.1	19.3	53.6–280	577	104.6	16.1	66.8–210
Current BMI (kg/m^2)	684	35.7	6.8	20.4–91.2	570	33.3	4.6	18.5–69.4
Highest lifetime weight (kg)	684	102.3	23.8	56.4–336	573	112.7	19.7	70–230
Highest BMI (kg/m^2)	683	38.8	8.0	21.2–92.6	566	35.8	5.8	18.8–79.4
Lowest lifetime weight (kg)	685	68.5	18.2	42.7–200	558	83.2	14.9	41.8–156
Lowest BMI (kg/m^2)	684	26.0	6.4	16.2–72.6	551	26.5	4.6	14.1–55.5

Gender data missing for 23 participants. Highest lifetime weight excludes pregnancy

($t_{(1226)} = 1.7$, $p < 0.001$). Around a third (31%) of the sample reported that their weight had stayed the same (+/−2 kg) over the past 12 months; equivalent numbers reported weight loss (16%) and weight gain (16%), and 36% said their weight had fluctuated during this time.

Almost two thirds (62%) of the sample reported that they were currently trying to lose weight. Among these participants, this current attempt had lasted anywhere from 1 day to more than 50 years (median = 1 year; IQR = 17–104 weeks). Only 7% of participants reported having never attempted weight loss, while for the remainder, their most recent attempt was within the last 3 months (3.2%), within the last 6 months (2.7%), within the last 12 months (9.1%), or more than 12 months ago (15.1%). A greater proportion of the women (70%) were currently attempting weight loss than men (53%; $\chi^2_{(2)} = 45.7$, $p < 0.001$); women also reported a greater number of weight loss attempts in their lifetimes (16 ± 34 attempts) than men (9 ± 21 attempts; $t_{(1004)} = -3.9$, $p < 0.001$). Participants currently trying to lose weight were significantly younger (57.6 ± 14.8 years) than those who were not (61.1 ± 13.4 years; $t_{(1243)} = 4.1$, $p < 0.001$).

Weight loss: Importance, perceived success, and confidence

Table 2 shows the mean values for, and associations amongst, participants' ratings of global importance, confidence, and perceived success for weight loss and weight loss maintenance, BMI, number of previous weight loss attempts, and number of self-reported health conditions. Overall, participants considered that weight loss and weight loss maintenance were extremely important. They perceived themselves to have been slightly successful at weight loss in the past, but unsuccessful at previous weight loss maintenance. Their confidence to lose

Table 2 Importance, success, and confidence ratings, and correlations with BMI, weight loss attempts, and number of health conditions

		Correlations [99% confidence intervals]		
	Mean (SD)	Current BMI	No. WL attempts	No. health conditions
Importance: WL	5.09 (1.14)	0.19 [0.12 to 0.26]	0.12 [0.05 to 0.19]	.06 [−0.01 to 0.13]
Importance: WLM	5.15 (1.11)	0.18 [0.11 to 0.25]	0.11 [0.4 to 0.18]	.07 [0.0 to 0.14]
Success: WL	3.63 (1.40)	−0.07 [−0.14 to 0.0]	0.01 [−0.08 to 0.06]	−.08 [−0.15 to −0.01]
Success: WLM	2.43 (1.30)	−0.23 [−0.3 to −0.16]	−0.15 [−0.22 to −0.08]	−.06 [−0.13 to 0.01]
Confidence: WL	3.34 (1.43)	−0.15 [−0.22 to −0.08]	−0.05 [−0.12 to 0.02]	−.15 [−0.22 to −0.08]
Confidence: WLM	2.82 (1.36)	−0.23 [−0.3 to −0.16]	−0.14 [−0.21 to −0.07]	−.07 [−0.14 to 0.0]

Note. 99% confidence intervals. All scales from 1 to 6. All correlations Pearson's *r*. *WL* weight loss, *WLM* weight loss maintenance

weight was slightly low, but their confidence to keep weight off after losing it was significantly lower ($t_{(1183)}$ = 15.33, $p < 0.001$).

Participants with higher BMIs considered that weight loss and weight loss maintenance were more important than participants with lower BMIs did. However, participants with higher BMIs were also less confident in their ability to lose weight and to keep it off. BMI was not related to perceptions of past weight loss success, but higher BMI was linked to lower perceived weight loss maintenance success. Participants with higher numbers of previous lifetime weight loss attempts considered weight loss and weight loss maintenance to be more important than those with fewer weight loss attempts. In contrast, perceptions of success and confidence were negatively related to these same factors, such that participants with more numerous lifetime previous weight loss attempts felt less successful and confident at keeping weight off. Participants with greater numbers of health conditions felt less confident at losing weight.

Motivating factors for weight loss

Participants were asked whether specific motivating factors prompted their decision to lose weight in their current or most recent attempt. Most participants reported that a wish to improve their overall health was a motivating factor (77%), followed by unhappiness with body shape/size (64%), unhappiness with appearance (61%), wishing to reduce health risks (60%), wishing to improve physical fitness (55%), and unhappiness with clothes fitting poorly (52%). Advice from a primary care professional (GP/nurse) was reported as a motivating factor by 30% of participants. Other motivating factors included being inspired by others who had recently lost weight (17%), wanting to lose weight for an upcoming event (16%), losing weight in response to comments from other people (14%), and advice from a non-primary care health professional (7%).

Participants who were motivated by primary care advice to lose weight tended to be older and have a greater number of health conditions ($r = 0.12$ and $r = 0.13$ respectively, both $p < 0.001$), but they did not tend to have a higher BMI ($r = 0.08$, $p = 0.005$). Instead, participants with a higher BMI were more likely to identify a health scare as a motivating factor ($r = 0.12$, $p < 0.001$). Younger participants and those with a higher BMI were more likely to be motivated by unhappiness with appearance ($r = 0.11$ and $r = -0.27$ respectively, both $p < 0.001$). Younger participants were also more likely to be motivated by unhappiness with body size/shape ($r = -0.22$, $p < 0.001$), wishing lose weight for a special event ($r = -0.20$, $p < 0.001$), poor fit of clothing ($r = -0.14$, $p < 0.001$) and wishing to improve fitness ($r = -0.11$, $p < 0.001$). Participants with higher numbers of previous weight loss attempts were more likely to cite unhappiness with appearance as a motivating factor ($r = -0.12$, $p < 0.001$) but were no more likely to endorse any of the other motivating factors.

Weight loss strategies and self-weighing

Participants were asked whether they had used specific weight loss strategies in the previous 12 months. Figure 1 shows the proportion of participants who reported using each strategy. Self-directed lifestyle modifications were most commonly used, including increasing fruit and vegetable and water consumption (75% and 58% respectively), switching to lower calorie food/drink items (57%), reducing intake of unhealthy foods and drinks (junk food: 63%; sugary drinks: 54%; alcohol: 47%), reducing portion sizes (65%), and changing eating patterns (e.g., timing of meals: 39%). Physical activity was used by a smaller proportion of patients: 37% became more active, 27% reduced sedentary time, and 26% took up a sport. Participants used strategies involving professional support less frequently: these included membership of a commercial or local authority weight-loss programme (25%), using prescription weight loss pills (i.e., Orlistat: 4%) or using resources from primary care (12%). Bariatric surgery was used by only 2%. A minority of participants used self-regulatory strategies, which included behavioural self-monitoring using a food diary or phone app (e.g., My Fitness Pal: 11%) and setting goals (23%). Participants who used each of these strategies were significantly younger than those who had not used them (all p values <0.001). Most participants weighed themselves at least weekly (weekly: 30%; several times per week: 8%; daily: 11%). The others weighed themselves every couple of weeks (12%), once a month (20%), or

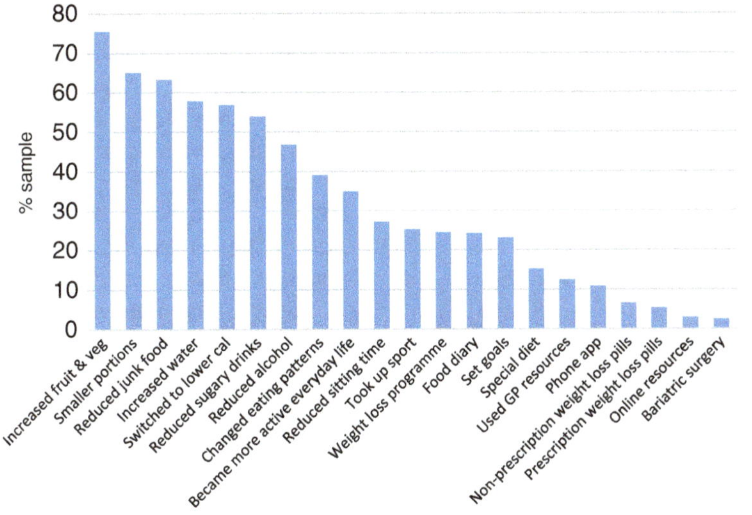

Fig. 1 Proportion of participants who used specific weight loss strategies ($N = 1309$)

never (11%). The majority of respondents weighed themselves at home (73%) rather than in another setting.

Professional weight loss support

A minority (40%) of the whole sample had sought some form of professional support in relation to their weight in the past 12 months: from a GP or practice nurse (20%), commercial weight loss consultant (13%), dietitian (9%) or exercise specialist (7%). Nutritionists, psychologists, and secondary care staff were rarely used for weight loss support (all <2%). Recent use of professional support was significantly higher amongst participants currently trying to lose weight (49%) than participants not currently trying (24%; $\chi^2_{(2)} = 54.7$, $p < 0.001$). Of the subgroup of participants trying to lose weight ($n = 810$), 25% had consulted a GP or practice nurse: these individuals were highly likely to use GP resources in their weight loss attempt ($r = 0.47$, $p < 0.001$) and likely to report that GP or practice nurse advice motivated their weight loss attempt ($r = 0.17$, $p < 0.001$).

Physical activity

Levels of physical activity that met current recommendations of at least 75 min of vigorous activity per week or 150 min of moderate activity per week were reported by 42% of participants. A greater proportion of men (49%) than women (37%; $\chi^2_{(2)} = 18.1$, $p < 0.001$) did so. Participants with recommended levels of physical activity had a slightly lower BMI than those who did not, but this did not reach the threshold for statistical significance ($r = 0.08$ $p < 0.01$). The majority (60%) of participants reported no vigorous physical activity at all, whilst 55% reported no moderate-intensity physical activity, and 15% reported doing no walking each week. The mean reported time spent walking per day was 15 min (median = 1 h).

Barriers to weight loss

Participants were asked whether they experienced specific barriers to weight loss during their most recent attempt. Commonly reported barriers included feeling tired (49%), stressed (41%), demotivated (38%) or low (37%). Participants reported feeling that they were missing out (30%), getting bored of routine (28%), did not have enough time (25%), and had competing priorities (17%). Thirty-seven percent of participants also reported that health conditions made it harder to lose weight: conditions perceived as barriers included arthritis (6% of total sample), diabetes (5%), joint/spinal problems (5%), thyroid problems (3%), cardiac problems (2%), and respiratory conditions (2%). Participants with greater numbers of barriers to weight loss had higher BMIs ($r = 0.22$, $p < 0.001$) and reported higher numbers of health conditions ($r = 0.16$, $p < 0.001$). They felt less confident about losing weight ($r = -0.15$, $p < 0.001$) and maintaining weight loss ($r = -0.23$, $p < 0.001$), and considered themselves less successful at weight loss maintenance ($r = -0.17$, $p < 0.001$).

Free-text comments about weight control

At the end of the survey, participants were invited to provide any additional comments in a free-text box. Comments were provided by 498 (38%) participants. Using a content analytic approach, we double-coded participant comments for common themes. Most provided further details of barriers to weight loss, including physical health ($n = 87$), pain ($n = 19$), limited mobility ($n = 19$), occupational demands ($n = 42$), family commitments ($n = 29$), poor psychological health ($n = 52$), and medication causing weight gain ($n = 11$). Participants stated that insufficient help was available to help them lose weight ($n = 23$), and highlighted the particular difficulty of maintaining weight loss once it had been achieved (n = 27). A smaller number described successful weight loss, all with commercial providers (n = 15). Others reflected on experiences in primary care that influenced their efforts to lose weight loss (n = 20): most participants described their experiences negatively, highlighting an absence of encouragement or advice.

Discussion

The results of this cross-sectional survey showed that primary care patients with objectively-recorded obesity were actively engaged in weight loss attempts, considered weight control to be important and had extensive previous experience of trying to lose weight and keep it off. However, participants' confidence and perceived success were low for weight loss and still lower for weight loss maintenance. Weight loss attempts tended to be self-guided (unsupported), using strategies without clear evidence of effectiveness, and were impeded by both psychological and physical health-related barriers. Overall, responses suggested an unmet need for informational support (particularly for weight loss maintenance), sign-posting to structured services, and recognition of the complex experiential and motivational context in which patients attempt weight control.

The majority of survey participants were actively trying to lose weight, indicating that guidance on *how* to lose weight is likely to be more useful to patients than advice to simply initiate weight loss. It appears more fruitful to capitalise upon and shape patients' existing efforts than to assume that they are currently disengaged. The proportion actively trying to lose weight (62%) resembled previous studies with participants with overweight and obesity [21–24] but was lower than in HSE participants with obesity (76%; [12]). Amongst those trying to lose weight, a minority had recently sought professional weight loss support and only a quarter had sought advice from primary care in the past 12 months, despite health concerns being the most common motivating factor for weight loss, in keeping with previous research [24, 25]. Those that did seek primary care advice were highly likely to go on to use primary care resources for weight loss and cite the advice received as a motivating factor in their weight loss attempt. Overall, this indicates that primary care advice and signposting has the potential to augment the activities of primary care patients not already using it, and complements existing evidence that such support is acceptable to, and would be viewed favourably by, patients [26, 27].

The most commonly-used weight loss strategies were those with inconclusive evidence for weight loss effectiveness, so providing information about the best-evidenced strategies may be useful to many primary care patients with obesity. Popular strategies were coherent with self-guided 'healthy lifestyle' advice but have not been shown to be effective weight loss interventions in isolation: these included increasing fruit and vegetable consumption [28, 29], reducing portion size [30] and drinking more water [31]. Strategies with stronger evidence bases, such as following a structured weight loss programme [32], using Orlistat [33], and goal setting and self-monitoring [34, 35] were used less frequently. Indeed, the finding that most participants' weight loss strategies were essentially self-guided (unsupported) is of particular concern given participants' limited confidence for weight loss and weight loss maintenance. Although we did not ask about participants' weight loss maintenance strategies, it is notable that overall confidence for maintenance was lower than that for weight loss, suggesting a greater need for support in this area. Overall, information that explicitly differentiates 'health' from 'weight loss' messages may be of particular benefit, as may recommendations for existing, supported weight loss programmes or drug regimens [32, 33].

Participants were less confident about maintaining weight loss than losing weight, and felt less successful at maintenance than loss, indicating the need for maintenance-specific advice and support. Whilst effective weight loss maintenance interventions exist [36], scalable interventions do not yet [37], and thus maintenance provision is limited in both commercial and local authority contexts. UK clinical guidelines contain minimal maintenance-specific content [5–7]. Maintenance confidence and success were lowest amongst those with higher BMIs and more previous weight loss attempts, possibly because repeated attempts and increasing weight ultimately reduced participants' belief that they are capable of keeping weight off over the longer term [38]. Similar relationships were not seen with confidence and success for weight loss. Overall, these findings highlight the importance of sign-posting patients to support, even if they have already achieved some weight loss independently, and of prompting patients to plan ahead for maintenance in discussions of weight loss strategies.

Participants at greatest apparent clinical risk, i.e., those with the highest BMIs and most numerous health conditions, were also those with the lowest confidence for weight loss and weight loss maintenance, indicating that this group of individuals may be in particular need of support. All the aforementioned factors have been shown to be prognostic of poor weight loss and weight loss maintenance in previous research [39, 40]. This group of participants also reported more numerous previous weight loss attempts and barriers, and lower perceived weight loss maintenance success. Health conditions were a key barrier to weight loss for participants, particularly those who were older, had higher BMIs, and lower weight loss confidence. However, this group still considered weight loss and weight loss maintenance to be important and were more likely to seek primary care support than others. These findings underscore the need to proactively discuss weight loss with patients with high BMI and multimorbidity, even though primary care staff may avoid doing so when they perceive there are other priorities such as health conditions [41].

Concerns about bodily appearance, size, and shape were particularly pertinent motivating factors to younger patients, as was the wish to become fitter, whereas health concerns were reported as motivating factors by patients of all ages. The latter finding is inconsistent with prior research indicating that health-related motivation for weight loss increases with age, particularly in men [42], but it may be attributable to the comparatively higher mean participant age in the current study. The former finding suggests that primary care staff should be particularly sensitive to the importance of body image and drive to improve fitness amongst younger patients. Counter-intuitively, but in keeping with recent meta-analytic findings [24], younger participants had higher numbers of previous weight loss attempts than older participants, potentially a consequence of greater social pressure to lose weight in this group [43]. Such pressure may also explain our finding that those with greater numbers of weight loss attempts were more likely to be motivated by appearance concerns.

A key strength of the study was the recruitment of participants with recently-recorded objective obesity from systematic searches of GP lists. Weight studies reliant upon self-selection tend to disproportionately attract women [44], whereas men and women were more equally represented in the current sample. Surveys using self-reported BMI data as a determinant of eligibility are vulnerable to the effects of systematic underreporting of weight and over-reporting of height [45]. Here, eligibility was determined using objective data from practice records. The aforementioned underreporting of current weight and height may explain the finding that, according to the self-report survey data, only 83% of the sample was classified as obese, with 17% reporting a BMI in the overweight range, and 0.5% in the healthy weight range. Alternatively, inaccuracies in patient records may explain this, as found in a previous study [46]; a consequent study limitation is that patients with a BMI in the eligible range may have been missed because their weight status has not been correctly coded. The response rate achieved (23%) is comparable to that of similar ad hoc surveys asking about health and lifestyle behaviours [47–49], but lower than other, larger surveys such as the GP Patient Survey [50]. More than 90% of participants in the current study self-identified as white. This limits the extent to which the study findings are generalizable to more diverse populations, although it accurately reflects the ethnic composition of the geographical area in which the survey was distributed [51]. The data presented are cross-sectional and, as such, causal inferences are precluded. Finally, data were not available regarding individual participants' frequency of primary care usage, and the sample's demographic composition (e.g., approximately equal numbers of men and women) differs from the typical composition of patients utilising UK primary care consultations [52] although the mean participant age is broadly consistent with it.

Conclusion

We examined the weight loss support needs of GP patients with objectively-recorded obesity in North East England, and identified the need for informational, structural, and weight loss maintenance-specific support. Study participants were motivated to lose weight and keep it off, but lacked the confidence and understanding of effective strategies required to do this. A minority had sought structured weight management support and fewer still advice from primary care, but those that did found it motivating and useful. GP provision of demonstrably-effective brief referral interventions to structured weight loss support [8] may be acceptable to these patients, to augment their current weight management activities and to optimise limited GP time and resources.

Abbreviations

BMI: Body mass index; GP: General practitioner

Acknowledgements

The authors wish to thank the staff of the North East and Cumbria Clinical Research Network for their invaluable assistance in communicating with practices about the study and coordinating the study distribution process. We are extremely grateful to the partners and other staff of the medical practices involved for agreeing to be involved in the study and for conducting the practice list searches, writing to patients, and labelling questionnaires for distribution. We would like to especially thank the participants who so generously gave their time and effort to completing the weight management survey. We hugely appreciate the contribution of Dr. Stephan Dombrowski (University of Stirling) to the pilot study for this work.

Funding

The study was partially funded by the UK National Prevention Research Initiative (NPRI) Phase 4 (grant MR/J000477/1). The NPRI includes the following Funding Partners (in alphabetical order): Alzheimer's Research Trust, Alzheimer's Society, Biotechnology and Biological Sciences Research Council, British Heart Foundation, Cancer Research UK, Chief Scientist Office, Scottish Government Health Directorate, Department of Health, Diabetes UK, Economic and Social Research Council, Health and Social Care Research and Development Division of the Public Health Agency (HSC & R&D Division), Medical Research Council, The Stroke Association, Wellcome Trust, Welsh Assembly Government and World Cancer Research Fund. FFS is funded by Fuse, the Centre for Translational Research in Public Health, a UKCRC Public Health Research Centre of Excellence based on funding from the British

Heart Foundation, Cancer Research UK, Economic and Social Research Council, Medical Research Council, and the National Institute for Health Research, under the auspices of the UK Clinical Research Collaboration. The funding body had no role in the study design, data collection, analysis, data interpretation or writing of this manuscript.

Authors' contributions

FFS and VAS conceived of the study. FFS and EE designed the study and VAS, EE and DK developed questionnaire items. EE and DK implemented the study under the supervision of FFS and VAS. KS, DK and AB transcribed study data and KS, EE and AB carried out data analysis. EE and KS drafted the manuscript and all authors read and approved the final manuscript.

Consent for publication

Not applicable.

Competing interests

The authors declare that they have no competing interests.

Author details

[1]Institute of Health & Society, Newcastle University, Newcastle upon Tyne NE2 4AX, UK. [2]School of Psychology and Speech Pathology, Curtin University, GPO Box U1987, Perth, WA 6845, Australia.

References

1. Ng M, Fleming T, Robinson M, Thomson B, Graetz N, Margono C, Mullany EC, Biryukov S, Abbafati C, Abera SF, et al. Global, regional, and national prevalence of overweight and obesity in children and adults during 1983-2013: a systematic analysis for the global burden of disease study 2013. Lancet. 2014;384(9945):766–81.
2. Guh DP, Zhang W, Bansback N, Amarsi Z, Birmingham CL, Anis AH. The incidence of co-morbidities related to obesity and overweight: a systematic review and meta-analysis. BMC Public Health. 2009;9:88.
3. The Global BMI Mortality Collaboration. Body-mass index and all-cause mortality: individual-participant-data meta-analysis of 239 prospective studies in four continents. Lancet. 2016;388(10046):776–86.
4. Avenell A, Broom J, Brown TJ, Poobalan A, Aucott L, Stearns SC, Smith WCS, Jung RT, Campbell MK, Grant AM. Systematic review of the long-term effects and economic consequences of treatments for obesity and implications for health improvement. Health Technol Assess. 2004;8(21): 1–182.
5. National Institute of Health and Care Excellence. Obesity: identification, assessment and management of overweight and obesity in children, young people and adults. CG189. London: National Institute of Health and Care Excellence; 2014.
6. National Institute of Health and Care Excellence. Obesity in adults: prevention and lifestyle weight management programmes (QS111). London: National Institute of Health and Care Excellence; 2016.
7. Scottish Intercollegiate Guidelines Network. Management of Obesity: a national clinical guideline (115): Scottish Intercollegiate Guidelines Network; 2010.
8. Aveyard P, Lewis A, Tearne S, Hood K, Christian-Brown A, Adab P, Begh R, Jolly K, Daley A, Farley A, et al. Screening and brief intervention for obesity in primary care: a parallel, two-arm, randomised trial. Lancet. 2016; 388(10059):2492–500.
9. Rose SA, Poynter PS, Anderson JW, Noar SM, Conigliaro J. Physician weight loss advice and patient weight loss behavior change: a literature review and meta-analysis of survey data. Int J Obes. 2013;37(1):118–28.
10. Blackburn M, Stathi A, Keogh E, Eccleston C. Raising the topic of weight in general practice: perspectives of GPs and primary care nurses. BMJ Open. 2015;5(8):e008546.
11. Shiffman S, Sweeney CT, Pillitteri JL, Sembower MA, Harkins AM, Wadden TA. Weight management advice: what do doctors recommend to their patients? Prev Med. 2009;49(6):482–6.
12. Piernas C, Aveyard P, Jebb SA. Recent trends in weight loss attempts: repeated cross-sectional analyses from the Health Survey for England. Int J Obes. 2016;40:1754–9.
13. Jackson SE, Wardle J, Johnson F, Finer N, Beeken RJ. The impact of a health professional recommendation on weight loss attempts in overweight and obese British adults: a cross-sectional analysis. BMJ Open. 2013;3(11): e003693.
14. Bastien M, Poirier P, Lemieux I, Després J-P. Overview of epidemiology and contribution of obesity to cardiovascular disease. Prog Cardiovasc Dis. 2014; 56(4):369–81.
15. Frost GS, Lyons GF. Obesity impacts on general practice appointments. Obes Res. 2005;13(8):1442–9.
16. Puhl R, Peterson JL, Luedicke J. Fighting obesity or obese persons? Public perceptions of obesity-related health messages. Int J Obes. 2013;37(6):774–82.
17. Puhl RM, Heuer CA. Obesity stigma: important considerations for public health. Am J Public Health. 2010;100(6):1019–28.
18. Booth ML, Ainsworth BE, Pratt M, Ekelund U, Yngve A, Sallis JF, Oja P. International physical activity questionnaire: 12-country reliability and validity. Med Sci Sport Exerc. 2003;195(9131/03):3508–1381.
19. IBM Corp. IBM SPSS statistics for windows. Version 21.0. Armonk, NY: IBM Corp; 2012.
20. O'Cathain A, Thomas KJ. "Any other comments?" Open questions on questionnaires–a bane or a bonus to research? BMC Med Res Methodol. 2004;4(1):25.
21. Johnston DW, Lordan G. Weight perceptions, weight control and income: an analysis using British data. Econ Hum Biol. 2014;12:132–9.
22. Anderson LA, Eyler AA, Galuska DA, Brown DR, Brownson RC. Relationship of satisfaction with body size and trying to lose weight in a national survey of overweight and obese women aged 40 and older, United States. Prev Med. 2002;35(4):390–6.
23. Bish CL, Blanck HM, Maynard LM, Serdula MK, Thompson NJ, Khan LK. Health-related quality of life and weight loss practices among overweight and obese US adults, 2003 Behavioral Risk Factor Surveillance System. MedGenMed. 2007;9(2):35.
24. Santos I, Sniehotta FF, Marques MM, Carraça EV, Teixeira PJ. Prevalence of personal weight control attempts in adults: a systematic review and meta-analysis. Obes Rev. 2016;18(1):32–50.
25. Visram S, Crosland A, Cording H. Triggers for weight gain and loss among participants in a primary care-based intervention. Br J Community Nurs. 2009;14(11):495–501.
26. Potter MB, JD V, Croughan-Minihane M. Weight management: what patients want from their primary care physicians. J Fam Pract. 2001;50(6):513.
27. Tan D, Zwar NA, Dennis SM, Vagholkar S. Weight management in general practice: what do patients want? Med J Australia. 2006;185(2):73–5.
28. Mytton OT, Nnoaham K, Eyles H, Scarborough P, Mhurchu CN. Systematic review and meta-analysis of the effect of increased vegetable and fruit consumption on body weight and energy intake. BMC Public Health. 2014; 14(1):1.
29. Kaiser KA, Brown AW, Brown MMB, Shikany JM, Mattes RD, Allison DB. Increased fruit and vegetable intake has no discernible effect on weight loss: a systematic review and meta-analysis. Am J Clin Nutr. 2014;100(2):567–76.
30. Rolls BJ. What is the role of portion control in weight management? Int J Obes. 2014;38(Suppl 1):S1–8.
31. Muckelbauer R, Sarganas G, Grüneis A, Müller-Nordhorn J. Association between water consumption and body weight outcomes: a systematic review. Am J Clin Nutr. 2013; ajcn. 055061
32. Jolly K, Lewis A, Beach J, Denley J, Adab P, Deeks JJ, Daley A, Aveyard P. Comparison of range of commercial or primary care led weight reduction programmes with minimal intervention control for weight loss in obesity: lighten up randomised controlled trial. BMJ. 2011;343:d6500.
33. Franz MJ, VanWormer JJ, Crain AL, Boucher JL, Histon T, Caplan W, Bowman JD, Pronk NP. Weight-loss outcomes: a systematic review and meta-analysis of weight-loss clinical trials with a minimum 1-year follow-up. J Am Diet Assoc. 2007;107(10):1755–67.
34. Burke LE, Wang J, Sevick MA. Self-monitoring in weight loss: a systematic review of the literature. J Am Diet Assoc. 2011;111(1):92–102.
35. Greaves CJ, Sheppard KE, Abraham C, Hardeman W, Roden M, Evans PH, Schwarz P. Systematic review of reviews of intervention components associated with increased effectiveness in dietary and physical activity

interventions. BMC Public Health. 2011;11(1):1.
36. Dombrowski SU, Knittle K, Avenell A, Araujo-Soares V, Sniehotta FF. Long term maintenance of weight loss with non-surgical interventions in obese adults: systematic review and meta-analyses of randomised controlled trials. BMJ. 2014;348:g2646.
37. Evans EH, Araújo-Soares V, Adamson A, Batterham AM, Brown H, Campbell M, Dombrowski SU, Guest A, Jackson D, Kwasnicka D. The NULevel trial of a scalable, technology-assisted weight loss maintenance intervention for obese adults after clinically significant weight loss: study protocol for a randomised controlled trial. Trials. 2015;16(1):421.
38. Teixeira PJ, Going SB, Sardinha LB, Lohman TG. A review of psychosocial pre-treatment predictors of weight control. Obes Rev. 2005;6(1):43–65.
39. Teixeira PJ, Going SB, Houtkooper LB, Cussler EC, Metcalfe LL, Blew RM, Sardinha LB, Lohman TG. Pretreatment predictors of attrition and successful weight management in women. Int J Obes Relat Metab Disord. 2004;28(9): 1124–33.
40. Elfhag K, Rössner S. Who succeeds in maintaining weight loss? A conceptual review of factors associated with weight loss maintenance and weight regain. Obes Rev. 2005;6(1):67–85.
41. Jochemsen-Van Der Leeuw HGA, Van Dijk N, Wieringa-de Waard M. Attitudes towards obesity treatment in GP training practices: a focus group study. Fam Pract. 2011;28(4):422–9.
42. Hankey C, Leslie WS, Lean MEJ. Why lose weight? Reasons for seeking weight loss by overweight but otherwise healthy men. Int J Obes. 2002;26:880–2.
43. Evans EH, Boothroyd LG, Muscariello E, Stephan BCM, Nasti G, Colantuoni A, Siervo M. Lower weight loss expectations and healthier eating attitudes in older overweight and obese women attempting weight loss. Clin Obes. 2015;5(3):136–44.
44. Pagoto SL, Schneider KL, Oleski JL, Luciani JM, Bodenlos JS, Whited MC. Male inclusion in randomized controlled trials of lifestyle weight loss interventions. Obesity. 2012;20(6):1234–9.
45. Shiely F, Perry IJ, Lutomski J, Harrington J, Kelleher CC, McGee H, Hayes K. Temporal trends in misclassification patterns of measured and self-report based body mass index categories-findings from three population surveys in Ireland. BMC Public Health. 2010;10(1):1.
46. Sniehotta FF, Dombrowski SU, Avenell A, Johnston M, McDonald S, Murchie P, Ramsay CR, Robertson K, Araujo-Soares V. Randomised controlled feasibility trial of an evidence-informed Behavioural intervention for obese adults with additional risk factors. PLoS One. 2011;6(8):e23040.
47. Sahlqvist S, Song Y, Bull F, Adams E, Preston J, Ogilvie D. Effect of questionnaire length, personalisation and reminder type on response rate to a complex postal survey: randomised controlled trial. BMC Med Res Methodol 2011, 11(1):1.
48. Coombes E, Jones AP, Hillsdon M. The relationship of physical activity and overweight to objectively measured green space accessibility and use. Soc Sci Med. 2010;70(6):816–22.
49. Sharpe RA, Thornton CR, Nikolaou V, Osborne NJ. Higher energy efficient homes are associated with increased risk of doctor diagnosed asthma in a UK subpopulation. Environ Int. 2015;75:234–44.
50. Warren FC, Abel G, Lyratzopoulos G, Elliott MN, Richards S, Barry HE, Roland M, Campbell JL. Characteristics of service users and provider organisations associated with experience of out of hours general practitioner care in England: population based cross sectional postal questionnaire survey. BMJ. 2015;350:h2040.
51. Office for National Statistics. Ethnicity and national identity in England and Wales: 2011. London, UK: Office for National Statistics; 2012.
52. Hobbs FDR, Bankhead C, Mukhtar T, Stevens S, Perera-Salazar R, Holt T, Salisbury C. Clinical workload in UK primary care: a retrospective analysis of 100 million consultations in England, 2007–14. Lancet. 2016;387(10035): 2323–30.

12

Identification, description and appraisal of generic PROMs for primary care

Mairead Murphy*, Sandra Hollinghurst and Chris Salisbury

Abstract

Background: Patients attend primary care with many types of problems and to achieve a range of possible outcomes. There is currently a lack of patient-reported outcome measures (PROMs) designed to capture these diverse outcomes. The objective of this systematic review was to identify, describe and appraise generic PROMs suitable for measuring outcomes from primary care.

Methods: We carried out a systematic Medline search, supplemented by other online and hand-searches. All potentially relevant PROMs were itemised in a long-list. Each PROM in the long-list which met inclusion criteria was included in a short-list. Short-listed PROMs were then described in terms of their measurement properties and construct, based on a previously published description of primary care outcome as three constructs: health status, health empowerment and health perceptions. PROMs were appraised in terms of extent of psychometric testing (extensive, moderate, low) and level of responsiveness (high, medium, low, unknown).

Results: More than 5000 abstracts were identified and screened to identify PROMs potentially suitable for measuring outcomes from primary care. 321 PROMs were long-listed, and twenty PROMs were catalogued in detail. There were five PROMs which measured change directly, without need for a baseline. Although these had less strong psychometric properties, they may be more responsive to change than PROMs which capture status at a point in time. No instruments provided coverage of all three constructs. Of the health status questionnaires, the most extensively tested was the SF-36. Of the health empowerment instruments, the PEI, PAM and heiQ provided the best combination of responsiveness and psychometric testing. The health perceptions instruments were all less responsive to change, and may measure a form of health perception which is difficult to shift in primary care.

Conclusions: This systematic review is the first of its kind to identify papers describing the development and validation of generic PROMs suitable for measuring outcomes from primary care. It identified that: 1) to date, there is no instrument which comprehensively covers the outcomes commonly sought in primary care, and 2) there are different benefits both to PROMs which measure status at a point in time, and PROMs which measure change directly.

Keywords: Systematic review, Patient-reported outcomes, Primary care, Questionnaires, Generic PROMs, Transitional PROMs

* Correspondence: mairead.murphy@bristol.ac.uk
Population Health Sciences, Bristol Medical School, University of Bristol, Canynge Hall, 39 Whatley Road, Bristol BS8 2PS, UK

Background

Introduction

Patient-reported outcome measures (PROMs) are self-report questionnaires designed to capture information on patients' health. An 'outcome' is change in health status, knowledge or behaviour which is attributable to preceding healthcare [1], and PROMs provide important evidence about this change as it is experienced by the patient [2]. There are thousands of PROMs in existence, with new PROMs being developed every day [3]. Experts in the field have called for harmonisation in this area [4], including research into existing instruments before development of new ones [5].

PROMs were originally developed to aid in evaluating and comparing the effectiveness of healthcare interventions [3]. By comparing patients' PROM scores before and after an intervention, the outcome of the intervention can be assessed. Numerous primary care interventions have been developed in recent years to meet changing population and service needs (including an aging population and increasing numbers of people with multi-morbidity [6, 7]). While there are a number of disease and problem-specific PROMs which can be used in primary care, many primary care interventions are targeted at people with a range of conditions or problems. Examples include electronic consultations [8], health coaching and behavioural change therapies [9, 10], and new approaches to address the needs of frequent attenders in general practice [11, 12]. Assessing the effectiveness of such interventions from a patient perspective requires a *generic* PROM, which can be administered across a population, regardless of presenting problem. Such a PROM should cover multi-layered outcomes encompassing aspects of enablement, resilience, symptoms and function, and health perceptions.

We conjectured that there was no such suitable PROM for primary care and undertook to investigate this through a review of the literature. We identified existing structured reviews of PROMs on related topics: for example PROMs for mental health [13], empowerment [14, 15], integrative medicine [16], patient experience [17] patient safety in primary care [18] and generic health status in older people [19]. However, an initial search of the literature found there was no structured review for generic PROMs specific to the measurement of outcome across all primary care patients.

We firstly carried out a qualitative study to delineate the domains which should be captured by a Primary Care PROM [20]. We then conducted a systematic review of PROMs suitable for primary care, which captured these domains.

Prior qualitative study

In our prior Qualitative study, we identified and categorised inter-related outcomes into ten groups occupying three domains:

1. **Health Status**: This involves both symptoms and medication side-effects and the impact of symptoms on patients' lives.
2. **Health Empowerment**: These are the internal and external resources which enable patients to improve their health. The internal resources include an understanding of health conditions, and an ability to self-care, stay healthy and follow a clinician-patient agreed plan. The external resources include patients' confidence in seeking healthcare, and ability to access suitable health-related supports. Although these external aspects are closely related to the patient experience of the consultation, they are the enduring impacts of the consultation that have a direct influence on patient's overall health status and are qualitatively different from measures of patient experience [20].
3. **Health Perceptions**: This involves health concerns and satisfaction, and confidence in their health for the future.

This study reports on a systematic review of PROMs suitable for use in primary care to measure these outcomes.

Methods

Search strategy

We designed a customised search strategy for Medline Ovid SP, following PRISMA guidelines where appropriate [21]. This was peer-reviewed by a University of Bristol librarian and included indexed papers from 1950 to 8th March 2014. The PICO framework normally used in systematic reviews (population, intervention, comparator and outcomes) [22] was adapted in order to identify primary care PROMs; the framework used was: Population, Aim, Subject and Construct (PASC). Four filters were developed using these PASC categories combined with an AND operator. The population filter was designed to retrieve papers relevant to primary care; the aim and subject filters combined were designed to retrieve papers describing development and validation of PROMs; and the construct filter was aimed at the domains of interest (health status, health empowerment, and health perceptions). Search terms for each category were developed through an iterative process of adjusting filters and performing test searches. A full description of the four filters is shown in Additional file 1.

We recognised that limiting the search to the Medline database meant some relevant papers may have been missed. We therefore followed-up all PROMs referred to in screened abstracts, contacted eighteen experts in the field, hand-searched three compilations of PROMs (McDowell [23], Bowling [24], and PROQOLID [25]) and screened all abstracts on the Oxford University PROMs group database using the keywords "individualised", "generic", "utility" or "primary care". (This a database of papers relating to patient-reported outcome measures, which contains references to more than 14,000 papers, last updated in 2005) [26]. A backwards reference search was carried out on all twenty original papers included in the final review, and a forward reference search for sixteen of the twenty original papers. (The four exceptions were those which had been cited more than 600 times).

Selection of PROMs

All abstracts identified in the electronic searches were screened. During this process, any PROMs named in the abstract were listed, apart from those which did not meet the inclusion criteria.

For each of the PROMs in the long list, a copy of the instrument was obtained from either a PROMs compilation [23, 24, 26, 27] or the initial development paper. Selection was based on inclusion and exclusion criteria on the *PROMs*, as opposed to the *papers* (see Table 1). To ensure decisions were made consistently, reasons for exclusion were documented against each PROM. (See Additional file 2).

Abstract screening and data extraction was done by a single reviewer (MM). The other two reviewers (CS/SH) independently checked the extracted data (shown in Figs. 1, 2 and 3), and reviewed the long-list of PROMs excluded from the review. (Additional file 2).

Data extraction

The selected PROMs were described in a tabular format (see Figs. 1 to 3). Data was extracted on their measurement properties, construct and psychometric properties.

The measurement properties extracted were adapted from an existing PROM classification framework [25], and included the number of items, the nature of the scale, the recall period, the level of PROM adaptability and the dimensionality.

The construct categories extracted were based on the prior qualitative study [20]. Where a construct was explicitly covered, this was block-highlighted in the tabular description. Where it was implicit (for example, an individualised questionnaire which asks about symptoms covers pain, but not explicitly) it was shaded.

The review of psychometric properties was limited to the *extent* of psychometric testing, and the *level* of responsiveness. PROMs were categorised as having an extensive, moderate or low extent of psychometric testing, depending on the number of validation studies published, whether the authorship of these papers extended beyond the original authors, and on number of times the original development paper has been cited. (see additional file 3 for details). With the exception of responsiveness, we chose not to provide categorical ratings for individual psychometric properties (for example, validity, reliability, interpretability) because these are actually properties of PROMs *as administered in a particular population*, not of property of a PROM in and of itself [28]. Although some structured reviews of PROMs have provided such categorical ratings[16], leading textbook compilations appraise these properties descriptively [23, 27] and we also took this approach. We made an exception for responsiveness, because the current study was based on the hypothesis that there is no suitably responsive PROM for testing interventions in primary care, so it was necessary to test this hypothesis. We categorised responsiveness as: unknown (responsiveness not known or tested); low (responsiveness shown in at least one study); medium (repeated evidence for responsiveness, including in primary care); high (responsiveness shown in primary care studies where other leading PROMs are not responsive).

PROM compilations [23, 24, 26, 27] were reviewed to extract psychometric information relating to the most common PROMs (e.g. the SF-36). Where the PROM was not listed in a complication, a forward

Table 1 Inclusion and exclusion criteria for long-listed PROMs

	Inclusion criteria	Exclusion criteria
Construct	1. PROMs which provide wide coverage of at least one domain as specified from the Qualitative Study.	1. Construct: PROMs excluded on the basis of construct may be: a) unrelated constructs – e.g. adjustment to illness, b) related, but covering only a single sub-domain (e.g. pain, adherence), c) related, but mostly comprising of constructs which were not identified in the Qualitative Study (e.g. quality of life, personality traits).
Population	2. PROMs which have been used in primary care, or for patients with chronic conditions / minor illness. 3. PROMs suitable for use in adults, across both sexes, any disease and any presenting health problems.	2. Disease Specific (e.g. asthma). 3. Population-specific (e.g. the elderly, the functionally limited, children). 4. Intervention-specific (e.g. occupational health, social care).
Administration	4. PROMs which can be self-administered, and are self-reported.	5. Not patient-reported (e.g. clinician-reported, proxy-reported and strictly interview administered).
Other Criteria	5. Instruments in English which can be completed in ten minutes or less.	6. Not available in English. 7. Too long (longer than 50 items).

Instrument Details					Measurement Properties				Construct: Health Status – symptoms				Health Status – symptom affects			Health Empowerment – Internal				Health Empowerment – External	Health Perceptions			Psychometric properties	
	Tool Name	Author	Date	Items	Scale: (a) Status(S)/Transitional(T)	Recall Period	Adaptability: (b) Standard(S)/Individual(I)	Dimensionality: (c) Profile(P)/Index(I)/Utility(U)	1a.Pain	1b. Anxiety/depression	1c. Other symptoms	1d. Side-effects	2a. Normal activities	2b. Can enjoy life	2c. Impact on others	3.Understanding	4. Self-care/stay healthy	5. Plan/adherence	6. Confidence seeking care	7. Access to support	8. Health satisfaction	9. Health concerns	10. On track for future	Extent of psychometric testing (d)	Responsiveness (e)
1	SF-36	Ware	1992	36	S	1/4 weeks	S	P/U	■	■	■		■	■							■		■	extensive	Medium
2	SF-12	Ware	1996	12	S	1/4 weeks	S	P/U		■	■		■	■							■			extensive	Medium
3	EQ-5D	Brooks	1996	5	S	today	S	U	■	■			■	░										extensive	Medium
4	COOP	Nelson	1990	9	S	4 weeks	S	P	■	■			■	■						■	■			moderate	Medium
5	CMP	various		1	T	up to present	S	I	░	░	░	░	░	░	░	░	░			░		░		moderate	High
6	MYMOP	Paterson	1996	3	S	1 week	I	I	░	░	░	░	░	░	░									moderate	High
7	PPQ	Haddad	2000	5	T	last week	S	I	■	■	■		■				■	■		░		■		moderate	High
8	HowRU	Benson	2011	4	S	today	S	I	■	■			■											limited	Unknown
9	ORIDL	Reilly	2007	2	T	up to present	S	P	░	░	░	░	░	░										limited	High
10	CIMOS	Eton	2007	29	S	current self	S	P	■	■	■		■	■	■		■							limited	Unknown

Fig. 1 Health Status Instruments Reviewed. 1 (SF-36): MOS Short Form 36v2 [34, 35]; 2 (SF-12): MOS Short Form 12 [36]; 3 (EQ-5D): EuroQol 5D [39]; 4 (COOP): Dartmouth COOP Charts [37]; 5 (CMP) Change in Main Problem [45–47] 6 (MYMOP): Measure Yourself Medical Outcomes Profile v2 [43]; 7 (PPQ): Patient Perception of Quality [32] 8 (HowRU) HowRU [50]; 9 (ORIDL) Outcomes Related to Impact on Daily Living [33]; 10 (CIMOS) Complementary and Integrative Medical Outcomes Scale [52]. Scale (a) S = Status (capturing status at a point in time). T = Transitional (capturing change over a period of time). Adaptability (b) S = Standardised (standard list of items) I = Individualised (respondents can select, identify or weight items). Dimensionality (c) P = Profile of scores. I = Index (single score). U = Utility (single preference-based score which can generate a QALY). Extent of psychometric testing (d) Extensive (Widespread validation in different populations/countries and/or > 1000 citations). Moderate (Independent validation and/or > 100 citations). Low (Validation by original authors and/or < 100 citations). Responsiveness (e) Unknown (responsiveness not known or tested). Low (responsiveness shown in at least one study). Moderate (Repeated evidence for responsiveness, including in primary care). High (responsiveness shown in primary care studies where other leading PROMs are not responsive)

reference search on the original PROM development paper was used.

A fuller description of the data extraction sheet is shown in Additional file 3.

Results

Search and selection of PROMs

Figure 4 shows the number of papers screened and PROMs identified. Many PROMs were excluded at short-listing stage because of the construct or the population. For example, the Sickness Impact Profile was excluded because it is most suitable for very ill populations [27]. Although several preference-based instruments were long-listed, only the *EQ-5D* and *SF-36*/*SF-12* were included in the final review. ICECAP [29] and AQoL-4D [30] were excluded because of their focus on general quality of life, which was not part of the construct under consideration. The Health Utilities Index was excluded because of its deliberately narrow focus on specific aspects of function [27].

The twenty selected PROMs are described in the following three sections by domain: Health Status, Health Empowerment and Health Perceptions. Where a PROM covered more than one domain, it is presented under the domain with which it has most overlap. A referenced list of the twenty PROMs can be found in Additional file 4.

Health status PROMs

Construct and measurement properties

Ten instruments which measure some form of health status were included. As shown in Fig. 1, nine of the ten instruments contain a standard list of questions. One of the instruments (*MYMOP*) is individualised, such that patients define the outcomes of interest in their own words [31]. Three of the PROMs contain transitional items: the *CMP*, *PPQ* [32] and *ORIDL* [33].

Five of the instruments result in a profile of scores. The most widely used and well-validated of these is the SF-36, which measures physical and emotional function [34, 35]. The second profile PROM (the *SF-12)* was designed as a short version of the *SF-36* [36] and was validated based on assessing how well the twelve-item scale scores predicted the 36-item scale scores [36]. The third most commonly cited profile instrument listed is the Dartmouth *COOP charts*. These were designed as a

	Instrument Details				Measurement Properties				Construct: Health Status – symptoms				Health Status – symptom affects			Health Empowerment – Internal			Health Empowerment – External		Health Perceptions			Psychometric properties	
	Tool Name	Author	Date	Items	Scale: (a) Status(S)/Transitional(T)	Recall Period	Adaptability: (b) Standard(S)/Individual(I)	Dimensionality: (c) Profile(P)/Index(I)/Utility(U	1a.Pain	1b. Anxiety/depression	1c. Other symptoms	1d. Side-effects	2a. Normal activities	2b. Can enjoy life	2c. Impact on others	3.Understanding	4. Self-care/stay healthy	5. Plan/adherence	6. Confidence seeking care	7. Access to support	8. Health satisfaction	9. Health concerns	10. On track for future	Extent of psychometric testing (d)	Responsiveness (e)
11	PAM-13	Hibbard	2005	13	S	current self	S	I								■	■	■						moderate	Low
12	PEI	Howie	1998	6	T	today	S	I					░			■	■					░	░	moderate	High
13	HeiQ	Osborne	2007	40	S	current self	S	P					■	■		■	■	░	■	■	■	■	■	moderate	Medium
14	EC-17	Kristjans	2007	17	S	current self	S	I								■	■	░	■					limited	Low
15	PE-LTCs	Small	2013	47	S	current self	S	I	░	░	░		■	■		■	■	■					■	limited	Unknown
16	Barriers	Bayliss	2005	41/36	S	current self	S	P					■	■		■	■	■	■		■			limited	Unknown
17	CAM-3	Bann	2010	22	T/S	current self	S	P								■	■	░	░				■	limited	Unknown

Fig. 2 Health Empowerment Instruments Reviewed11 (PAM-13): Patient Activation Measure [55]; 12 (PEI): Patient Enablement Instrument [58]; 13 (heiQ): Health Education Impact Questionnaire [56]; 14 (EC-17): Effective Consumer Scale [59]; 15 (PE-LTCs): Patient Empowerment in Long-Term Conditions [61]; 16 (Barriers): Barriers to Self-Care in Multiple Long-Term Conditions [62]; 17 (CAM-3) Three scales for Complementary and Alternative Medicine [63]. Scale (a) S = Status (capturing status at a point in time). T = Transitional (capturing change over a period of time). Adaptability (b) S = Standardised (standard list of items) I = Individualised (respondents can select, identify or weight items). Dimensionality (c) P = Profile of scores. I = Index (single score). U = Utility (single preference-based score which can generate a QALY). Extent of psychometric testing (d) Extensive (Widespread validation in different populations/countries and/or > 1000 citations). Moderate (Independent validation and/or > 100 citations). Low (Validation by original authors and/or < 100 citations). Responsiveness (e) Unknown (responsiveness not known or tested). Low (responsiveness shown in at least one study). Moderate (Repeated evidence for responsiveness, including in primary care). High (responsiveness shown in primary care studies where other leading PROMs are not responsive)

	Instrument Details				Measurement Properties				Construct: Health Status – symptoms				Health Status – symptom affects			Health Empowerment – Internal			Health Empowerment – External		Health Perceptions			Psychometric properties	
	Tool Name	Author	Date	Items	Scale: (a) Status(S)/Transitional(T)	Recall Period	Adaptability: (b) Standard(S)/Individual(I)	Dimensionality: (c) Profile(P)/Index(I)/Utility(U	1a.Pain	1b. Anxiety/depression	1c. Other symptoms	1d. Side-effects	2a. Normal activities	2b. Can enjoy life	2c. Impact on others	3.Understanding	4. Self-care/stay healthy	5. Plan/adherence	6. Confidence seeking care	7. Access to support	8. Health satisfaction	9. Health concerns	10. On track for future	Extent of psychometric testing (d)	Responsiveness (e)
18	SRHS	various		1	S/T	current self	S	I													■			moderate	low
19	HPQ	Ware	1976	33	S	current self	S	P/I					░								■	■	■	moderate	low
20	IPQ	Broadbe	2006	9	S	current self	S	P/I	░	■		░	■	■		■	░					■	■	moderate	low

Fig. 3 Health Perceptions Instruments Reviewed. 18 (SRHS): Single item indicator of self-rated health status [27]; 19 (HPQ): RAND Health Perceptions Questionnaire [73]; 20 (IPQ): Illness Perceptions Questionnaire [74]. Scale (a) S = Status (capturing status at a point in time). T = Transitional (capturing change over a period of time). Adaptability (b) S = Standardised (standard list of items) I = Individualised (respondents can select, identify or weight items). Dimensionality (c) P = Profile of scores. I = Index (single score). U = Utility (single preference-based score which can generate a QALY). Extent of psychometric testing (d) Extensive (Widespread validation in different populations/countries and/or > 1000 citations). Moderate (Independent validation and/or > 100 citations). Low (Validation by original authors and/or < 100 citations). Responsiveness (e) Unknown (responsiveness not known or tested). Low (responsiveness shown in at least one study). Moderate (Repeated evidence for responsiveness, including in primary care). High (responsiveness shown in primary care studies where other leading PROMs are not responsive)

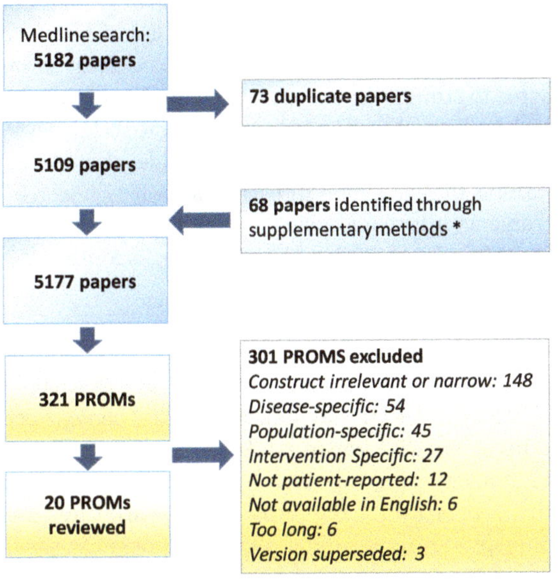

* Supplementary methods included a forward and backward reference search, the Oxford University PROMs group database,[24] and a review of three compilations of PROMs (McDowell,[25] Bowling,[26] and PROQOLID[27])

Fig. 4 Papers and PROMs identified through the systematic review

rapid way to assess functional health routinely in clinical practice [37] and consist of a set of nine charts, each with a title, a question, and a five-point pictorial response scale. The fourth profile reviewed is the transitional *ORIDL*. This consists of two scores designed to be comparable across different people and diseases [33]. The last profile is the Complementary and Integrative Medicine Outcome Scales (*CIMOS*) [38]. This instrument was developed to measure the outcomes typically experienced by people receiving complementary and alternative medicine. Four of the instruments generate index (but not utility) scores. These are the *CMP*, *howRU*, *MYMOP* and *PPQ*. Three instruments generate utility scores: the, SF-36, SF-12 and the EQ-5D [39–41] (which is recommended by NICE as the tool of choice for economic evaluation [42]).

Psychometric properties

The *SF-36*, *SF-12* and the *EQ-5D* have been extensively used and tested, with the original papers describing each cited approximately 21,000, 9000 and 3000 times respectively. The *COOP Charts*, the *CMP* and *MYMOP* have undergone moderate levels of psychometric testing. The original *PPQ* French version has also had moderate testing, but testing of the English version has been more limited. The remaining three instruments have had limited testing.

The most responsive to change are the individualised instrument (*MYMOP*), and the three transitional instruments (*PPQ*, *CMP* and *ORIDL*). *MYMOP* shows change when the *SF-36* does not [31, 43, 44]. Various formats of the *CMP* have been used in primary care trials [45–47]. However, as a single-item, this has lower reliability than multi-item instruments [28]. *ORIDL* is also transitional. Although limited testing has been done of *ORIDL*, in the initial validation study, it showed good correlation with *MYMOP* and *PEI* [33]. One study showed that *ORIDL* continued to show change on repeated follow-up when *MYMOP* did not [48].

The *SF-36*, *SF-12*, *EQ-5D* and the *COOP charts* all have a medium level of responsiveness. However, there is considerable variability within this. The most responsive of these instruments is the *SF-36* profile scores [27]. The *COOP charts* show good reliability and validity in primary care populations. Unsurprisingly, given that each profile score is based on a single item, they are less reliable than the *SF-36*, have a ceiling effect, and are less responsive to change over time [27]. In terms of preference-based values, testing has showed that the recent *SF-12* value set is just as responsive to change and generates similar estimates to the *SF-36* preference-based index [49]. A study of patients with depression also showed the *SF-12* utility scores to be more responsive than the *EQ-5D-3 L* which suffers from ceiling effects in general [27].

HowRU [50], has not been tested for responsiveness. However, it has shown less of a ceiling effect than *EQ-5D-3 L*, despite being even shorter [51]. This may be because of wording e.g. "low or worried" (howRU) rather than "anxious or depressed" (EQ-5D). Responsiveness is also unknown in *CIMOS*, which has undergone very little psychometric testing, demonstrating acceptable levels of reliability and validity in only one study [52].

Summary

The *SF-36* is, by far, the most validated of the health status instruments and the most responsive of the moderately and extensively tested PROMs. *MYMOP* and *ORIDL* both represent good attempts to increase responsiveness, but the *ORIDL* detailed nine-point scale has not been widely validated, and, although it has been used in trials [47, 53], MYMOP is not recommended for self-completion, which is necessary for routine or trial use [31]. *EQ-5D* and *SF-12* have the benefits of brevity, and the ability to generate a preference-based score. *HowRU* shows that it is possible to have a valid instrument that is very short. Haddad's transitional scale provides another good option for increasing responsiveness while maintaining a standard list of items.

Health empowerment

Construct and measurement properties

Figure 2 shows the seven instruments which cover both internal and external aspects of the Health Empowerment construct.

The constructs measured by these seven instruments all include internal aspects of empowerment, with explicit items on understanding of health problems, and the ability to self-care, or stay healthy. External aspects of empowerment are less extensively covered, perhaps because these are traditionally seen as measures of patient experience, not outcome [54], and because we did not include measures which exclusively capture patient experience in our review. None of the instruments directly address symptoms. The three most widely used are *PAM-13, PEI* and the *heiQ*. *PAM-13* is based on a single construct of activation: which is being engaged in managing one's own health. Patients are measured on a four-stage Guttman scale of activation: from belief that an active role is important, to taking action and staying the course under stress [55]. The *heiQ* was developed to assess the impact of patient education programs across a broad range of chronic conditions [56]. It has a wider construct than the *PAM-13* and contains eight independent dimensions: positive and active engagement in life, health directed behaviour; constructive attitudes and approaches; self-monitoring and insight; health service navigation; social integration and support and emotional wellbeing [56, 57]. These domains overlap with both internal and external empowerment, and also with the other two domains. For example, "positive and active engagement in life" overlaps with Health Status. The instrument also includes aspects of Health Perceptions, including "satisfaction with health", and "health concerns". *PEI* was developed specifically for primary care, and asks the patient to retrospectively rate change in enablement, resulting from a single consultation. As well as understanding and self-care, it addresses concerns, and indirectly addresses the impact of symptoms (through questions on coping with illness, and coping with life) [58].

The four remaining instruments are less widely used. *EC-17* was developed to measure the skills and attributes of an effective consumer, for use in self-management interventions [59, 60]. *PE-LTCs* was developed to measure empowerment in long-term conditions [61]. The *Barriers* instrument does not purport to assess empowerment, rather barriers to self-management in long-term conditions [62]. However, the construct of "barriers" is related to empowerment, in that reducing barriers increases empowerment. *CAM-3* measures the quality of the therapeutic relationship as: 1) patient-centred care, 2) perceived provider support 3) empowerment. While this is described as an experience measure, it focuses on the consequences of a positive experience, for example, trust in the therapist and belief that the root causes are being identified and treated. In measuring patient-centred care and perceived provider support as well as empowerment, it includes some external aspects of empowerment in addition to internal [63].

All seven instruments contain a standard list of questions, asking about today, or a person's perception of their current self. Two of the instruments are, at least partly, transitional. The status instruments are based on a list of belief statements with a Likert (bipolar) response scale (e.g. strongly disagree to strongly agree) apart from the *EC-17*, which has behavioural statements with an adjectival scale (never to always). Four of the instruments provide a single index score, and the remaining three give a profile of scores. All instruments are scored using a summative method, apart from *PAM-13*, which uses a Rasch scoring algorithm [55].

Psychometric properties

The first three of the instruments (*PAM-13, PEI* and *heiQ*) have undergone moderate levels of testing. *PEI* has been used widely in UK general practice and has shown acceptable psychometric properties. As a transitional questionnaire, it measures change directly, and is thus responsive.

The properties of the *heiQ* were investigated using item response theory and structural equation modelling. It has demonstrated good construct validity, including, most recently, testing for measurement invariance [64]. Some of the *heiQ* sub-scores have shown responsiveness to change in randomised controlled trials [65–67].

PAM-13 has strong psychometric properties, and association with a number of other health outcomes [68]. Recent studies in the US found patient activation was influenced by community interventions [69, 70], suggesting it may be appropriate as an outcome measure in primary care.

The *EQ-17* has shown some preliminary evidence for responsiveness to change in arthritis patients [60, 71], although psychometric testing has been more limited. However, the authors of the instrument acknowledge that, while some skills of an effective consumer can be learned, others are a "part of personality" and not amenable to change [59]. (pg. 1932) When compared directly to *PAM-13* it was less responsive (standardised response mean 0.25/ 0.41).

Summary

All the health empowerment instruments reviewed could, in theory, be used to measure empowerment outcomes in primary care. However, as all except *PEI* and *CAM-3* were developed with long-term conditions in mind, they are less suitable for people without long-term conditions. This is most problematic with *EC-17, PE-LTCs* and the *Barriers* questionnaire, which all refer to a "disease". The first three instruments (*PAM-13, PEI* and *heiQ*), which are the most robust and responsive to change, make minimal reference to "your illness" or else refer to "health problems" in general. Of these three, only the *PEI* was developed specifically for primary care. The main weakness of this is that it only works at a single consultation level, through the words "as a result of your consultation today". A format of the *PEI* which asks patients to rate a longer episode of care has been tested for acupuncture. This adjusted the wording to "as a result of visiting the acupuncturist over the last few weeks or months." However, patients had difficulty attributing change directly to the intervention [72]. *PAM-13*, is more robust, but the construct is relatively narrow: its emphasis is on the internal, and it contains elements about control and responsibility which are not present in the construct described in Chapter 3. The *heiQ* has the widest construct. The main weakness of the *heiQ* for use in primary care is its length, and the fact that it does not explicitly address symptoms, which, for some patients, may be the primary reason for attendance.

Health perceptions

Construct and measurement properties

Three instruments which predominantly cover a Health Perceptions construct were identified (Fig. 3). The single *self-rated health status* item is based on empirical evidence that people possess insights into their own health, and that this can be captured through a single rating of how they perceive their health at a point in time [27]. *Self-rated health status* items ask for a general impression of health, rather than symptoms, function or health problems, and thus capture a Health Perceptions construct, specifically the "satisfaction with health" outcome. The *HPQ* is an important extension of single items, which covers six domains: prior health, current health, health outlook, resistance/susceptibility to illness, health worry/concern and sickness orientation. The developers of the *HPQ* contended that this subjective concept has as much to do with a person's feelings and beliefs as their actual health status [73]. The *IPQ* is based on a model of the cognitive representation of illness measured by eight domains: Consequences, Timeline, Personal control, Treatment control, Identity, Concern, Understanding, Emotional response [74].

All three instruments contain a standard list of questions, asking about a person's perception of their current self. All are status questions, although the *self-rated health status* item can also be asked as a transitional question. The *HPQ* can be scored as a profile, comprised of six subscores, or an overall index can be created from 22 of the 33 items. The *IPQ* can be reported as a profile (the responses to the nine questions) or a summative index.

Psychometric properties

The *self-rated health status* item is quick to administer. It consistently predicts long-term outcomes such as mortality. This suggests that it reflects health trajectory, and not merely current health status [27], which may make it less suitable for use over the short to medium term. A body of research has shown that general questions, self-rated health included, are answered less reliably than specific questions [75]. Single items are, by necessity, less precise than multiple items, and less responsive to change [76]. The *HPQ* has shown good reliability and validity. The high stability over time suggests that it may be more useful as a personality indicator than an outcome measure that is responsive to change [27]. The *IPQ* is most suitable for relatively ill populations [74]. The *IPQ* has shown good reliability and validity in populations with illness, but has generally been used as a variable which is associated with various outcome measures, rather than a measure in its own right [77]. Responsiveness to change in primary care has never been tested. One paper has shown the measure to be responsive to change in secondary care [78] and the authors suggest that the role of medical interventions in shifting illness perceptions is an important and under-researched area [77].

Summary

The three health perceptions instruments are among the least responsive in this review. The constructs captured by them are similar to the Health Perceptions construct which arose in the prior qualitative study but also has some important differences, in that the items capture more general perceptions about health, which are less likely to be shifted by intervention.

Discussion

Key findings

As far as we are aware, this is the first systematic review of its kind for generic PROMs for primary care. This review identified PROMs that are potentially suitable for measuring a wide-range of outcomes in any adult primary care patient, and twenty of these were reviewed in detail. The two key findings of the review were that: to date, there is no instrument which comprehensively covers the outcomes commonly sought in primary care; and there are different benefits both to PROMs which measure status at a point in time, and PROMs which measure change directly. These findings will inform researchers selecting or developing PROMs to test interventions in primary care, and should have a subsequent effect on policy and patient care, as the conclusions of clinical research studies which inform healthcare policy depend on the PROM selected as an endpoint. Confirming that a gap exists by reviewing existing PROMs is a necessary first step in any PROM development [5]. Our findings provided sufficient grounds for proceeding with development of a PROM for primary care; and, following completion of this review, we developed and tested the Primary Care Outcome Questionnaire and made it publicly available [79].

Strengths and limitations

Strengths of this review include a reproducible search strategy, developed in collaboration with a librarian, a set of clear inclusion and exclusion criteria, and publication of the longlist of excluded PROMs for transparency.

The search strategy successfully identified the twelve papers used in the iterative process of developing and testing. However, all systematic reviews have the potential of omitting relevant articles, including unpublished material. Our exclusion criteria omitted PROMs which captured a narrow construct, such as pain, fatigue, or anxiety. This limited the scope of the review to generic measures, and meant that modular measures, such as PROMIS [80], were excluded. The electronic search was limited to the Medline database, and one of the filters relied on keywords assigned by authors. Some papers describing the development and validation of PROMs for primary care may not have been picked up by this strategy. However, although the use of keywords in a filter is not usually recommended in systematic reviews [81], it can be justified when the unit of analysis is the PROM, not the paper, because all PROMs alluded to in abstracts were followed up, which meant that even if the original development paper of a PROM was not identified by the search strategy, it could be identified through other means. Moreover, the search was supplemented by forward and backward reference searching, review of the Oxford PROMs Bibliography, and consultation with experts. Lastly, the decision on which PROMs to include and exclude at abstract screening stage, and any data extraction was carried out by a single researcher. Independent screening and extraction would have helped to identify and minimise error. We have attempted to be as transparent as possible by describing inclusion and exclusion criteria and by publishing a longlist of all potential PROMs identified in Additional file 2.

Comparison with the literature

Systematic reviews of health status measurement instruments are often poorly conducted with many studies having a poorly described search strategy, using only a single database and failing to report whether data extraction was done by two independent reviewers [82].

We followed PRIMSA and COSMIN guidelines in this review, diverging from these only where there were clear reasons. For example, we did not use the existing search strategy for measurement properties published by the COSMIN group [83], because it was highly sensitive (therefore over-inclusive) and did not fit the purposes of this review. The approach we took had much in common with other systematic reviews of PROMs on related topics (such as empowerment [14, 15], integrative medicine [16], and patient experience) [17]. For example, in their review of patient experience measures, Hudon et al. similarly relied on keywords for one filter, and took a similar approach to mapping the constructs captured by the instruments reviewed onto their defined construct of "patient-centred care", excluding instruments which measured only a narrow part of this construct [17].

This review identified various benefits and downsides to standardised, transitional and individualised PROMs respectively. Standardised PROMs are most successful in terms of their psychometric properties. Item wording and selection of a scale for standardised strongly affect interpretation. The review contained five PROMs with transitional questions. As anticipated [84], these were more responsive than the status measures. Only one individualised PROM, *MYMOP* was included in the review. As with other individualised PROMs [85–88] this is recommended for completion only through interview.

None of the instruments reviewed provided coverage of all outcome groups identified in the prior qualitative study. Of the Health Status questionnaires, the most extensively tested is the *SF-36*. This is also the most responsive of the standardised status instruments reviewed. Individualised and transitional questionnaires show greater responsiveness to change. Of the Health Empowerment instruments, the *PEI*, *PAM* and *heiQ* provide the best combination of responsiveness to change and psychometric testing. The Health Perceptions instruments reviewed are all less responsive to change, and may measure a form of health perception which is difficult to shift in primary care.

Conclusions

This systematic review is the first of its kind to identify papers describing the development and validation of generic PROMs suitable for measuring outcomes from primary care. It identified that, to date, there is no instrument which comprehensively covers the outcomes primary care patients seeks and primary care clinicians seek to deliver, and thus provided grounds for proceeding with development of a PROM for primary care. It also provides a reusable search strategy for the identification of papers describing primary care PROMs. Finally, it presents information on a range of instruments which measure health status, health empowerment and health perceptions, and a critique of their strengths and limitations for use in primary care, which will be of benefit to other researchers in this field.

Additional files

Additional file 1: Medline Search Strategy. Reproducible Medline search strategy, including the contents of all four filters.

Additional file 2: Long-list of PROMs identified. Long-list of all PROMs identified through the first review of abstracts, as potentially meeting the inclusion criteria. The reasons for excluding these after the PROMs was reviewed are also documented.

Additional file 3: Data extraction sheet column headings description. Description of the column headings and possible categories for the data extraction sheet, used to create Figs. 1–3.

Additional file 4: List of instruments reviewed. Referenced list of the twenty instruments reviewed with a short description of each instrument.

Abbreviations

CAM-3: Three scales for Complementary and Alternative Medicine; CIMOS: Complementary and Integrative Medical Outcomes Scale; CMP: Change in Main Problem; EC-17: Effective Consumer Scale – 17 items; EQ-5D: European Quality of Life-5 Dimensions; heiQ: Health Education Impact Questionnaire; HPQ: Health Perceptions Questionnaire; ICECAP: ICEpop CAPability measure; IPQ: Illness Perceptions Questionnaire; MYMOP: Measure Yourself Medical Outcomes Profile; NICE: National Institute for Health and Care Excellence; ORIDL: Outcome in Relation to Impact on Daily Living; PAM: Patient Activation Measure; PEI: Patient Enablement Instrument; PE-LTCs: Patient Empowerment in Long-Term Conditions; PPQ: Patient Perception of Quality; PRISMA: Preferred Reporting Items for Systematic Reviews and Meta-Analyses; PROM: Patient-reported outcome measure; SF-12: Short Form 12; SF-36: Short Form 36; SRHS: Self-Rated Health Score

Acknowledgements

The authors would like to thank Sarah Dawson for advice on developing systematic reviews for PROMs and Cath Borwick for reviewing the search strategy.

Funding

This study was funded by a capacity building grant from the NIHR School for Primary Care Research (SPCR). The Avon Primary Care Research Collaborative funded time to write the paper. Neither funding body had any role in the study design, data collection, analysis, or interpretation or in writing the manuscript. The NIHR SPCR is a partnership between the Universities of Bristol, Cambridge, Keele, Manchester, Newcastle, Nottingham, Oxford, Southampton and University College London. The views expressed are those of the author(s) and not necessarily those of the NHS, the NIHR or the Department of Health.

Authors' contributions

MM, SH and CS designed the study. MM collected the data. MM carried out the data analysis, and CS/SH reviewed and validated it. MM drafted the manuscript. CS/SH reviewed and revised the manuscript. All authors approved the final manuscript.

Consent for publication

Not applicable

Competing interests

The authors declare that they have no competing interests.

References

1. Donabedian A. The quality of care. How can it be assessed? J Am Med Assoc. 1988;260(12):1743–8.
2. Fitzpatrick R. Patient-reported outcomes and performance measurement. In: Performance Measurement for Health System Improvement: Experiences, Challenges and Prospect, smith P, et al. Cambridge: Cambridge University Press; 2009. p. 63–86.
3. Black N, et al. Patient-reported outcomes: pathways to better health, better services, and better societies. Qual Life Res. 2016;25(5):1103–12.
4. Center for Drug Evaluation and Research (CDER), Guidance for Industry Patient-Reported Outcome Measures: Use in Medical Product Development to Support Labeling Claims, US Food and Drug Administration. 2009: http://www.fda.gov/downloads/Drugs/.../Guidances/UCM193282.pdf.
5. Garratt A, et al. Quality of life measurement: bibliographic study of patient assessed health outcome measures. Br Med J. 2002;324(7351):1417.
6. Barnett K, et al. Epidemiology of multimorbidity and implications for health care, research, and medical education: a cross-sectional study. Lancet. 2012;380(9836):37–43.
7. Salisbury C, et al. Epidemiology and impact of multimorbidity in primary care: a retrospective cohort study. Br J Gen Pract. 2011;61(582):e12–21.
8. Olayiwola JN, et al. Electronic consultations to improve the primary care-specialty care Interface for cardiology in the medically underserved: a cluster-randomized controlled trial. Ann Fam Med. 2016;14(2):133–40.
9. Thom DH, et al. A qualitative study of how health coaches support patients in making health-related decisions and behavioral changes. The Annals of Family Medicine. 2016;14(6):509–16.
10. Sharma AE, et al. What happens after health coaching? Observational study 1 year following a randomized controlled trial. Ann Fam Med. 2016;14(3):200–7.
11. Hudon C, et al. Case Management in Primary Care for frequent users of health care services with chronic diseases: a qualitative study of patient and family experience. Ann Fam Med. 2015;13(6):523–8.
12. Barnes R. ISRCTN registry: Footprints in Primary Care. study registered 2015. https://doi.org/10.1186/ISRCTN62939408, http://www.isrctn.com/ISRCTN62939408.
13. Fitzpatrick R, Garratt A, Schmidt L. Instruments for mental health: a review., report from the patient-reported health instruments group to the Department of Health. 2000.
14. Herbert RJ, et al. A systematic review of questionnaires measuring health-related empowerment. Research & Theory for Nursing Practice. 2009;23(2):107–32.
15. Hudon C, et al. Assessing enablement in clinical practice: a systematic review of available instruments. J Eval Clin Pract. 2010;16(6):1301–8.
16. Hunter J, Leeder S. Patient questionnaires for use in the integrative medicine primary care setting—a systematic literature review. European Journal of Integrative Medicine. 2013;5(3):194–216.
17. Hudon C, et al. Measuring patients' perceptions of patient-centered care: a systematic review of tools for family medicine. Ann Fam Med. 2011;9(2):155–64.
18. Ricci-Cabello I, et al. Measuring experiences and outcomes of patient safety in primary care: a systematic review of available instruments. Fam Pract. 2015;32(1):106–19.
19. Haywood KL, Garratt AM, Fitzpatrick R. Quality of life in older people: a structured review of self-assessed health instruments. Expert Review of Pharmacoeconomics & Outcomes Research. 2006;6(2):181–94.
20. Murphy M, et al. Patient and practitioners' views on the most important outcomes arising from primary care consultations: a qualitative study. BMC Fam Pract. 2015;16:108.
21. Liberati A, et al. The PRISMA statement for reporting systematic reviews and meta-analyses of studies that evaluate healthcare interventions: explanation and elaboration. Br Med J. 2009;339:b2700.
22. Centre for Reviews and Dissemination, University of York. York: CRD's guide for undertaking reviews in health care; 2009.
23. McDowell I. Measuring Health. 2 ed. 2006, New York: Oxford University Press.
24. Bowling A. Measuring Health: A review of quality of life measurement scales. 3 ed. Vol. 1. Maidenhead: Open University Press; 2004.
25. MAPI Research Trust. *PROQOLID*. 2014 [cited 2014 17/10/2014]; Available from: https://eprovide.mapi-trust.org/about/about-proqolid.
26. Valderas JM, Alonso J. Patient reported outcome measures: a model-based classification system for research and clinical practice. Qual Life Res. 2008;17(9):1125–35.
27. University of Oxford. Oxford PROMs bibliography. 2005 [cited 2014 17/10/2014]; Available from: http://phi.uhce.ox.ac.uk/instruments.php.
28. Streiner DL, Norman GR. Health measurement scales: a practical guide to their development and use. New York: Oxford University Press; 2008.
29. Al-Janabi H, Flynn TN, Coast J. Development of a self-report measure of capability wellbeing for adults: the ICECAP-A. Qual Life Res. 2012; 21(1):167–76.
30. Richardson JR, et al. Construction of the descriptive system for the assessment of quality of life AQoL-6D utility instrument. Health Qual Life Outcomes. 2012;10:38.
31. Paterson C. University of Bristol website, PHC section, MYMOP. 2012 [cited 2014 25/04/2014]; Available from: http://www.bristol.ac.uk/primaryhealthcare/resources/mymop/strengthsandweaknesses/.

32. Haddad S, et al. Patient perception of quality following a visit to a doctor in a primary care unit. Fam Pract. 2000;17(1):21–9.
33. Reilly D, et al. Outcome related to impact on daily living: preliminary validation of the ORIDL instrument. BMC Health Serv Res. 2007;7:139.
34. Ware, J.E., Jr. And C.D. Sherbourne, The MOS 36-item short-form health survey (SF-36). I. Conceptual framework and item selection. Med Care, 1992. 30(6): p. 473–483.
35. Ware J, et al. In: Metric Q, editor. *Chapter 1*, in User's Manual for the SF-36v2 Health Survey. Lincoln: Quality Metric; 2007.
36. Ware J Jr, Kosinski M, Keller SD. A 12-Item Short-Form Health Survey: construction of scales and preliminary tests of reliability and validity. Med Care. 1996;34(3):220–33.
37. Nelson EC, et al. The functional status of patients. How can it be measured in physicians' offices? Med Care. 1990;28(12):1111–26.
38. Eton DT, et al. Developing a self-report outcome measure for complementary and alternative medicine. Explore (NY). 2005;1(3):177–85.
39. Brooks R. EuroQol: the current state of play. Health Policy. 1996;37(1):53–72.
40. Herdman M, et al. Development and preliminary testing of the new five-level version of EQ-5D (EQ-5D-5L). Qual Life Res. 2011;20(10):1727–36.
41. Devlin NJ, Parkin D, Browne J. Patient-reported outcome measures in the NHS: new methods for analysing and reporting EQ-5D data. Health Econ. 2010;19(8):886–905.
42. National Institute of Clinical Excellence Guide to the methods of technology appraisal 2013. 2013.
43. Paterson C. Measuring outcomes in primary care: a patient generated measure, MYMOP, compared with the SF-36 health survey. Br Med J. 1996;312(7037):1016–20.
44. Mirza S, et al. Comparing sensitivity to change of two patient-reported outcome measures in a randomised trial of patients referred for physiotherapy services. Trials. 2013;14(Suppl 1):O50. https://doi.org/10.1186/1745-6215-14-S1-O50.
45. Campbell JL, et al. Telephone triage for management of same-day consultation requests in general practice (the ESTEEM trial): a cluster-randomised controlled trial and cost-consequence analysis. Lancet. 2014;384(9957):1859–68.
46. Kamper SJ, Maher CG, Mackay G. Global rating of change scales: a review of strengths and weaknesses and considerations for design. The Journal of Manual & Manipulative Therapy. 2009;17(3):163–70.
47. Salisbury C, et al. Effectiveness of PhysioDirect telephone assessment and advice services for patients with musculoskeletal problems: pragmatic randomised controlled trial. Br Med J. 2013;346(jan29 3):f43.
48. Higgins M, et al. Evaluation report of wellness enhancement Learning,Piloted for people with CFS/ME. 2009, TheWEL Programme: www.thewel.org.
49. Brazier JE, Roberts J. The estimation of a preference-based measure of health from the SF-12. Med Care. 2004;42(9):851–9.
50. Benson T, et al. Evaluation of a new short generic measure of health status: howRu. Informatics in Primary Care. 2011;18:89–101.
51. Benson T, et al. Comparison of howRU and EQ-5D measures of health-related quality of life in an outpatient clinic. Informatics in Primary Care. 2013;21(1):12–7.
52. Eton DT, Temple LM, Koffler K. Pilot validation of a self-report outcome measure of complementary and alternative medicine. Explore: The Journal of Science & Healing. 2007;3(6):592–9.
53. Flower A, Lewith GT, Little P. A feasibility study exploring the role of Chinese herbal medicine in the treatment of endometriosis. J Altern Complement Med. 2011;17(8):691–9.
54. Ahmed S, et al. The use of patient-reported outcomes (PRO) within comparative effectiveness research: implications for clinical practice and health care policy. Med Care. 2012;50(12):1060–70.
55. Hibbard JH, et al. Development and testing of a short form of the patient activation measure. Health Serv Res. 2005;40(6 Pt 1):1918–30.
56. Osborne RH, Elsworth GR, Whitfield K. The health education impact questionnaire (heiQ): an outcomes and evaluation measure for patient education and self-management interventions for people with chronic conditions. Patient Education & Counseling. 2007;66(2):192–201.
57. Elsworth GR, Nolte S, Osborne RH. Factor structure and measurement invariance of the health education impact questionnaire: does the subjectivity of the response perspective threaten the contextual validity of inferences? SAGE Open Medicine. 2015;3:1–13.
58. Howie JG, et al. A comparison of a patient enablement instrument (PEI) against two established satisfaction scales as an outcome measure of primary care consultations. Fam Pract. 1998;15(2):165–71.
59. Kristjansson E, et al. Development of the effective musculoskeletal consumer scale. J Rheumatol. 2007;34(6):1392–400.
60. Santesso N, et al. Responsiveness of the effective consumer scale (EC-17). J Rheumatol. 2009;36(9):2087–91.
61. Small N, et al. Patient empowerment in long-term conditions: development and preliminary testing of a new measure. BMC Health Serv Res. 2013;13:263.
62. Bayliss EA, Ellis JL, Steiner JF. Barriers to self-management and quality-of-life outcomes in seniors with multimorbidities. Ann Fam Med. 2007;5(5):395–402.
63. Bann CM, Sirois FM, Walsh EG. Provider support in complementary and alternative medicine: exploring the role of patient empowerment. Journal of Alternative & Complementary Medicine. 2010;16(7):745–52.
64. Nolte S, et al. Tests of measurement invariance failed to support the application of the "then-test". J Clin Epidemiol. 2009;62(11):1173–80.
65. Cadilhac DA, et al. A phase II multicentered, single-blind, randomized, controlled trial of the stroke self-management program. Stroke. 2011;42(6):1673–9.
66. Francis KL, et al. Effectiveness of a community-based osteoporosis education and self-management course: a wait list controlled trial. Osteoporos Int. 2009;20(9):1563–70.
67. Stone GR, Packer TL. Evaluation of a rural chronic disease self-management program. Rural Remote Health. 2010;10(1):1203.
68. Mosen DM, et al. Is patient activation associated with outcomes of care for adults with chronic conditions? Journal of Ambulatory Care Management. 2007;30(1):21–9.
69. McDonald EM, et al. Improvements in health behaviors and health status among newly insured members of an innovative health access plan. J Community Health. 2013;38(2):301–9.
70. Deen D, et al. Asking questions: the effect of a brief intervention in community health centers on patient activation. Patient Education and Counselling. 2011;84(2):257–60.
71. Kennedy CA, et al. A prospective comparison of telemedicine versus in-person delivery of an interprofessional education program for adults with inflammatory arthritis. J Telemed Telecare. 2016;3:1–10.
72. Paterson C. Measuring changes in self-concept: a qualitative evaluation of outcome questionnaires in people having acupuncture for their chronic health problems. BMC Complement Altern Med. 2006;6:7.
73. Ware J. Scales for measuring general health perceptions. Health Serv Res. 1976;11:396–415.
74. Broadbent E, et al. The brief illness perception questionnaire. J Psychosom Res. 2006;60(6):631–7.
75. Herrmann D. Reporting current, past, and changed health status. What we know about distortion. Med Care. 1995;33(4 Suppl):AS89–94.
76. Bowling A. Just one question: if one question works, why ask several? J Epidemiol Community Health. 2005;59(5):342–5.
77. Petrie KJ, Jago LA, Devcich DA. The role of illness perceptions in patients with medical conditions. Current Opinion in Psychiatry. 2007;20(2):163–7.
78. Petrie KJ, et al. Changing illness perceptions after myocardial infarction: an early intervention randomized controlled trial. Psychosom Med. 2002;64(4):580–6.
79. Murphy, M., S. Hollinghurst, and C. Salisbury. The primary care outcomes questionnaire. 2017 [cited 2017 22/05/2017].
80. National Institutes of Health. Patient reported outcomes measurement information system (PROMIS). 2016; Available from: http://www.healthmeasures.net/explore-measurement-systems/promis#2.
81. Higgins, J. and S. Green, Cochrane handbook for systematic reviews of interventions version 5.1.0 The Cochrane Collaboration, Editor. updated March 2011.
82. Mokkink LB, et al. Evaluation of the methodological quality of systematic reviews of health status measurement instruments. Qual Life Res. 2009;18(3):313–33.
83. Terwee CB, et al. Development of a methodological PubMed search filter for finding studies on measurement properties of measurement instruments. Qual Life Res. 2009;18(8):1115–23.
84. Lloyd H, et al. Patient reports of the outcomes of treatment: a structured review of approaches. Health Qual Life Outcomes. 2014;12:5.
85. O'Boyle CA, et al. Individual quality of life in patients undergoing hip replacement. Lancet. 1992;339(8801):1088–91.

13

Shifting hospital care to primary care: An evaluation of cardiology care in a primary care setting in the Netherlands

Tessa C. C. Quanjel[1*], Jeroen N. Struijs[2], Marieke D. Spreeuwenberg[3], Caroline A. Baan[4] and Dirk Ruwaard[1]

Abstract

Background: In an attempt to deal with the pressures on the healthcare system and to guarantee sustainability, changes are needed. This study is focused on a cardiology Primary Care Plus intervention in which cardiologists provide consultations with patients in a primary care setting in order to prevent unnecessary referrals to the hospital. This study explores which patients with non-acute and low-complexity cardiology-related health complaints should be excluded from Primary Care Plus and referred directly to specialist care in the hospital.

Methods: This is a retrospective observational study based on quantitative data. Data collected between January 1 and December 31, 2015 were extracted from the electronic medical record system. Logistic regression analyses were used to select patient groups that should be excluded from referral to Primary Care Plus.

Results: In total, 1525 patients were included in the analyses. Results showed that male patients, older patients, those with the referral indication 'Stable Angina Pectoris' or 'Dyspnoea' and patients whose reason for referral was 'To confirm disease' or 'Screening of unclear pathology' had a significantly higher probability of being referred to hospital care after Primary Care Plus.

Conclusions: To achieve efficiency one should exclude patient groups with a significantly higher probability of being referred to hospital care after Primary Care Plus.

Keywords: Substitution, Primary care, Referrals, Hospital care

Background

In an attempt to rein in rising healthcare costs, policy reforms have altered healthcare systems in many Western countries [1, 2]. A considerable number of these reforms focus on limiting the volume growth of more costly hospital care by stimulating substitution of care [3–5]. Substitution of care can be defined as the continual regrouping of resources across and within care settings to exploit the best and least costly solutions in the face of changing needs and demands [6, 7]. Internationally well-known concepts related to substitution such as joint consultations and specialist outreach services concentrate on providing specialist services in primary care settings, improving access to specialist services to enhance the efficiency and quality of health care, and reduce referrals to specialist services in hospital outpatient departments [8–14]. These concepts aim to integrate care by intensifying collaboration and communication between specialists and general practitioners (GP). Previous studies have shown that these kinds of interventions could result in improved patient satisfaction, improved access to specialist care, fewer diagnostic actions and reduced referrals to hospital care [8–11, 13]. Despite these positive findings some studies show that specialist outreach services could lead to higher healthcare costs [12–14].

Also, in the Netherlands, the healthcare sector is focused on substitution of care. For example, to limit the volume growth of more costly specialised care in the

* Correspondence: t.quanjel@maastrichtuniversity.nl
[1]Department of Health Services Research, Care and Public Health Research Institute, Faculty of Health Medicine and Life Sciences, Maastricht University, Maastricht, The Netherlands
Full list of author information is available at the end of the article

hospital setting, all involved healthcare providers have agreed upon shifting less complex treatments from hospital care to primary care [4, 15]. Consequently, several pioneering regions started experiments with a concept called Primary Care Plus (PC+). PC+ is concentrated on the substitution of specialist care in the hospital setting with specialist care in the primary care setting. As GPs act as gatekeepers of the Dutch healthcare system, secondary care provided by specialists is only accessible through GP referral [3]. PC+ initiatives strengthen the gatekeeping and coordinating role of the GP by intensifying collaboration and communication between GPs and specialists. Besides intensifying collaboration between the primary and secondary care sector, PC+ is designed to enhance the connectivity and alignment of care between these sectors [16]. Moreover, it is aimed at improving the health of the population and patients' experience of care, while at the same time reducing the number of unnecessary referrals to hospital care in order to reduce medical spending [17].

Previous research on PC+ has shown that it is essential to select an appropriate patient population to achieve efficient substitution of care [18]. It should not be designed as an intermediate station between the GP and the hospital. To achieve efficiency it is a precondition that PC+ interventions should exclude patients who need hospital care anyway.

In this study, we focus on a cardiology PC+ centre. Currently, GPs can refer all non-acute and low-complexity patients with cardiology-related complaints to this PC+ centre. Based on certain cardiology-related referral indications and reasons for referral the GP refers a patient to the cardiologist at the centre. After the consultation of a patient, the cardiologist provides the GP a comprehensive description of the results of the test diagnosis and his recommendation regarding further treatment (if needed). This study intends to explore which cardiology-related referral indications and reasons for referral are appropriate for PC+ and which are more appropriate for immediate specialist care in the hospital setting. Hence, patient groups that are more often referred to hospital care after a consultation at the PC+ centre are assumed to be less appropriate for PC+ and preferably should be referred directly to hospital care. The research question is as follows: '*Which patients with non-acute and low-complexity cardiology-related health complaints should be excluded from Primary Care Plus and referred directly to specialist care in the hospital?*'

Methods

Design

This is a retrospective observational study based on register data. It is part of an extensive practice-based, mixed-methods study focusing on the effects of a cardiology PC+ intervention. The study is approved by the Medical Research and Ethics Committee of the Maastricht University Medical Centre (METC 15-4-032).

Setting

This study was conducted in a geographically demarcated region located in the most southern part of the Netherlands. The region consists of 11 municipalities, covering 277,000 residents, approximately 135 GPs and one general hospital. Compared to the overall population of the Netherlands, the region is characterised by a relatively unhealthy population with a low socio-economic status [19, 20]. In 2013, the Minister of Health appointed nine regions in the Netherlands as so-called pioneer sites aimed at restructuring health services based on population management. This means focusing on addressing health needs at all points along the continuum of health and well-being for a specified population by integrating services across health care, prevention, social care and welfare [21, 22]. This study is focused on the pioneer site called MyCare. MyCare is a regional partnership between the care group (a legal entity exclusively owned by GPs), the hospital, the patient representative foundation and the dominant health insurance company in the region, CZ. One of the interventions of MyCare is the cardiology PC+ centre.

Intervention

In the cardiology PC+ centre cardiologists provide consultations in a primary care setting. All GPs in the region are able to refer non-acute and low-complexity patients with cardiology-related complaints to the centre. A consultation at the centre consists of the following diagnostic tests: a blood test, an ECG, an echo and an exercise test. After the tests, patients meet the cardiologist, who explains the results of the tests. The cardiologist sends a comprehensive description of the results of the tests, the diagnosis and his recommendation regarding further treatment (if needed) to the GP. The two overall recommendations are: 1) the patient may remain in the primary care setting; 2) the patient needs to be referred to hospital care. The patients who may remain in the primary care setting can either need no care or low-complexity care, e.g. medication. The flow of patients is visualised in Fig. 1.

The study population consisted of adult patients (≥18 years) with non-acute and low-complexity cardiology-related health complaints who visited the cardiologist at the PC+ centre between January 1 and December 31, 2015.

Data collection

Data were collected between January 1 and December 31, 2015 and were extracted from the electronic medical

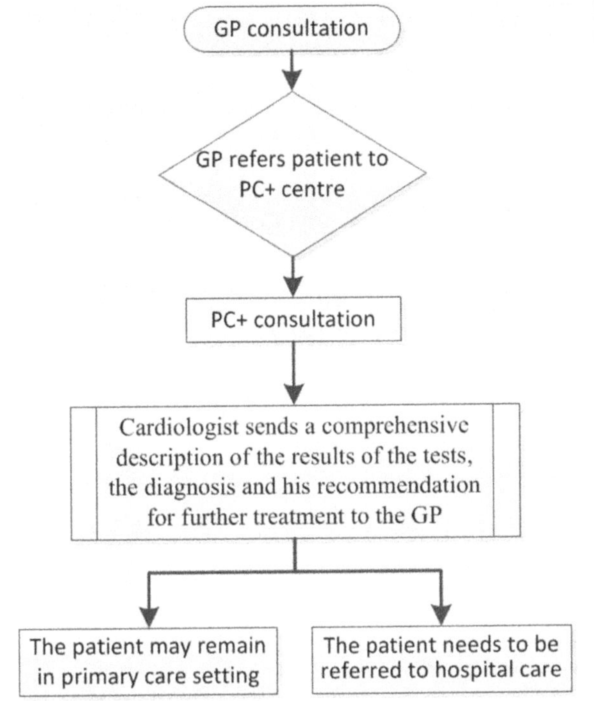

Fig. 1 The flow of patients

Table 1 Overview of the variables and categories

Variables	Categories
Gender	Male Female
Age	-
Referral indication given by the general practitioner*	Heart palpitations Heart murmur Cardiac screening Suspected arrhythmia Atypical chest pain Reduced exercise capacity Collapse Abnormal ECG Dyspnoea Suspected heart failure Suspected coronary sclerosis Analyses of atrial fibrillation Stable Angina Pectoris
Reason for referral given by the general practitioner*	To reassure the patient Upon patient request Upon specialist advice or request To exclude disease Screening of unclear pathology Checking the unknown To confirm disease
Advice given by the cardiologist after PC+	Follow-up in primary care setting Follow-up in hospital care setting

**Categories are included as separate variables in the analysis*

record system of the PC+ centre. The data consisted of all patients referred by the GPs to the PC+ centre during the above-mentioned time period, including information about the patient characteristics (i.e. age and gender), the referral characteristics (i.e. the referral indication and reason for referral both given by the GP), and the advice of the cardiologist regarding follow-up after PC+ of each patient (see Table 1). The referral indication categories were based on the standardised cardiology referral procedure that was set up by the cardiologists and the regional care group. The categories of the variable reason for referral were based on previous research by Van Hoof et al. [23].

Data analysis

Descriptive statistics were computed to provide information about the study population. Data were described using absolute counts and percentages for categorical variables, and means and standard deviations for continuous variables. Statistical model assumptions were examined before conducting further analyses.

Logistic regression analyses were performed to investigate the predictive value of the independent variables on the dependent variable. The dependent variable, the advice of the cardiologist regarding the follow-up of the patient, consists of two possibilities: 1) follow-up in primary care setting; 2) follow-up in hospital care setting. Gender, age, referral indication (13 categories) and reason for referral (7 categories) are the independent variables. Age was rescaled such that one unit (year) is equal to ten years. The categories of the 13 indications for referral and seven reasons for referral were used as separate variables with dichotomous coding. An overview of the variables is provided in Table 1. Only people with no missing data were included in the analyses.

First, univariate logistic regression analyses were performed to identify the independent predictors of the outcome of PC+ and to perform a pre-selection for the multivariable logistic regression analyses. Odds ratios (ORs), 95% confidence intervals (CIs) and p-values were reported. A p-value cut-off point of 0.15 was used to select the candidate variables for the multivariable analyses. This is also called purposeful selection of covariates [24–26].

Second, multivariable logistic regression analyses were performed using a stepwise backward method. Model selection was based on likelihood ratio test statistics. The validity was assessed using a Hosmer Lemeshow goodness-of-fit Chi-square analysis. Odds ratios (ORs), 95% confidence intervals (CIs) and p-values were reported; p-values < 0.05 were considered statistically significant. Analyses were performed using IBM SPSS Statistics, version 24.

Results

The data extracted from the electronic medical record system resulted in 1681 cases. Of these, 1525 cases were included for analyses as 156 cases contained missing values on the variables referral indication ($n = 116$), reason for referral ($n = 36$) or both ($n = 4$). The patients' average age was 57.6 years (SD ± 14.6), with a minimum and maximum age of 18 and 97, respectively, and 46.4% of the patients were male. In 23.1% ($n = 352$) of the cases the cardiologist advised referring the patient to hospital care, while in all other cases ($n = 1173$; 76.9%) the cardiologists' advice was to keep the patient in primary care. See Table 2 for an overview of the descriptive analyses.

Table 3 shows the results of the univariate analyses. Gender, age, four referral indications and five reasons for referrals were independent predictors of the advice 'follow-up in hospital care setting'. The referral indication 'Stable Angina Pectoris' was the most predictive variable (OR = 5.000, 95% CI = 2.885–8.666). The reason for referral 'To confirm disease' was the strongest predictor of the advice of the cardiologist (OR = 4.786, 95% CI = 3.006–7.618). The variables gender, age, 'Atypical chest pain', 'Dyspnoea', 'Heart palpitations', 'Abnormal ECG', 'Cardiac screening', 'Stable Angina Pectoris', 'Suspected heart failure', 'To exclude disease', 'Screening of unclear pathology', 'To confirm disease', 'Reassurance' and 'Checking the unknown' had p-values smaller than the cut-off point of 0.15 and were included in the multivariable logistic regression analysis.

Table 4 presents the independent variables that were significant multivariable predictors of the advice of the cardiologist regarding follow-up after PC+. 'Stable Angina Pectoris' (OR = 3.360; 95% CI = 1.850–6.100) and 'To confirm disease' (OR = 3.807; 95% CI = 2.307–6.284) are the two strongest predictors. The reason for referral 'To reassure the patient' (OR = 0.223; 95% CI = 0.069–0.718) is the only significant predictor with an OR < 1. This implies that patients referred with the reason 'To reassure the patient' were more likely to get the advice 'follow-up in primary care setting' after the PC+ consultation.

Table 2 Description of study population ($N = 1525$)

Variables	Mean (SD±) or n (%)
Gender:	
Female	818 (53.6%)
Male	707 (46.4%)
Age	57.6 (±14.6)
Referral indication given by the general practitioner:	
Atypical chest pain	630 (41.3%)
Dyspnoea	202 (13.2%)
Heart palpitations	192 (12.6%)
Abnormal ECG	103 (6.8%)
Cardiac screening	102 (6.7%)
Reduced exercise capacity	67 (4.4%)
Collapse	60 (3.9%)
Stable Angina Pectoris	55 (3.6%)
Suspected arrhythmia	32 (2.1%)
Suspected heart failure	31 (2.0%)
Heart murmur	25 (1.6%)
Suspected coronary sclerosis	16 (1.0%)
Analyses of atrial fibrillation	10 (0.7%)
Reason for referral given by the general practitioner	
To exclude disease	1193 (81.4%)
Screening of unclear pathology	132 (8.7%)
To confirm disease	78 (5.1%)
To reassure the patient	67 (4.4%)
Checking the unknown	29 (1.9%)
Upon patient request	20 (1.3%)
Upon specialist advice or request	6 (0.4%)
Advice given by the cardiologist after PC+:	
Follow-up in primary care setting	1173 (76.9%)
Follow-up in hospital care setting	352 (23.1%)

Discussion

Main findings

The study objective was to explore which cardiology-related referral indications and reasons for referral are appropriate for specialist care in PC+ and which are more appropriate for specialist care in the hospital setting. Results showed that significant predictors of the advice 'follow-up in hospital care setting' are gender (male), age (per ten years), the referral indications 'Stable Angina Pectoris' or 'Dyspnoea' and the reasons for referral 'To confirm disease' or 'Screening of unclear pathology'.

Interpretation of the main findings

Patients with one or more of the significant predictors have a higher probability of being referred to hospital care after a consultation at the PC+ centre. For example, a patient with an age of 30 years with the referral indication 'Stable Angina Pectoris' has a probability of 22.4% of getting the advice 'Follow-up in hospital care setting', and when in this case the reason for referral is 'To confirm disease' the probability is 51.1%, and if this patient is 70 years (instead of 30 years) it is even 72.2%. The reason for referral 'To reassure the patient' is a significant predictor of the advice 'Follow-up in primary care setting'. The probability of these patients getting the advice 'Follow-up in hospital care setting' is only 1%.

The aim of PC+ is to substitute specialist care in the hospital setting with specialist care in the primary care setting. To achieve this it is crucial that PC+ is not designed as an intermediate station and thus it is important to select the appropriate patient groups for PC+. However, the results of this observational explorative study based on quantitative data of the PC+ centre need further interpretation. The results provide only

Table 3 Univariate association between independent variables and the advice of the cardiologist: follow-up in hospital care setting after PC+

Independent variables	Advice of the cardiologist: follow-up in hospital care setting after PC+[A]		
	OR	*95% CI*	*P-value*
Gender[B]*	1.694	1.332–2.155	< .001
Age[C]*	1.352	1.236–2.478	< .001
Referral indication			
Atypical chest pain*	0.683	0.533–0.876	.003
Dyspnoea*	1.667	1.206–2.304	.002
Heart palpitations *	0.581	0.386–0.875	.009
Abnormal ECG*	1.477	0.952–2.291	.082
Cardiac screening*	0.650	0.380–1.109	.114
Reduced exercise capacity	0.795	0.429–1.474	.466
Collapse	0.919	0.491–1.718	.791
Stable Angina Pectoris*	5.000	2.885–8.666	< .001
Suspected arrhythmia	0.765	0.312–1.874	.558
Suspected heart failure*	1.860	0.882–3.920	.103
Heart murmur	0.631	0.215–1.849	.401
Suspected coronary sclerosis	2.017	0.728–5.588	.177
Analyses of atrial fibrillation	2.236	0.627–7.967	.215
Reason for referral			
To exclude disease*	0.477	0.365–0.623	< .001
Screening of unclear pathology*	2.368	1.633–3.435	< .001
To confirm disease *	4.786	3.006–7.618	< .001
To reassure the patient*	0.149	0.047–0.477	.001
Checking the unknown*	2.400	1.135–5.075	.022
Upon patient request	0.367	0.085–1.588	.180
Upon specialist advice or request	0.666	0.077–5.715	.711

*Note:[A] The advice was coded as: 0 = Follow-up in primary care setting, 1 = Follow-up in hospital care setting setting;[B] Gender was coded as 0 = female and 1 = male;[C] Age was rescaled such that one unit is equal to ten years; * Selected variable for multivariable logistic regression analyses. Predictor with a p < .15*

Table 4 Multivariable logistic regression analysis: significant predictive variables on the advice of the cardiologist: follow-up in hospital care setting after PC+

Independent variables	Advice of the cardiologist: follow-up in hospital care setting after PC+[A]			
	b	OR	*95% CI*	*P-value*
Gender[B]	0.617	1.854	1.437–2.393	< .001
Age[C]	0.228	1.256	1.143–1.381	< .001
Referral indication				
Dyspnoea	0.458	1.581	1.120–2.231	.009
Stable Angina Pectoris	1.203	3.331	1.847–6.009	< .001
Reason for referral				
Screening of unclear pathology	0.845	2.328	1.580–3.430	< .001
To confirm disease	1.282	3.604	2.180–5.959	< .001
To reassure the patient	−1.475	0.229	0.071–0.739	.014

Note: [A] The advice was coded as: 0 = Follow-up in primary care setting, 1 = Follow-up in hospital care setting;[B] Gender was coded as 0 = female and 1 = male; [C]Age was rescaled such that one unit is equal to ten years insight which patients are more likely to be referred from PC+ to hospital care. This insight can be used as an input and can provide guidance for the healthcare professionals to improve the referral patterns (e.g. list of inclusion criteria for PC+). GPs and cardiologists should deliberate and collaborate to improve the referring procedures in order to enhance the connectivity between the different healthcare providers and the alignment of care. In addition to the characteristics taken into account in this study, more factors will probably influence which patient groups are appropriate for PC+, such as clinical information and specialist characteristics (e.g. level of expertise, experience and confidence). Hence, further research is needed to find out more precisely which patients are appropriate for PC+ and which patients should be excluded from PC+.

Reflection with existing literature

Previous studies have shown that outreach clinics could lead to increased healthcare costs [15, 27]. This is also a pitfall of PC+. Focusing on the appropriate patient groups and preventing PC+ from becoming an intermediate station increase its chances of success. Additionally, previous research showed that GPs experienced difficulty and uncertainty in referring eligible patients to PC+ [18]. Medical specialists sometimes saw patients in PC+ who should have been referred directly to hospital care or who could have been treated by the GP him–/herself [18]. Selecting the appropriate patient groups seemed to be essential for achieving efficient substitution. Moreover, PC+ is related to the concept integrated care as described by Kodner and Spreeuwenberg [16]. Intensifying the communication and collaboration between GPs and medical specialists in order to connect and align multiple services, providers and settings is one of its core features. Additionally, it is aimed at enhancing population health, quality of care as experienced by patients and reducing the number of unnecessary and inappropriate referrals in order to achieve efficiency. Hence, to improve the referral procedures it is recommended that GPs and cardiologists deliberate and collaborate. The patient groups that have a significantly higher probability of receiving the advice 'Follow-up in hospital care setting' should not be referred first to PC+. Additionally, they should deliberate about the patients who are referred with the reason 'To reassure the patient'. Previous research indicated that perceived medical need is the strongest predictor but not the only predictor of GPs' behaviour: perceived pressure from patients is also a strong independent predictor of GPs' behaviour that affects the referral behaviour [28, 29]. It is plausible that some of the patients with the reason for referral 'To reassure the patient' were not referred to PC+ based on a medical need but on perceived pressure from the patients. With reference to efficiency, the results indicate that GPs should refer patients with a medical need and as few patients as possible with only a 'To reassure the patient' need. The strengthened collaboration and intensified communication generates knowledge transfer between the GPs and cardiologists. In the long term it is expected that this will induce a learning-effect for the GPs, which will probably result in less inappropriate referrals.

Strengths and limitations

This study used quantitative data extracted from the electronic medical record system of a cardiology PC+ centre. The study is based on a large sample size, namely on almost all referrals to the centre over one year. The results provide insight into which patients are less appropriate for PC+. Eventually this will lead to an increased number of appropriate referrals and fewer inappropriate referrals, in order to contribute to containing the rising healthcare costs.

A limitation of this study concerns the generalizability of the findings. The findings are context-bound, and generalizability to other countries (e.g. countries where GPs do not have a gatekeeping role), specialties (as this study is focused on cardiology) and/or other PC+ models is limited.

Future research

The results of this study are based on traditional statistical analyses providing insight into the appropriate patient groups for cardiology PC+ centres. This research is limited to quantitative data, and complementary (qualitative) research may be helpful for interpreting the findings in more detail.

The results showed a gender difference in the probability of being referred to specialist care in the hospital setting after a consultation at PC+; male patients have a significantly higher probability. This gender difference should be further investigated because previous studies demonstrated that the risk of heart disease in women has been underestimated. The awareness of the cardiovascular disease health risk in women among healthcare providers is relatively low and women are often misunderstood in terms of their symptoms [30, 31].

The results of this study can provide guidance for further research. To be better able to select the appropriate patient groups for PC+ it is recommend to investigate the influence of other factors and characteristics, and to perform complementary qualitative research to interpret and clarify the quantitative results. Future research could, for example, focus on the specialist characteristics (e.g. level of expertise, experience and confidence) and it should also include clinical outcomes (e.g. including follow-up data after a consult at the PC+ centre).

Additionally, regarding the cost-effectiveness of this PC+ intervention it is supposed that the introduction of PC+ will lead to reduced healthcare costs by lower costs in PC+ than in hospital care due to lower overhead costs, fewer referrals to hospital care, and less use of additional hospital-based services. Future research will take into account the effects on the health of the population, patients' experiences of care and healthcare costs and will specifically focus on the cost-effectiveness of PC+ [17].

Conclusions

Although the success of PC+ does not only depend on selecting the appropriate patient groups, this is important for achieving efficiency. The results of this study can be used to improve the referral pattern and to enhance the connectivity and alignment of care. Patients with the referral indication 'Stable Angina Pectoris' or 'Dyspnoea', and reason for referral 'To confirm disease' or 'Screening of unclear pathology', seem to be more appropriate for specialist care in the hospital setting instead of PC+. Additionally, the reason for referral 'To reassure the patient' is a significant predictor of the advice 'Follow-up in primary care setting'.

Abbreviations

GP: General practitioner; PC+: Primary Care Plus

Acknowledgements

We gratefully acknowledge the PC+ centre for participating in this research and providing the data.

Funding

This research did not receive any specific grant from funding agencies in the public, commercial, or not-for-profit sectors.

Authors' contributions

TCCQ, JNS, MDS, CAB and DR designed the study. TCCQ and MDS collected and analysed the data. TCCQ and JNS wrote the first draft of the paper. TCCQ, JNS, MDS, CAB and DR read and revised and approved the manuscript. All authors agree to be accountable for all aspects of the study.

Competing interests

The authors declare that they have no competing interests.

Author details

[1]Department of Health Services Research, Care and Public Health Research Institute, Faculty of Health Medicine and Life Sciences, Maastricht University, Maastricht, The Netherlands. [2]Department for Quality of Care and Health Economics, Centre for Nutrition, Prevention and Health Services, National Institute for Public Health and the Environment, Bilthoven, The Netherlands. [3]Research Centre for Technology in Care, Zuyd University of Applied Sciences, Heerlen, The Netherlands. [4]Scientific Centre for Transformation in Care and Welfare (Tranzo), University of Tilburg, Tilburg, The Netherlands.

References

1. Porter ME, Lee TH. The strategy that will fix healthcare. Harv Bus Rev. 2013; 91(10):50–70.
2. Van Ginneken E. Perennial health care reform – the long Dutch quest for cost control and quality improvement. N Engl J Med. 2015;373(10):885–9.
3. Schäfer W, Kroneman M, Boerma W, et al. The Netherlands: health system review. Health Systems in Transition. 2010;12(1):1–229.
4. Rijksoverheid. Naar beter betaalbare zorg. Rapport Taskforce Beheersing Zorguitgaven. [To more affordable care. Report Taskforce Control Healthcare Expenditures.] Ministerie van Volksgezondheid, Welzijn en Sport; Den Haag: Rijksoverheid; 2012. [in Dutch].
5. Saltman RB, Figueras J. Analyzing the evidence on European health care reforms. Health Aff. 1998;17(2):85–108.
6. Warner M. Re-designing health services. Reducing the zone of delusion. London: The Nuffield Trust; 1997.
7. Grone O. and Gracia-Barbero M. Integrated care. A position paper of the WHO European office for integrated health care services. International Journal of Integrated Care. 2001;1:e21.
8. Vlek JF, Vierhout WP, Knottnerus JA, et al. A randomised controlled trial of joint consultations with general practitioners and cardiologists in primary care. Br J Gen Pract. 2003;53(487):108–12.
9. Schulpen GJ, Vierhout WP, van der Heijde DM, Landewe RB, Winkens RA, van der Linden S. Joint consultation of general practitioner and rheumatologist: does it matter? Ann Rheum Dis. 2003;62(2):159–61.
10. Vierhout WP, Knottnerus JA, van Ooji A, Crebolder HF, et al. Effectiveness of joint consultation sessions of general practitioners and orthopaedic surgeons for locomotor-system disorders. Lancet. 1995;346(8981):990–4.
11. Bowling A, Stramer K, Dickinson E, Windsor J, Bond M. Evaluation of specialists' outreach clinics in general practice in England: process and acceptability to patients, specialists, and general practitioners. J Epidemiol Community Health. 1997;51(1):52–61.
12. Black M, Leese B, Gosden T, Mead N. Specialist outreach clinics in general practice: what do they offer? Br J Gen Pract. 1997;47(422):558–61.
13. Bowling A, Bond M. A national evaluation of specialists' clinics in primary care settings. Br J Gen Pract. 2001;51(465):264–9.
14. Powell J. Systematic review of outreach clinics in primary care in the UK. Journal of Health Services Research & Policy. 2002;7(3):177–83.
15. van Volksgezondheid M. Welzijn en Sport (2013), Onderhandelingsresultaten Schippers met ziekenhuizen, medisch specialisten, zelfstandige behandelcentra, GGZ en huisartsen. [Negotiation results of Minister Schippers with hospitals, medical specialists, independent treatment centres, mental health care and general practitioners.], vol. 2013. Den Haag: Ministerie van Volksgezondheid, Welzijn en Sport. [Ministry of Health, Welfare and Sport]. [in Dutch]
16. Kodner DL, Spreeuwenberg C. Integrated care: meaning, logic, applications, and implication - a discussion paper. International Journal of Integrated Care. 2002;2(14):1–6.
17. Berwick DM, Nolan TW, Whittington J. The triple aim: care, health, and cost. Health Aff. 2008;27(3):759–69.
18. Van Hoof SJM, Kroese MEAL, Spreeuwenberg MD, et al. Substitution of hospital care with primary care: defining the conditions of Primary Care Plus. International Journal of Integrated Care. 2016;16(1):1–11.
19. Steenbakkers M, Vermeer AJM, Janssen-Goffin MJH, Hajema KJ. Een nieuwe kijk op gezondheid in Zuid-Limburg. Regionaal rapport Volksgezondheid Toekomst Verkenning 2014. [A new look at health in South-Limburg Regional report Public Health Future Exploration]. Limburg: Geleen: GGD Zuid; 2014. [in Dutch]
20. Drewes HW, Heijink R, Struijs JN, Baan CA. Samen werken aan duurzame zorg; Landelijke monitor proeftuinen. [Working together towards sustainable healthcare; National monitor pioneer sites]. Bilthoven: Rijksinstituut voor Volksgezondheid en Milieu; 2015. [in Dutch]
21. Struijs JN, Drewes HW, Heijink R, Baan CA. How to evaluate population management? Transforming the Care Continuum Alliance population health guide toward a broadly applicable analytical framework. Health Policy. 2015; 119(4):522–9.
22. Hendrikx RJ, Drewes HW, Spreeuwenberg M, Ruwaard D, Struijs JN, Baan CA. Which triple aim-related measures are being used to evaluate population management initiatives? An international comparative analysis. Health Policy. 2016;120(5):471–85.
23. van Hoof SJ, Spreeuwenberg MD, Kroese ME, et al. Substitution of outpatient care with primary care: a feasibility study on the experiences

among general practitioners, medical specialists and patients. BMC Fam Pract. 2016;17(108):1–9.
24. Twisk JWR. Inleiding in de toegepaste biostatistiek. [Introduction in the applied biostatistics] Amsterdam: Reed Business Education; 2014. [in Dutch].
25. Hosmer DW, Lemweshow S. Applied Logistic Regression. New York: Wiley; 2000.
26. Bursac Z, Gauss CH, Williams DK, Hosmer DW. Purposeful selection of variables in logistic regression. Source Code for Biology and Medicine. 2008;3(17):1–8.
27. Gruen RL, Weeramanthri TS, Knight SS and Bailie RS. Specialist outreach clinics in primary care and rural hospital settings. Cochrane Database Syst Rev. 2003;(4):1–71.
28. Little P, Dorward M, Warner G, Stephens K, Senior J, Moor M. Importance of patient pressure and perceived pressure and perceived medical need for investigations, referral, and prescribing in primary care: nested observational study. Br Med J. 2004;328(7437):444–8.
29. Armstrong D, Fry J, Armstrong P. Doctors' perceptions of pressure from patients for referral. Br Med J. 1991;302(11):1186–8.
30. Mosca L, Linfante AH, Benjamin EJ, et al. National study of physician awareness and adherence to cardiovascular disease prevention guidelines. Circulation. 2005;111(4):499–510.
31. Healy B. The Yentl Syndrome. N Engl J Med. 1991;325(4):274–6.

14

Burnout syndrome and its prevalence in primary care nursing

Carolina S. Monsalve-Reyes[1,2], Concepción San Luis-Costas[3], Jose L. Gómez-Urquiza[4,8*], Luis Albendín-García[5], Raimundo Aguayo[6] and Guillermo A. Cañadas-De la Fuente[7]

Abstract

Background: burnout syndrome is a significant problem in nursing professionals. Although, the unit where nurses work may influence burnout development. Nurses that work in primary care units may be at higher risk of burnout. The aim of the study was to estimate the prevalence of emotional exhaustion, depersonalization and low personal accomplishment in primary care nurses.

Methods: We performed a meta-analysis. We searched Pubmed, CINAHL, Scopus, Scielo, Proquest, CUIDEN and LILACS databases up to September 2017 to identify cross-sectional studies assessing primary care nurses' burnout with the Maslach Burnout Inventory were included. The search was done in September 2017.

Results: After the search process, $n = 8$ studies were included in the meta-analysis, representing a total sample of $n = 1110$ primary care nurses. High emotional exhaustion prevalence was 28% (95% Confidence Interval = 22–34%), high depersonalization was 15% (95% Confidence Interval = 9–23%) and 31% (95% Confidence Interval = 6–66%) for low personal accomplishment.

Conclusions: Problems such as emotional exhaustion and low personal accomplishment are very common among primary care nurses, while depersonalization is less prevalent. Primary care nurses are a burnout risk group.

Keywords: Burnout, Primary care nursing, Nursing, Family nursing, Meta-analysis, Epidemiology, Prevalence

Background

The development of burnout among healthcare professionals has been widely studied in recent years, since the large number of stress-inducing factors in the hospital environment heightens the risk of presenting burnout syndrome [1–3]. In addition, relationships and continued contact with patients and their families can be difficult, which fosters the development of chronic stress that can provoke burnout among healthcare staff [4].

The burnout syndrome has been extensively studied, even though the most widely accepted definition of burnout is that proposed by Maslach & Jackson [5], who identified it as a three-dimensional syndrome involving emotional exhaustion (EE), cynical treatment and negative thoughts towards patients and the healthcare team (or depersonalisation, DP), and a low degree of personal accomplishment (PA) regarding the own work performed. The study of burnout is important because its negative effects can impact both on the professional who suffers it, causing different signs and symptoms [6], and also on the health institution itself, by increasing staff absenteeism, and on the quality of care provided by increasing medical errors and diminishing patient safety [7, 8].

In hospital settings, nurses are among the professionals most affected by burnout [9] and for this reason numerous studies have been conducted to identify protective factors and elements of risk. For example, some sociodemographic factors such as age, gender or marital status and its influence have been assessed [10, 11]. Psychological factors like the big five personality traits [12]

* Correspondence: jlgurquiza@ugr.es
[4]Nursing Department, University of Granada, Granada, Spain
[8]Faculty of Health Sciences, University of Granada, Cortadura del Valle Street S/N, 51001 Ceuta, Spain
Full list of author information is available at the end of the article

or occupational factors, such as job seniority or job satisfaction, have been also studied [13–15].

However, one key factor that may be associated with burnout syndrome is the hospital service in which nurses work; the tasks performed and the role played by the healthcare staff, as well as the type of patients treated, all vary according to the type of service provided, and this difference could influence the development of the syndrome. For example, nurses working in oncology [16], accident and emergency units [17] or intensive care [18], due to their different daily tasks, are likely to experience different levels and prevalence rates of burnout.

Primary healthcare units differ in many respects from the attention provided in hospital units, in that preventive and remedial treatment is provided for chronic diseases, to pre-assigned groups of patients. Primary healthcare is provided in the community itself, and may take place over a prolonged period [19]. By contrast, in the hospital environment the medical treatment is of a shorter-term nature, and there is greater variability among the patients. Although burnout and its risk factors in nursing primary care professionals, such as age, job seniority, anxiety and depression, have been studied previously [20], the prevalence results reported by the studies vary widely, with some authors reporting a high EE of 5,2% [21] while others report 31,3% [22]. Similar situations occur with high DP and low PA, where some authors find 92,8% of the sample with low PA [23] and others find a 4,3% of the sample with low PA [22]. So, it is difficult to ascertain the real impact of burnout syndrome on primary healthcare nurses. To our knowledge, no previous meta-analysis has been undertaken to address this question, as has been done in the case of nurses working in services such as Accident & Emergency [24] or oncology [25].

Taking into account the above considerations, we aimed to conduct a systematic review and meta-analysis of the prevalence of high levels of EE, high levels of DP and low levels of PA among primary care nurses. Thus, the question that guided this meta-analysis was: What is the prevalence rate of high EE, high DP and low PA in primary care nurses?

Method

This study consists of a meta-analysis, performed in accordance with the PRISMA recommendations [26].

Literature search and study selection

The following search terms were used: "burnout AND primary care nursing", "burnout AND family nursing", "burnout AND community health nursing" and "burnout AND district nursing". The search was carried out in September 2017, consulting the following research databases: Pubmed, CUIDEN, CINAHL, LILACS, Proquest, Scopus and Scielo.

Conditions for inclusion were that the papers should be primary studies, of a quantitative type, based on a sample of primary healthcare nurses and providing data on the prevalence of any burnout dimension (EE, DP or PA), measured by the Maslach Burnout Inventory (MBI) [5]. The studies should have been published in English, Spanish or Portuguese, but no restriction was placed regarding the date of publication.

The search and study selection process was conducted by two members of the research team, working independently, to ensure the reliability of the process. If they disagreed regarding the inclusion or otherwise of a paper, a third member of the research team was consulted. The selection process involved an initial reading, of the title and abstract. The papers initially selected were then read in full, and those considered a priori suitable for inclusion were then subjected to a critical reading to detect possible methodological bias. From the papers finally selected, backward and forward citation checking was then performed.

Critical reading

All of the studies included were cross-sectional, and their methodological quality was evaluated by the checklist suggested by Ciapponi [27], using the items corresponding to the studies internal validity: numbers 2, 3, 4, 5, 6, 11, 12, 13, 14,2 15, 16, 17 and 18. The critical reading results are shown in Additional file 1.

Data coding

The following study variables were collected: a) surname of the first author; b) date of publication; c) language of the study; d) country where the research was carried out; e) study methodology; f) type of sampling; g) MBI type (Human Services Survey vs. General Survey); h) sample of primary healthcare nurses; i) sample of primary healthcare nurses with high EE; j) sample of primary care nurses with high DP; k) sample of primary healthcare nurses with low PA. These data were compiled using a Coding Manual.

The intraclass correlation coefficient and Cohen's kappa coefficient were calculated to evaluate the reliability of the data coding, producing mean values of 0.99 (minimum = 0.98, maximum = 1) and 0.97 (minimum = 0.95, maximum = 1), respectively.

Data analysis

Data analysis was performed using StatsDirect software, with the meta-analysis package, and the possibility of publication bias was tested by Egger's linear regression method. Finally, a sensitivity analysis was carried out to detect whether exclusion of any of the studies would have produced significant changes in the results obtained.

The prevalence and the confidence interval of each dimension of burnout were calculated by three independent random-effects meta-analyses. Sample heterogeneity was analysed with the Cochran Q test and the I^2 index.

Results

The search process initially obtained $n = 1430$ results, which after reading title and abstract, full-text and the application of the inclusion and exclusion criteria were reduced to $n = 8$ for high EE and $n = 7$ for high DP and low PA [21–23, 28–32]. The selection process is illustrated in Fig. 1.

All of the included studies were transversal and descriptive, and used the HSS version of the MBI. Only one study used random sampling, and 75% were conducted in Europe. The characteristics of these studies are listed in Table 1.

The sensitivity analysis performed, of the influence of each study on the overall result, revealed no statistically significant changes in the prevalence rates. Neither was any significant publication bias detected, being Egger's linear regression score 1.66 ($p = 0.43$) for high EE, 1.09 ($p = 0.77$) for high DP and 5.29 ($p = 0.67$) for low PA.

Cochran's Q value was 33.10 ($p < 0.001$) for EE, 46.31 ($p < 0.001$) for DP and 697.45 ($p < 0.001$) for low PA.

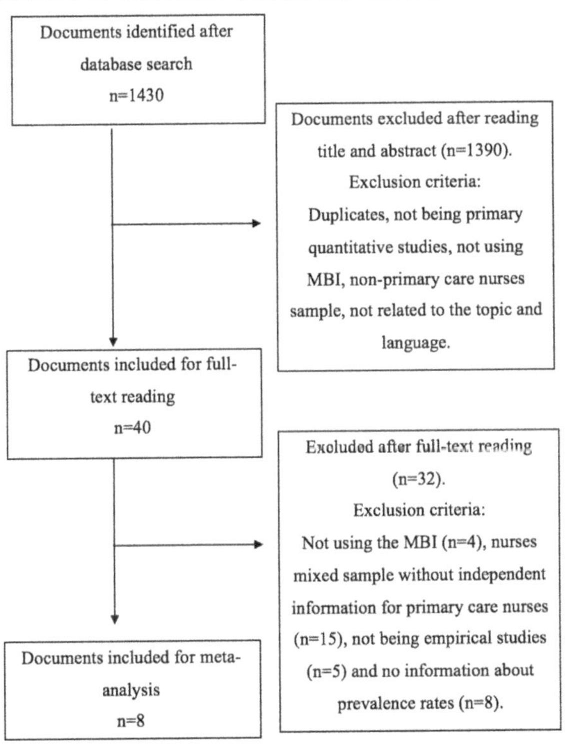

Fig. 1 Documents search flow diagram

The I^2 index revealed a high level of heterogeneity, at 78.9% for EE, 87% for DP and 99.1% for low PA.

The total population for the meta-analysis was composed of $n = 1110$ primary care nurses. The prevalence rate obtained for high emotional exhaustion was 28% (95% CI: 22–34%). Figure 2 shows the forestplot of high EE.

In depersonalization dimension the prevalence rate was 15% (95% CI: 9%–23%). The forestplot of high DP is shown in Fig. 3.

Finally, a 31% (95% CI: 6–66%) was found for low personal accomplishment. Figure 4 show illustrate the forestplot of low PA.

Discussion

Our meta-analysis shows that low personal accomplishment is the most widely affected dimension of burnout in primary care nurses, being present in 31% of the sample. This is followed by emotional exhaustion, which was observed in 28% of the nurses in the sample. The lowest level of prevalence corresponded to depersonalisation, which affected 15% of these nurses.

To our knowledge, no previous meta-analysis has been performed regarding the prevalence of burnout in primary care nurses. The number of studies included in the present meta-analysis is lower than in those with A&E nurses [24] or oncology nurses [25]. Meta-analytical studies of the prevalence of burnout among A&E nurses have reported values similar to our own for EE and low PA, with prevalence rates of 31% and 29%, respectively. However, these previous papers measured a much higher presence of DP (36%) than in our sample of primary care nurses [24]. On the other hand, a meta-analysis focusing on burnout among oncology nurses observed higher levels of EE, lower levels of DP and PA, than in the primary care nurses in our sample [25]. Nevertheless, it is foreseeable that primary care nurses will experience less DP than A&E nurses, because they often follow the evolution of chronic patients for years, perhaps visiting patients in their homes and in their community. This situation favours empathy and the formation of a close relationship with the patient, which is of crucial importance to the quality of care [33].

The important degree of EE and low PA observed among primary care nurses may be due, among other factors, to their sometimes encountering difficult patients, who can be very demanding and may continually seek medical attention, necessary or otherwise. Such persons disrupt the routines of the service and have a negative impact on medical professionals [34–36]. In addition, the importance that primary care is gaining in health services, and the growing demand for services in this area, forces nurses to meet the new challenges and requests that are generated, adding more pressure to

Table 1 Characteristics of included studies ($n = 8$)

Author, year. Country	Study type; Sampling method	Type of MBI	Sample size (Females%; Response rate%)	n with high EE	n with high DP	n with low PA
Das Merces et al., 2016. Brasil [28]	O; Intentional	HSS	$n = 28$ (100%; 90,32%)	8	6	13
Faura et al., 1995. Spain [29]	O; Intentional	HSS	$n = 116$ (90.5%; ND)	27	–	–
Hayter, 1999. England [30]	O; Intentional	HSS	$n = 30$ (80%; 94%)	8	0	6
Holmes et al., 2014. Brasil [31]	O; Random	HSS	$n = 45$ (100%; 100%)	24	5	5
Navarro-Gonzalez et al., 2005. Spain [21]	O; Intentional	HSS	$n = 178$ (73,3%; 48%)	28	33	84
Soto Cámara et al., 2005. Spain [23]	O; Intentional	HSS	$n = 208$ (86.5%: 83,87%)	60	67	193
Tomas-Sabado et al., 2010. Spain [32]	O; Intentional	HSS	$n = 160$ (89.7%; 67%)	35	19	14
Vila Faguera et al., 2015. Spain [22]	O; Intentional	HSS	$n = 345$ (80.2%; 44.5%)	108	51	15

DP Depersonalization, *EE* Emotional exhaustion, *HSS* Human Services Survey, *MBI* Maslach Burnout Inventory, *ND* No Data, *O* Observational, *PA* Personal Accomplishment

their work [37]. To all this, we must add the difficulties of nursing work, such as contact with vulnerable people and families in consultation and in patients´ homes [38], the increasing workload, or the lack of control over their own work environment [39], which may favour EE and decrease PA.

Some limitations of this study should be acknowledged. The number of studies included is low, because not all studies of burnout in primary care nurses provide prevalence data. Moreover, the studies included are all cross-sectional and descriptive, which accounts for their low level of evidence (although this design is usually considered appropriate for prevalence studies). Furthermore, the included studies, despite meeting almost all the items of the critical reading guide, have small sample sizes. To this, we must add the high heterogeneity found in the results, which may be due to the different countries where the studies have been done, because the healthcare systems of each country have different workplace conditions, salary, shifts and competencies for the nursing workforce [40], which may influence nurses´ burnout and should be taken into account when interpreting the results.

Future research in this area should include a longitudinal evaluation of the sociodemographic, occupational, and psychological factors that may influence the development of burnout syndrome among primary care nurses. It would be interesting to examine interventions aimed at preventing and/or reducing emotional exhaustion in this occupational group. Finally, in view of the results obtained in this meta-analysis, action should be taken to enhance feelings of personal accomplishment

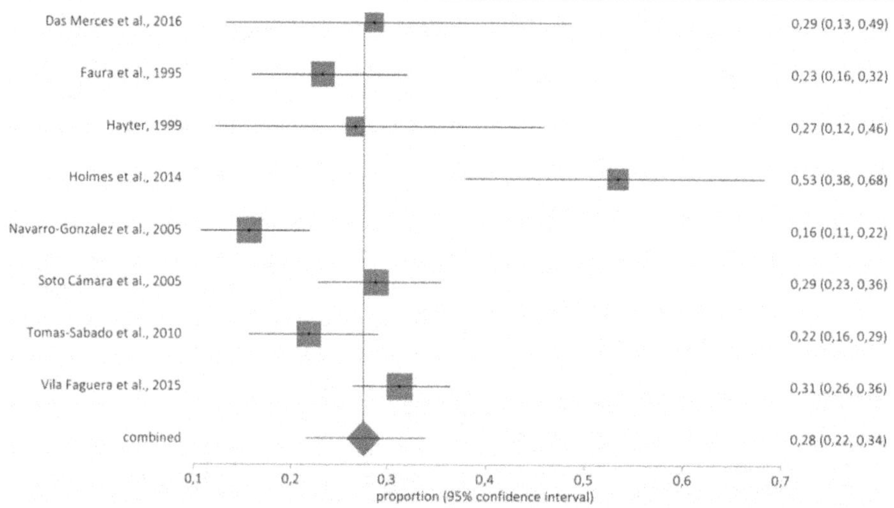

Fig. 2 Forestplot of high emotional exhaustion

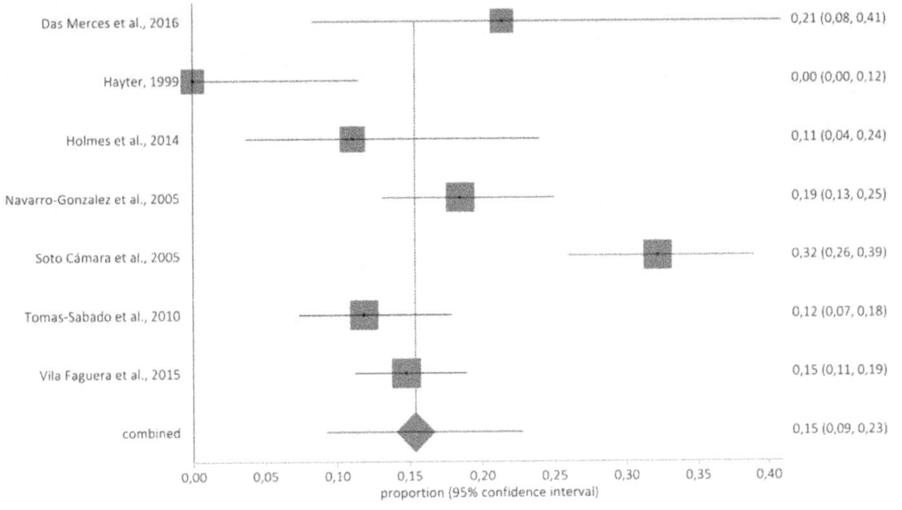

Fig. 3 Forestplot of high depersonalization

among primary care nurses, for example by fostering professional empowerment, by establishing primary care nurses' groups so they can express their feeling [41], promoting leadership capabilities and positive psychological capacities [42] or improving the workplace conditions.

Conclusions

Problems such as emotional exhaustion and low personal accomplishment are very common among primary care nurses from the countries included in the meta-analysis, with a prevalence between 22 and 34% and around 31% respectively. Depersonalisation is less prevalent in this population, at around 15%, which indicates that primary care nurses included in the meta-analysis relate well with their patients.

Abbreviations

CI: Confidence Interval; DP: Depersonalization; EE: Emotional Exhaustion; MBI: Maslach Burnout Inventory; PA: Personal Acomplishment

Funding

This work was funded by the Excellence Research Project P11HUM-7771 (Junta de Andalucía-Spain).

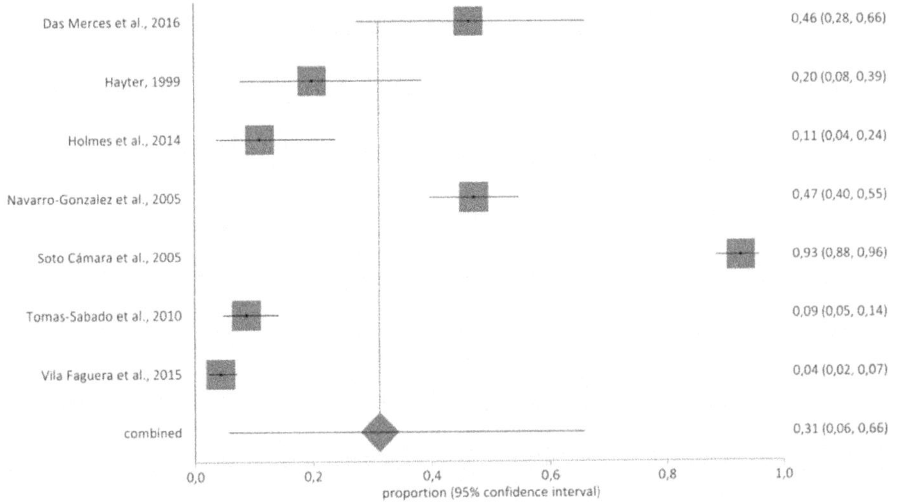

Fig. 4 Forestplot of low personal accomplishment

Authors' contributions

CSM-R (design of the meta-analysis, creation of database, analysis and interpretation of data, and elaboration of the manuscript). CSL-C (design of the meta-analysis, creation of database, analysis and interpretation of data, and elaboration of the manuscript). JLG-U (design of the meta-analysis, search of studies, creation of database, analysis and interpretation of data, and elaboration of the manuscript). LA-G (search of studies, creation of database, analysis and interpretation of data, and elaboration of the manuscript). RA (creation of database, analysis and interpretation of data, and elaboration of the manuscript). GAC-DF (creation of database, analysis and interpretation of data, and elaboration of the manuscript). All authors read and approved the final manuscript.

Competing interests

The authors declare that they have no competing interests.

Author details

[1]Departamento de Ciencias Sociales, Universidad Católica de La Santísima Concepción, Concepción, Chile. [2]Doctorado en Psicología de la Salud, Facultad de Psicología, Universidad Nacional de Educación a Distancia (UNED), Madrid, Spain. [3]Spanish University of Distance Education, Madrid, Spain. [4]Nursing Department, University of Granada, Granada, Spain. [5]Andalusian Health Service and University of Granada, Granada, Spain. [6]Psychology Department, University of Granada, Granada, Spain. [7]Nursing Department, University of Granada, Granada, Spain. [8]Faculty of Health Sciences, University of Granada, Cortadura del Valle Street S/N, 51001 Ceuta, Spain.

References

1. Maslach C, Schaufeli W, Leiter MP. Job burnout. Annu Rev Psychol. 2001;52: 397–422.
2. Peterson U, Demerouti E, Bergström G, Samuelsson M, Asberg M, Nygren A. Burnout and physical and mental health among Swedish healthcare workers. J Adv Nurs. 2008;62(1):84–95.
3. Wood BD, Killion JB. Burnout among healthcare professionals. Radiology Manag. 2007;29:30–4.
4. Sablik Z, Samborska-Sablik A, Drozdz J. Universality of physicians´ burnout syndrome as a result of experiencing difficulty in relationship with patients. Arch Med Sci. 2013;9(3):398–403.
5. Maslach C, Jackson SE. The measurement of experienced burnout. J Organizational Behav. 1981;2:99–113.
6. Schaufeli WB, Leiter MP, Maslach C. Burnout: 35 years of research and practice. Career Development International. 2009;14:204–20.
7. Shanafelt TD, Balch CM, Bechamps G, Russell T, Dyrbye L, Satele D, et al. Burnout and medical errors among American surgeons. Ann Surg. 2010; 251(6):995–1000.
8. Teng CI, Shuy YI, Chiou WK, Fan HC, Lam SM. Interactive effects of nurse-experienced time pressure and burnout on patient safety: a cross-sectional survey. Int J Nurs Stud. 2010;47(11):1442–50.
9. Cañadas-De la Fuente GA, Vargas C, San Luis C, García I, Cañadas GR, De La Fuente EI. Risk factors and prevalence of burnout syndrome in the nursing profession. Int J Nurs Stud. 2015;52(1):240–9.
10. Gómez-Urquiza JL, Vargas C, De la Fuente EI, Fernández-Castillo R. Cañadas-De la Fuente GA. Age as a risk factor for burnout syndrome in nursing professionals: a meta-analytic study. Res Nurs Health. 2017;40(2):99–110.
11. Ayala E, Carnero AM. Determinants of burnout in acute and critical care military nursing personnel: a cross-sectional study from Peru. PLoS One. 2013;8(1):e54408. https://doi.org/10.1371/journal.pone.00544081.
12. Hudek-Knezevic J, Kalebic Maglica B, Krapic N. Personality, organizational stress, and attitudes toward work as prospective predictor of professional burnout in hospital nurses. Croat Med J. 2011;52(4):538–49.
13. Cañadas-De la Fuente GA, Albendín-García L, De la Fuente EI, San Luis C, Gómez-Urquiza JL, Cañadas GR. Síndrome de burnout en profesionales de enfermería que realizan jornada física complementaria en servicios de cuidados críticos y urgencias. Rev Española de Salud Pública. 2016;90:e1–9.
14. Dickinson T, Wright KM. Stress and burnout in forensic mental health nursing: a literatura review. Br J Nurs. 2008;17(2):82–7.
15. Vargas C, Cañadas GA, Aguayo R, Fernández R, De la Fuente EI. Which occupational risk factors are associated with burnout in nursing? A meta-analytic study. Int J Clin Health Psychol. 2014;14(1):28–38.
16. Gómez-Urquiza JL, Aneas-López AB, De la Fuente-Solana EI, Albendín-García L, Díaz-Rodríguez L. Cañadas-De la Fuente GA. Prevalence, risk factors and levels of burnout among oncology nurses: a systematic review. Oncol Nurs Forum. 2016;43(3):E104–20.
17. Albendín L, Gómez JL. Cañadas-De la Fuente GA, Cañadas GR, San Luis C, Aguayo R. Bayesian prevalence and burnout levels in emergency nurses. A systematic review. Rev Latinoam Psicol. 2016;48(2):137–45.
18. Chuang CH, Tseng PC, Lin CY, Lin KH, Chen YY. Burnout in the intensive care unit professionals: a systematic review. Medicine 2016; 95(50):e5629. https://doi.org/10.1097/MD.0000000000 005629.
19. Girard A, Hudon C, Poitras M, Roberge P, Chouinard M. Primary care nursing activities with patients affected by physical chronic disease and common mental disorders: a qualitative descriptive study. J Clin Nurs. 2017;26(9–10):1385–94.
20. Gómez-Urquiza JL, Monsalve-Reyes CS, San Luis-Costas C, Fernández-Castillo R, Aguayo-Estremera R. Cañadas-De la Fuente GA. Factores de riesgo y niveles de burnout en enfermeras de atención primaria: una revision sistemática. Aten Primaria. 2017;49(2):77–85.
21. Navarro González D, Ayechu-Díaz A, Huarte-Labiano I. Prevalence of burnout syndrome and its associated factors in primary care staff. SEMERGEN. 2015;41:191–8.
22. Vilá Falgueras M, Cruzate Muñoz C, Orfila Pernas F, Creixell Sureda J, González López MP, Davins MJ. Burnout and teamwork in primary care team. Aten Primaria. 2015;47(1):25–31.
23. Soto Camara R, Santamaría CI. Prevalence of burnout in primary care nurses. Enferm Clin. 2005;15(3):123–30.
24. Gómez-Urquiza JL, De la Fuente-Solana EI, Albendín-García L, Vargas-Pecino C, Ortega-Campos E. Cañadas-De la Fuente GA. Prevalence of burnout syndrome in emergency nurses: a meta-analytic study. Crit Care Nurse. 2017;37(5):e1–9.
25. Cañadas-De la Fuente GA, Gómez-Urquiza JL, Ortega-Campos EM, Cañadas GR, Albendín-García L, De la Fuente-Solana EI. Prevalence of burnout syndrome in oncology nursing: a meta-analytic study. Psychooncology. 2018; In press. doi:https://doi.org/10.1002/pon.4632
26. Urrútia G, Bonfill X. PRISMA declaration: a proposal to improve the publication of systematic reviews and meta-analysis. Med Clín. 2010;135:507–11.
27. Ciapponi A. Guía de lectura crítica de estudios observacionales en epidemiología (primera parte). Evidencia: actualización en la práctica Ambulatoria. 2010;13:135–40.
28. Das Merces MC, Cordeiro TM, Santana AI, Lua I, Silva DS, Alves MS, et al. Burnout syndrome in nursing workers of the primary health care. Rev Baiana Enferm. 2016;39(3):1–9.
29. Faura T, Roige M, Serra R, Ortega C, Monegal M, et al. Prevalencia del síndrome de burnout en enfermeras de hospitalización y de atención primaria. Enferm Clin. 1995;5(3):105–10.
30. Hayter M. Burnout and AIDS care-related factors in HIV community clinical nurse specialists in the north of England. J Adv Nurs. 1999;29:984–93.
31. Holmes ES, Santos SR, Farias JA, Costa MB. Burnout syndrome in nurses acting in primary care: an impact on quality of life. J Res Fundam Care Online. 2014;6(4):1384–95.
32. Tomás-Sábado J, Maynegre-Santaularia M, Pérez-Bartolomé M, Alsina-Rodríguez M, Quinta-Barbero R, Granell-Navas S. Burnout syndrome and suicide risk among primary care nurses. Enferm Clín. 2010;20(3):173–8.
33. Bikker AP, Fitzpatric B, Murphy D, Mercer SW. Measuring empathic, person-centred communication in primary care nurses: validity and reliability of the consultation and relational empathy (CARE) measure. BMC Fam Pract. 2015; 16:149. https://doi.org/10.1186/s12875-015-0374-y.
34. Mas Garriga X, Cruz Doménech JM, Fañanás Lanau N, Allué Buil A, Zamora Casas I, Viñas VR. Difficult patients in primary care: a quantitative and qualitative study. Aten Primaria. 2003;31(4):214–21.
35. Smits FT, Mohrs JJ, Beem EE, Bindels PJ, Van Weert HC. Defining frequent attendance in general practice. BMC Fam Pract. 2008;9:21. https://doi.org/10.1186/1471-2296-9-21.
36. Zoboli EL, Santos DV, Schveiter MC. Adaptation of the inventory of ethical problems to the child health context. Acta Paulista Enfermagem. 2016;29(5): 586–94.

37. Duhoux A, Menear M, Charron M, Lavoie-Tremblay M, Alderson M. Interventions to promote or improve the mental health of primary care nurses: a systematic review. J Nurs Manag. 2007;25:597–607.
38. Souto Silva CC, De Carvalho Lira ALB, Rodrigues Feijao A, Fernandes Costa IK, De Medeiros SM. Burnout and health technologies in the context of primary health care nursing. Escola Anna Nery. 2017;21(2):e20170031.
39. Regina Lorenz V. De Brito Guirardello E. The environment of professional practice and burnout in nurses in primary healthcare. 2014;22(6):926–33.
40. Van der Schoot E, Oginska H, Estryn-Behar M. Burn- out in the nursing profession in Europe. In: Hasselhorn HM, Tackbenberg P, Müller BH, editors. working conditions and intent to leave the profession among nursing staff in Europe (pp. 53–57). Stockholm, Sweden: National Institute for Working Life and Authors; 2003.
41. Jennings BM. Work stress and burnout among nurses: role of the work environment and working conditions. In: Hughes RG, editor. Patient Safety and Quality: an evidence based handbook for nurses. Rockville (MD): Agency for Healthcare Research and Quality (US); 2008.
42. Spence Laschinger HK, Fida R. New nurses burnout and workplace wellbeing: the influence of authentic leadership and psychological capital. Burnout Research. 2014;1(1):19–28.

15

Development and validation of the Evidence Based Medicine Questionnaire (EBMQ) to assess doctors' knowledge, practice and barriers regarding the implementation of evidence-based medicine in primary care

Ranita Hisham[1*], Chirk Jenn Ng[1], Su May Liew[1], Pauline Siew Mei Lai[1], Yook Chin Chia[1,5], Ee Ming Khoo[1], Nik Sherina Hanafi[1], Sajaratulnisah Othman[1], Ping Yein Lee[2], Khatijah Lim Abdullah[3] and Karuthan Chinna[4]

Abstract

Background: Evidence-Based Medicine (EBM) integrates best available evidence from literature and patients' values, which then informs clinical decision making. However, there is a lack of validated instruments to assess the knowledge, practice and barriers of primary care physicians in the implementation of EBM. This study aimed to develop and validate an Evidence-Based Medicine Questionnaire (EBMQ) in Malaysia.

Methods: The EBMQ was developed based on a qualitative study, literature review and an expert panel. Face and content validity was verified by the expert panel and piloted among 10 participants. Primary care physicians with or without EBM training who could understand English were recruited from December 2015 to January 2016. The EBMQ was administered at baseline and two weeks later. A higher score indicates better knowledge, better practice of EBM and less barriers towards the implementation of EBM. We hypothesized that the EBMQ would have three domains: knowledge, practice and barriers.

Results: The final version of the EBMQ consists of 80 items: 62 items were measured on a nominal scale, 22 items were measured on a 5 point Likert-scale. Flesch reading ease was 61.2. A total of 343 participants were approached; of whom 320 agreed to participate (response rate = 93.2%). Factor analysis revealed that the EBMQ had eight domains after 13 items were removed: "EBM websites", "evidence-based journals", "types of studies", "terms related to EBM", "practice", "access", "patient preferences" and "support". Cronbach alpha for the overall EBMQ was 0.909, whilst the Cronbach alpha for the individual domain ranged from 0.657–0.940. The EBMQ was able to discriminate between doctors with and without EBM training for 24 out of 42 items. At test-retest, kappa values ranged from 0.155 to 0.620.

Conclusions: The EBMQ was found to be a valid and reliable instrument to assess the knowledge, practice and barriers towards the implementation of EBM among primary care physicians in Malaysia.

Keywords: Evidence-based medicine, Primary care physicians, Attitudes, Questionnaire

* Correspondence: ranita@um.edu.my
[1]Department of Primary Care Medicine, Faculty of Medicine, University of Malaya, Kuala Lumpur, Malaysia
Full list of author information is available at the end of the article

Background

Evidence-based medicine (EBM) is defined as the integration of best available evidence in a conscientious, explicit and judicious manner from literature and patients' values which then informs clinical decision making [1]. Practicing EBM in clinical practice helps doctors make a proper diagnosis and selects the best treatment available to treat or manage a disease [2]. The use of EBM in clinical setting is thought to provide the best standard of medical care at the lowest cost [3].

Evidence-based medicine has an increasing impact in primary care over recent years [4]. It involves patients in decision making and influences the development of guidelines and quality standards for clinical practice [4]. Primary care physicians are the first person of contact for patients [5]. They have high workload and at the same time they need to uphold the quality of healthcare [6]. Therefore, it is important for them to treat patients based on research evidence, clinical expertise and patient preferences [7]. However, integrating EBM into clinical practice in primary care is challenging as there are variations in team composition, organisational structures, culture and working practices [8].

A search from literature revealed that the international main barriers were lack of time, lack of resources, negative attitudes towards EBM and inadequate EBM skills [9]. A recent qualitative study conducted in 2014 found that the unique barriers in implementing EBM among primary care physicians in Malaysia were lack of awareness and attention toward patient values. Patient values forms a key element of EBM and they still preferred obtaining information from their peers and interestingly, they used WhatsApp—a smart phone messenger [10].

Therefore, we need an instrument to determine the knowledge, practice and barriers of the implementation of EBM among the primary care physicians. It is important to have an instrument to identify the gaps on a larger scale and improve the implementation of EBM in their clinical practice. A systematic review by Shaneyfelt et al. [11] reported that 104 instruments have been developed to evaluate the acquisition of skills by healthcare professionals to practice EBM. These instruments assessed one or more of the following domains on EBM: knowledge, attitude, search strategies, frequency of use of evidence sources, current applications, intended future use and confidence in practice. However, only eight instruments were validated: four instruments assessed the competency in EBM teaching and learning [12–16], whilst four assessed knowledge, attitude and skills [16–19]. However, no instrument has assessed the knowledge, practice and barriers in the implementation of EBM. Therefore, this study aimed to develop and validate the English version of the Evidence-Based Medicine Questionnaire (EBMQ), which was designed to assess knowledge, practice and barriers of primary care physicians regarding the implementation of EBM.

Methods

Development of the evidence-based medicine questionnaire

A literature search was conducted in PubMed; using keywords such as "Evidence-based medicine", "general practioners", "primary care physicians" and "survey/questionnaire" from this search, nine relevant studies were identified [12–16, 19, 20]. However, only one instrument [20] evaluated the attitude and needs of primary care physicians. Twenty four items from this questionnaire and findings from two previous qualitative studies in rural and urban primary care settings in Malaysia [10, 21] were used to develop the EBMQ (version 1). The EBMQ was developed in English, as English is used in the training of doctors in medical schools and also taught as a second language in all public schools in Malaysia.

Face and content validity of the EBMQ was verified by an expert panel which consisted of nine academicians (a nurse, a pharmacist and seven primary care physicians). Each item was reviewed, and the relevance and appropriateness of each item was discussed (version 2). A pilot test was then conducted on ten medical officers with a minimum of one year working experience wihout any postgraduate qualification. They were asked to evaluate verbally if any items were difficult to understand. Feedback received were that the font was too small and that there was no option for "place of work" for those working in a University hospital. Changes were made based on these comments to produce version 3, which was then pilot tested in another two participants. No difficulties were encountered. Hence, version 3 was used as the final version.

The evidence based medicine questionnaire (EBMQ)

The EBMQ consists of 84 items and 6 sections as shown in Table 1. Only 55 items (33 items in the "knowledge" domain, 9 items in the "practice" domain and 13 items in the "barriers" domain) were measured on a Likert-scale, and could be validated. The final version of the EBMQ is added in Additional file 1. A higher score indicates better knowledge and better practice of EBM and less barriers in practicing EBM.

Participants took 15 to 20 min to complete the EBMQ. We hypothesized that the EBMQ would have 3 domains: knowledge, practice and barriers.

Table 1 The initial version of the Evidence-Based Medicine Questionnaire (version 3)

Section	Description	No. of items	Domain	Type of data	Response options	Response combined for analysis
A	Demographic profile	6	NA	Nominal scale		
B	Frequencies in looking for medical information	20	NA	Nominal scale		
C	Knowledge regarding evidence-based medicine	17	Knowledge regarding information sources	4-point Likert scale[a]	1 = Unaware 2 = Aware but not used in clinical decision making 3 = Have read it but not used in clinical decision making 4 = Read and used in clinical decision making	
		16	Knowledge regarding terms related to EBM	5-point Likert scale[a]	1 = Never heard this term before 2 = Heard of this term but do not understand what this term but would like to 3 = Do not understand this term but would like to 4 = Have some understanding of this term 5 = Understand this term well and able to explain what it means to others	1 = Never heard and do not understand 2 = Do not understand but would like to 3 = Understand
D	Practice of evidence-based medicine	9	Practice	5-point Likert scale[a]	1 = Strongly disagree 2 = Disagree 3 = Neither agree nor disagree 4 = Agree 5 = Strongly agree	1 = Disagree 2 = Neutral 3 = Agree
E	Barriers in practicing evidence-based medicine	13	Barriers	5-point Likert scale[a]	1 = Strongly disagree 2 = Disagree 3 = Neither agree nor disagree 4 = Agree 5 = Strongly agree	1 = Disagree 2 = Neutral 3 = Agree
F	Needs for evidence-based medicine	3	Needs	Nominal scale		
	Total	80				

NA Not applicable
[a]Only items in these domain were tested for construct validity

Validation of the evidence-based medicine questionnaire

Participants

Primary care physicians with or without EBM training, who could understand English and who attended a Diploma in Family Medicine workshop, were recruited from December 2015 to January 2016.

Sample size

Sample size calculation was based on a participant to item ratio of 5:1 to perform factor analysis [22]. There are 55 items in the EBMQ. Hence, the minimum number of participants required was 55*5 = 275.

Procedure

Permission was obtained from the Academy of Family Physicians Malaysia to recruit participants who attended their workshops. For those who agreed, written informed consent was obtained. Participants were then asked to fill in the EBMQ at baseline. Two weeks later, the EBMQ was mailed to each participant, with a postage-paid return envelope. If a reply was not obtained within a week, participants were contacted via email and/or SMS, and reminded to send in their completed EBMQ form as soon as possible.

Data analysis

Data were analyzed using the Statistical Package for Social Sciences (SPSS) version 22 software (Il, Chicago, USA). Normality could not be assumed, hence non-parametric tests were used. Categorical variables were presented as percentage and frequencies, while continuous variables were presented as median and interquartile range (IQR).

Validity

Flesch reading ease

The readability of the EBMQ was assessed using Flesch reading ease. This was calculated based on the average number of syllables per word and the average number of words per sentence [23]. An average document should have a score of 60–70 [23].

Exploratory factor analysis

Exploratory factor analysis (EFA) was used to test the underlying structures within the EBMQ. EFA is a type of factor analysis that is utilised to identify the number of latent variables that underlies an entire set of items [24]. EFA was performed to explore the factors appropriateness that can be grouped into specific factors and also to provide information about the validity of each item in each domain. It is important to ensure that the items in each domain of the EBMQ are connected to their basic factors.

Factor loadings were assessed using the Keiser-Meyer-Olkin (KMO) and Bartlett's test of sphericity. The principal components variance with promax variation were used for data reduction purposes, and eigenvalues > 1 was selected to see the variances of the principal components. KMO value of > 0.6, individual factor loadings > 0.5, average variance extracted (AVE) > 0.5 and composite reliability (CR) > 0.7, indicate good structure within the domains [25, 26].

Discriminative validity

To assess discriminative validity, participants were divided into those with or without EBM training. We hypothesized that the knowledge and practice of participants with EBM training would have better knowledge, better practice and less barriers than those without EBM training. The Chi-square test was used to determine if there was any difference between the two groups. A p-value < 0.05 was considered as statistically significant.

Reliability

Internal consistency

Internal consistency was performed to test the consistency of the results and estimates the reliability of the items in the EBMQ. The internal consistency of the EBMQ was assessed using Cronbach's α coefficient. A Cronbach's alpha value of 0.5–0.69 is acceptable, while values of 0.70–0.90 indicate a strong internal consistency [27]. Corrected item-total correlations should be > 0.2 for it to be considered acceptable [28]. If omitting an item increases the Cronbach's α significantly, the item will be excluded.

Test-retest reliability

The test-retest was performed to measure the reliability and stability of the items in the EBMQ over a period of time. It is also important to administer the same test twice to measure the consistency of the answers by the participants. The intra-class correlation coefficient (ICC) was used to assess the total score at test-retest. A ICC agreement value of 0.7 was considered acceptable [29]. ICC values between 0.75 and 1.00 indicate high reliability, 0.60 and 0.74 indicate good reliability, 0.40–0.59 has fair reliability and those below 0.40 indicate low reliability [30].

Results

A total of 343 primary care doctors were approached; of whom 320 agreed to participate (response rate = 93.2%). The majority of them were female (69.4%) with a median age of 32.2 years [IQR = 4.0]. Nearly all (97.2%) were medical officers, working in government health clinics (54.4%) and possessed no postgraduate qualifications after their basic medical degree (78.4%). All participants had heard about EBM, but only 222 (69.7%) had attended an EBM course (Table 2).

Validity

Flesch reading ease of the EBMQ was 61.2. Initially, we hypothesized that the "knowledge" domain would have two factors. However, EFA found that the "knowledge" domain had four factors: ("evidence-based medicine websites", "evidence-based journals", "type of studies" and "terms related to EBM") after 9 items (item C1: "Clinical Practice Guidelines", item C7: "Dynamed", item C11: "InfoPoems", item C4: "Cochrane", item C8: "TRIP database", item C15: "BestBETs", item C9: "MEDLINE", item C17: "Medscape" and item C16: "UpToDate") were removed. This model explained 54.3% of the variation (Table 3).

EFA found that the "practice" domain had only one factor with eight items after one item (item 9: "I prefer to manage patients based on my experience") was removed. This model explained 49.0% of the variation (Table 3).

We hypothesized that the 'barriers' domain would only have one factor. However, EFA revealed that the 'barriers' domain has three factors ("access", "support" and "patient's preferences") after three items were removed (item 7: "I can consult the specialist anytime to answer my queries", item 10: "I have the authority to change the management of patients in my clinic" and item 11: "There are incentives for me to practice EBM"). This model explained 49.9% of the variation (Table 3).

Discriminative validity

In the "knowledge" domain, doctors who had EBM training had significant higher scores in 13 out of 24 items compared to those without training. In the "practice" domain, doctors who had EBM training had significant higher scores in 5 out 8 items compared to those without training. In the "barriers" domain, doctors who had EBM training had significant higher scores in 5 out of 10 items compared to those without training (Table 4).

Table 2 Demographic characteristics of participants

	n (%)
Median age [IQR]	32.2 [4.0]
Female	222 (69.4)
Male	98 (30.6)
No. of participants with postgraduate qualifications	
None	251 (78.4)
Diploma	58 (18.1)
Masters	11 (3.4)
Current designation	
Medical Officer	311 (97.2)
Family Medicine Specialist	9 (2.8)
Current Work Place	
Government health clinics	174 (54.4)
Private clinic	81 (25.3)
Government hospital	42 (13.1)
Others[a]	13 (4.1)
Private hospital	5 (1.6)
University hospital	5 (1.6)
Have heard of the term "evidence-based medicine"	319 (99.7)
Have attended EBM courses	222 (69.7)
Have received formal trainings in literature search	156 (48.8)
Have received formal trainings in questions formulation	121 (37.8)
Have received formal trainings in critical appraisal	111 (34.7)
Have conducted research after graduating from medical school	111 (34.7)
Have published any article in a journal	36 (11.3)

IQR Interquartile range
[a]Others: Military health clinic ($n = 6$), Private Polyclinic($n = 1$), Private University($n = 1$), Traditional & Complimentary Medicine Division($n = 1$), University Health Clinic($n = 4$)

Reliability

Cronbach alpha for the overall EBMQ was 0.909, whilst individual domains ranged from 0.657 to 0.933 (Table 4). All corrected item-total correlation (CITC) values were > 0.2. At retest, 185 participants completed the EBMQ (response rate = 57.85%), as $n = 23$ (42%) were uncontactable. Thirty items had good and fair correlations ($r = 0.418–0.620$) while 12 items had low correlations (r = < 0.4). (Table 5).

Discussion

The EBMQ was found to be a valid and reliable instrument to assess the knowledge, practice and barriers of primary care physicians regarding the implementation of EBM. The final EBMQ consists of 42 items with 8 domains after 13 items were removed. The Flesch reading ease was 61.2. This indicates that the EBMQ can be easily understood by 13–15 years old students who study English as a first language [23].

Initially, we hypothesized that there were two factors in the "knowledge" domain: "sources related to EBM" and "terms related to EBM". However, EFA revealed that the EBMQ had four factors: "evidence-based medicine websites", "evidence-based journals", "terms related to EBM" and "type of studies" after 9 items were removed. This was because "sources related to EBM" was further divided into another three factors. It is not surprising because knowledge is a broad concept that can be further recategorized. EFA revealed that the "practice" domain had one factor which concurred with our initial hypothesis. One item (item P9: "I prefer to manage patients based on my experience") was removed as this was regarding doctors'experience rather than their practice. Initially, we hypothesized that there was one factor in the "barriers" domain. However, EFA revealed that there were three factors: 'access to resources', 'patient preferences towards EBM' and 'support from the management' after three items were removed. This may be because instead of one barrier, EFA had re-grouped into three factors that provided a better description of barriers encountered by the primary care physicians. As highlighted in literature [9, 31], there are many barriers to practice EBM and some of it were also categorized according the specific and types of barriers.

The EBMQ was able to discriminate the knowledge, practice and barriers between doctors with and without EBM training. In the knowledge domain, there were significant differences for all items in the "terms related to EBM". This is not surprising as doctors with EBM training would have been exposed to these terms. No differences was found between those with and without EBM training in "information sources related to EBM" as those who did not attend EBM training could still access online information resources. Several studies were found to improve knowledge but did not report in detail which areas on knowledge. Hence, we could not compare their findings to our studies [32–35].

Our findings also showed that doctors with EBM training had better practice of EBM. This differed from several studies which reported changes in practice [32, 36–39] and some reported no changes in practice [35, 40]. However, the authors commented that these findings were not meaningful as it was self-perceived. Other than that, in our findings, doctors who attended EBM training had less barriers regarding the implementation of EBM in their clinical practice. They seemed to have better access to

Table 3 Exploratory factor analysis of the evidence-based medicine questionnaire

Original domains	After EFA was performed	Item No.	Item	Factor 1	Factor 2	Factor 3	KMO	AVE (%)	Bartlett's test	CR
Knowledge	Evidence-based medicine websites ($n = 6$)	C6	Centre of Evidence-Based Medicine (CEBM)	0.605	–	–	0.834	43.0	< 0.001	0.662
		C10	ACP Journal Club	0.583	–	–				
		C5	Database of abstracts of reviews of effectiveness (DARE)	0.550	–	–				
		C13	InfoClinics	0.545	–	–				
		C2	Bandolier (published in Oxford)	0.495	–	–				
		C14	Centre of Reviews & Dissertation	0.477	–	–				
	Evidence-based journals ($n = 2$)	C12	BMJ Clinical Evidence	–	0.665	–	0.500	48.9	< 0.001	0.609
		C3	Evidence-Based Medicine (from BMJ publishing group)	–	0.658	–				
	Type of studies ($n = 4$)	K3	Case-control study	0.654	–	–	0.692	49.7	< 0.001	0.685
		K4	Randomized controlled trial	0.632	–	–				
		K1	Systematic review	0.622	–	–				
		K2	Meta-analysis	0.459	–	–				
	Terms related to EBM ($n = 12$)	K13	Publication bias	–	0.956	–	0.896	52.0	< 0.001	0.884
		K11	Confidence interval	–	0.817	–				
		K12	Heterogeneity	–	0.745	–				
		K16	Clinical effectiveness	–	0.642	–				
		K7	Odds ratio	–	0.607	–				
		K8	P-value	–	0.589	–				
		K15	Positive predictive value	–	0.569	–				
		K14	Test sensitivity and specificity	–	0.553	–				
		K10	Number needed to treat	–	0.531	–				
		K9	Level of evidence	–	0.524	–				
		K6	Absolute risk	–	0.436	–				
		K5	Relative risk	–	0.416	–				
Practice ($n = 9$)	Practice ($n = 8$)	P4	EBM improves my patient care	0.829	–	–	0.892	49.0	< 0.001	0.882
		P7	EBM guides my clinical decision making	0.817	–	–				
		P8	I prefer to manage patients based on EBM	0.759	–	–				
		P3	Reading research papers is important to me	0.739	–	–				
		P6		0.727	–	–				

Table 3 Exploratory factor analysis of the evidence-based medicine questionnaire *(Continued)*

Original domains	After EFA was performed	Item No.	Item	Factor 1	Factor 2	Factor 3	KMO	AVE (%)	Bartlett's test	CR
			I can implement EBM in my clinical practice							
		P2	I trust the findings from research studies	0.662	–	–				
		P5	EBM reduces my workload	0.521	–	–				
		P1	I support EBM	0.456	–	–				
Barriers ($n = 13$)	Access ($n = 6$)	B4	I have time to practise EBM in my clinic	0.686		–	0.818	36.8	< 0.001	0.774
		B5	My clinic facilities are adequate to support the practice of EBM	0.675	–	–				
		B3	I have time to read research papers	0.633	–					
		B6	Research articles are easily available to me	0.632	–	–				
		B1	I am able to assess the quality of research.	0.543	–	–				
		B2	I have access to internet to practice EBM	0.435						
	Patient preferences ($n = 2$)	B8	My patients prefers me to practise EBM	–	0.754	–				
		B9	My patient believes in information that is based on evidence	–	0.754	–	0.500	56.8	< 0.001	0.725
	Support ($n = 2$)	B12	My colleagues support the practice of EBM	–	–	0.786				
		B13	My organization supports the practice of EBM	–	–	0.786	0.500	61.7	< 0.001	0.764

EBM Evidence-based medicine, *EFA* Exploratory Factor Analysis, *KMO* Keiser-Meyer-Olkin, *AVE* Average Variance Extracted, *CR* Composite Reliability

Table 4 The discriminative validity of the Evidence-Based Medicine Questionnaire

Item	Details of item	With EBM training (*n* = 222) n(%)				Without EBM training (*n* = 98) n(%)				Chi-square	*p*-value
		Unaware	Aware but not used in clinical decision making	Have read it but not used in clinical decision making	Read and used in clinical decision making	Unaware	Aware but not used in clinical decision making	Have read it but not used in clinical decision making	Read and used in clinical decision making		
Knowledge Domain (Information sources related to EBM)											
C2	Bandolier	154(69.4)	35(15.8)	19(8.6)	14(6.3)	66(67.3)	13(13.3)	12(12.2)	7(7.1)	1.350	0.717
C5	DARE	155(18.9)	42(18.9)	16(7.2)	9(4.1)	71(72.4)	15(15.3)	12(12.2)	–	6.510	0.089
C6	CEBM	123(56.3)	69(31.1)	17(7.7)	11(5.0)	58(59.2)	22(22.4)	14(14.3)	4(4.1)	5.074	0.166
C10	ACP	147(66.2)	38(17.1)	24(10.8)	13(5.9)	63(64.3)	16(16.3)	14(14.3)	5(5.1)	0.825	0.844
C13	InfoClinics	152(68.5)	44(19.8)	18(8.1)	8(3.6)	63(64.3)	16(16.3)	10(10.2)	9(9.2)	4.946	0.176
C14	CRD	175(78.8)	31(14.0)	15(6.8)	1(0.5)	75(76.5)	12(12.2)	9(9.2)	2(2.0)	2.564	0.464
C3	EBM	10(4.5)	46(20.7)	66(29.7)	100(45.0)	4(4.1)	28(28.6)	24(24.5)	42(42.9)	2.577	0.462
C12	BMJ	26(11.7)	43(19.4)	73(32.9)	80(36.0)	10(10.2)	25(25.5)	22(22.4)	41(41.8)	4.442	0.218
Item	Details of item		With EBM training (*n* = 222) n(%)				Without EBM training (*n* = 98) n(%)			Chi-square	*p*-value
			Never heard and do not understand	Do not understand but would like to	Understand		Never heard and do not understand	Do not understand but would like to	Understand		
Knowledge Domain (Terms related to EBM)											
K1	Systematic review		6(2.7)	12(5.4)	204(91.9)		8(8.2)	8(8.2)	82(83.7)	5.975	0.050
K2	Meta-analysis		10(4.5)	14(6.3)	198(89.2)		6(6.1)	14(6.3)	198(89.2)	16.837	≤ 0.001*
K3	Case-control study		4(1.8)	8(3.6)	210(94.6)		5(5.1)	8(3.1)	90(91.8)	2.746	0.253
K4	Randomized controlled trial		4(1.8)	7(3.2)	211(95.0)		4(4.1)	1(1.0)	93(94.9)	2.651	0.266
K5	Relative risk		8(3.6)	25(11.3)	189(85.1)		9(9.2)	16(16.3)	73(74.5)	6.287	0.043*
K6	Absolute risk		8(3.6)	33(14.9)	181(81.5)		10(10.2)	15(15.3)	73(74.5)	5.699	0.058*
K7	Odds ratio		1(0.5)	60(27.0)	151(68.0)		14(14.3)	26(26.5)	58(59.2)	8.395	0.015*
K8	*P*-value		11(5.0)	38(17.1)	173(77.9)		14(14.3)	19(19.4)	65(66.3)	9.004	0.011*
K9	Level of evidence		7(3.2)	30(13.5)	185(83.3)		9(9.2)	19(19.4)	70(71.4)	7.686	0.021*
K10	Number needed to treat		11(5.0)	42(18.5)	170(76.6)		11(11.2)	20(20.4)	67(68.4)	4.640	0.098*
K11	Confidence interval		17(7.7)	61(27.5)	144(64.9)		21(21.4)	25(25.5)	52(53.1)	12.502	0.002*
K12	Heterogeneity		21(9.5)	74(33.3)	127(57.2)		22(22.4)	35(35.7)	41(41.8)	11.709	0.003*
K13	Publication bias		23(10.4)	65(29.3)	134(60.4)		23(23.5)	30(30.6)	45(45.9)	10.703	0.005*
K14	Test sensitivity and specificity		4(1.8)	25(11.3)	193(86.9)		11(11.2)	13(13.3)	74(75.5)	14.172	≤ 0.001*
K15	Positive predictive value		5(2.3)	36(16.2)	181(81.5)		5(2.3)	36(16.2)	181(81.5)	7.415	0.025*
K16	Clinical effectiveness		10(4.5)	48(21.6)	164(73.9)		16(16.3)	19(19.4)	63(64.3)	12.738	0.002*
Item	Details of item			With EBM training (*n* = 222) n(%)			Without EBM training (*n* = 98) n(%)			Chi-square	*p*-value

Table 4 The discriminative validity of the Evidence-Based Medicine Questionnaire *(Continued)*

		Disagree	Neutral	Agree	Disagree	Neutral	Agree		
Practice Domain									
P1	I support EBM	1(0.5)	8(3.6)	213(95.9)	2(2.0)	6(6.1)	90(91.8)	2.941	0.230
P2	I trust the findings from research studies	1(0.5)	37(16.7)	184(82.9)	3(3.1)	13(13.3)	82(83.7)	4.216	0.121
P3	Reading research papers is important to me	–	25(11.3)	197(88.7)	4(4.1)	20(20.4)	74(75.5)	14.511	0.001*
P4	EBM improves my patient care	–	19(8.6)	203(91.4)	3(3.1)	8(8.2)	87(88.8)	6.862	0.032*
P5	EBM reduces my workload	22(9.9)	87(39.1)	113(50.9)	21(9.4)	39(17.5)	38(17.1)	8.838	0.012*
P6	I can implement EBM in my clinical practice	2(0.9)	23(10.3)	197(88.7)	3(1.3)	16(7.2)	79(35.5)	4.537	0.103
P7	EBM guides my clinical decision making	–	11(5.0)	211(95.0)	3(3.1)	9(9.2)	86(87.8)	9.130	0.010*
P8	I prefer to manage patients based on EBM	2(0.9)	36(16.2)	184(82.9)	3(3.1)	25(25.5)	70(71.4)	6.235	0.044*
Barriers Domain									
B1	I am able to assess the quality of research.	35(15.8)	76(34.2)	111(50.0)	17(17.3)	40(40.8)	41(41.8)	1.871	0.392
B2	I have access to internet to practice EBM	4(1.8)	18(8.1)	200(90.1)	11(11.2)	12(12.2)	75(76.5)	15.573	< 0.001*
B3	I have time to read research papers	25(11.3)	93(41.9)	104(46.8)	22(22.4)	39(39.8)	37(37.8)	7.142	0.028*
B4	I have time to practise EBM in my clinic	18(8.1)	60(27.0)	144(64.9)	144(64.9)	17(17.3)	32(32.7)	8.545	0.014*
B5	My clinic facilities are adequate to support the practice of EBM	47(20.2)	85(38.2)	90(40.5)	34(15.3)	34(15.3)	120(54.0)	6.935	0.031*
B6	Research articles are easily available to me	50(22.5)	71(32.0)	101(45.5)	40(40.8)	29(29.6)	29(29.6)	12.447	0.002*
B8	My patients prefers me to practise EBM	28(12.6)	138(62.2)	56(25.2)	15(15.3)	59(60.2)	24(24.5)	0.424	0.809
B9	My patient believes in information that is based on evidence	35(15.8)	95(42.8)	92(41.4)	11(11.2)	47(48.0)	40(40.8)	1.391	0.499
B12	My colleagues support the practice of EBM	13(5.9)	84(37.8)	125(56.3)	12(12.2)	36(36.7)	50(51.0)	3.922	1.141
B13	My organization supports the practice of EBM	12(5.4)	72(32.4)	138(62.2)	8(8.2)	33(33.7)	57(58.2)	1.038	0.595

EBM **Evidence-based medicine**
***$p \leq 0.05$ is significant**

Table 5 The psychometric properties of the Evidence-Based Medicine Questionnaire

No.	Items	Test-Retest Reliability						
		Corrected Item-total Correlation	Cronbach's alpha if items is deleted	Test ($n = 320$)		Retest ($n = 184$)		ICC
				Mean (SD)	Median	Mean (SD)	Median	
Knowledge Domain								
C2	Bandolier (Published in Oxford)	0.487	0.811	1.31 (0.650)	1.00	1.68 (1.003)	1.00	0.567
C5	Database of abstracts of reviews of effectiveness(DARE)	0.630	0.778	1.54 (0.916)	1.00	1.67 (0.922)	1.00	0.485
C6	Centre of Evidence-Based Medicine (CEBM)	0.630	0.777	1.44 (0.769)	1.00	1.76 (0.937)	1.00	0.453
C10	ACP Journal Club	0.570	0.791	1.62 (0.844)	1.00	1.55 (0.886)	1.00	0.333
C13	InfoClinics	0.566	0.791	1.58 (0.907)	1.00	1.63 (0.913)	1.00	0.418
C14	Centre of Reviews & Dissertation (CRD)	0.650	0.780	1.52 (0.863)	1.00	1.48 (0.815)	1.00	0.396
C3	Evidence-based medicine (EBM)	0.492	–	1.52 (0.863)	3.00	3.21 (0.881)	3.00	0.416
C12	BMJ Clinical Evidence	0.492	–	3.23 (0.868)	3.00	2.90 (0.997)	3.00	0.379
K1	Systematic review	0.774	0.866	4.19 (0.775)	4.00	4.23(0.814)	4.00	0.421
K2	Meta-analysis	0.718	0.887	2.79(0.516)	3.00	4.10(0.793)	4.00	0.463
K3	Case-control study	0.826	0.848	2.91(0.373)	3.00	4.28(0.681)	4.00	0.497
K4	Randomized controlled trial	0.777	0.866	2.93(0.346)	3.00	4.37(0.686)	4.00	0.522
K5	Relative risk	0.747	0.927	2.77(0.535)	3.00	4.04(0.741)	3.00	0.450
K6	Absolute risk	0.763	0.926	2.74(0.554)	3.00	4.01(0.775)	4.00	0.561
K7	Odds ratio	0.742	0.926	2.58(0.634)	3.00	3.82(0.822)	4.00	0.506
K8	P-value	0.713	0.927	2.67(0.616)	3.00	4.00(0.803)	4.00	0.487
K9	Level of evidence	0.721	0.927	2.75(0.538)	3.00	4.06(0.846)	4.00	0.359
K10	Number needed to treat	0.676	0.929	2.67(0.599)	3.00	3.95(0.943)	4.00	0.528
K11	Confidence interval	0.757	0.926	2.49(0.699)	3.00	3.78(0.882)	4.00	0.529
K12	Heterogeneity	0.663	0.930	2.39(0.713)	3.00	3.54(0.950)	4.00	0.483
K13	Publication bias	0.686	0.929	2.42(0.729)	3.00	3.58(0.997)	4.00	0.580
K14	Test sensitivity and specificity	0.697	0.928	2.79(0.512)	3.00	4.24(0.734)	4.00	0.504
K15	Positive predictive value	0.707	0.928	2.74(0.522)	3.00	4.06(0.861)	4.00	0.503
K16	Clinical effectiveness	0.667	0.929	2.63(0.630)	3.00	2.89(0.938)	4.00	0.570
Practice Domain								
P1	I support EBM	0.417	0.875	2.94 (0.279)	3.00	4.43 (0.648)	4.00	0.605
P2	I trust the findings from research studies	0.618	0.854	4.02 (0.683)	4.00	4.09 (0.611)	4.00	0.323
P3	Reading research papers is important to me	0.684	0.846	4.06 (0.687)	4.00	4.06 (0.679)	4.00	0.477
P4	EBM improves my patient care	0.765	0.838	4.18 (0.642)	4.00	4.27 (0.626)	4.00	0.301
P5	EBM reduces my workload	0.499	0.877	3.44 (0.898)	3.00	3.43 (0.830)	3.00	0.532
P6	I can implement EBM in my clinical practice	0.682	0.846	4.04 (0.661)	4.00	3.90 (0.743)	4.00	0.532
P7	EBM guides my clinical decision making	0.748	0.841	4.18 (0.607)	4.00	4.10 (0.600)	4.00	0.344
P8	I prefer to manage patients based on EBM	0.699	0.844	4.01 (0.713)	4.00	4.02 (0.689)	4.00	0.422

Table 5 The psychometric properties of the Evidence-Based Medicine Questionnaire *(Continued)*

No.	Items	Test-Retest Reliability						
		Corrected Item-total Correlation	Cronbach's alpha if items is deleted	Test ($n = 320$)		Retest ($n = 184$)		ICC
				Mean (SD)	Median	Mean (SD)	Median	
Barrier Domain								
B1	I am able to assess the quality of research.	0.472	0.747	2.31 (0.736)	2.00	3.34 (0.808)	3.00	0.475
B2	I have access to internet to practice EBM	0.386	0.767	2.81 (0.497)	3.00	3.83 (0.874)	4.00	0.388
B3	I have time to read research papers	0.546	0.728	3.32 (0.803)	3.00	3.29 (0.795)	3.00	0.494
B4	I have time to practise EBM in my clinic	0.583	0.718	3.55 (0.810)	4.00	3.45 (0.774)	4.00	0.356
B5	My clinic facilities are adequate to support the practice of EBM	0.583	0.718	3.13 (0.894)	3.00	3.30 (2.367)	3.00	0.142
B6	Research articles are easily available to me	0.547	0.731	3.16 (0.982)	3.00	3.06 (0.942)	3.00	0.275
B8	My patients prefers me to practise EBM	0.569	–	3.14 (0.798)	3.00	3.24 (0.690)	3.00	0.323
B9	My patient believes in information that is based on evidence	0.569	–	3.29 (0.853)	3.00	3.41 (0.717)	3.00	0.547
B12	My colleagues support the practice of EBM	0.618	–	3.53 (0.795)	4.00	3.53 (0.752)	4.00	0.620
B13	My organization supports the practice of EBM	0.618	–	3.63 (0.756)	4.00	3.53 (0.771)	4.00	0.471

ICC Intraclass correlation
*Statistically significant at $p < 0.05$

resources, more patients had a positive attitude towards EBM, and better support from management to practice EBM compared to those without EBM training. This could be because doctors with EBM training knew how to overcome problems that would prevent them from practicing EBM. In the systematic review [41], the barriers in the implementation of EBM remains unclear as it was not reported.

The overall Cronbach's alpha as well as the individual domains were > 0.7. This indicates that the EBMQ has adequate psychometric properties, which was similar to previous studies [12, 14–16, 19, 42]. The majority (71.4%) of the items in EBMQ had good and fair correlation at test-retest, which indicates that the EBMQ has achieved adequate reliability. The reliability testing two weeks later did not affect the methodology as the acceptable time interval for test-retest reliability is approximately 2 weeks [28]. The discriminative validity was performed using the baseline data and not after retest which then impact on the methodology.

To our knowledge, this was the first validation study assessed the discriminative validity (i.e. between doctors with and without EBM training) that assessed their implementation of EBM. One of the limitations of this study was that participants were recruited whilst attending a Family Medicine module workshop. This may mean that participants that were recruited may be more interested in the practice of EBM as they are already interested in furthering their post-graduate studies. This cohort are likely to be more interested with the practice of EBM as they are more incline to further their studies rather than the normal general practitioners. Hence, our result may not be generalizable.

Conclusions

The EBMQ was found to be a valid and reliable instrument to assess the knowledge, practice and barriers of primary care physicians towards EBM in Malaysia. The EBMQ can be used to assess doctors' practices and barriers in the implementation of EBM. Information gathered from the administration of the EBMQ will assist policy makers to identify the level of knowledge, practice and barriers of EBM and to improve its uptake in clinical practice. Although the findings of this study are not generalizable, they may be of interest to primary care physicians in other countries.

Abbreviations

AVE: Average variance extracted; CITC: Corrected item-total correlation; CR: Composite reliability; EBM: Evidence-based medicine; EBMQ: Evidence-based medicine questionnaire; EFA: Exploratory factor analysis; ICC: Intra-correlation coefficient; IQR: Interquartile range; KMO: Kaiser-Meyer-Oklin; SPSS: Statistical Package for Social Sciences

Acknowledgements

We would like to thank the participants of this study.

Funding

This study was funded by University of Malaya Research Grant (RP037A-15HTM).

Authors' contributions

NCJ and LSM conceived the study and CYC, KEM, NSH, SO, LPY, KLA participated in its design and coordination. RH, NCJ, LSM and LSMP contributed to data analysis and interpretation. KC provided statistical advice, data analysis and interpretation. RH drafted the manuscript and all the authors critically revised it and approved the final manuscript.

Competing interests

The authors declare that they have no competing interests.

Author details

[1]Department of Primary Care Medicine, Faculty of Medicine, University of Malaya, Kuala Lumpur, Malaysia. [2]Department of Family Medicine, Faculty of Medicine and Health Sciences, Universiti Putra Malaysia, UPM Serdang, Selangor, Malaysia. [3]Department of Nursing Sciences, Faculty of Medicine, University of Malaya, Kuala Lumpur, Malaysia. [4]Department of Social and Preventive Medicine, Julius Centre University of Malaya, University of Malaya, Kuala Lumpur, Malaysia. [5]Department of Medical Sciences School of Healthcare and Medical Sciences Sunway University, Selangor, Malaysia.

References

1. Sackett DL, Rosenberg WMC, Gray JAM, Haynes RB, Richardson WS. Evidence based medicine: what it is and what it isn't. BMJ. 1996;312:71–2.
2. Saarni SI, Gylling HA. Evidence based medicine guidelines: a solution to rationing or politics disguised as science? J Med Ethics. 2004;30:171–5.
3. Lewis SJ, Orland BI. The importance and impact of evidence-based medicine. J Manag Care Pharm. 2004;10:S3–5.
4. Slowther A, Ford S, Schofield T. Ethics of evidence based medicine in the primary care setting. J Med Ethics. 2004;30:151–5.
5. Kumar R. Empowering primary care physicians in India. J Fam Med Prim Care. 2012;1:1–2.
6. Mohr DC, Benzer JK, Young GJJD. Provider workload and quality of care in primary care settings: moderating role of relational climate. Med Care. 2013;51:108–14.
7. Tracy CS, Dantas GC, Upshur REG. Evidence-based medicine in primary care: qualitative study of family physicians. BMC Fam Prac. 2003;4:6–6.
8. Craig P, Dieppe P, Macintyre S, Michie S, Nazareth I, Petticrew M. Developing and evaluating complex interventions: the new Medical Research Council guidance. BMJ. 2008;337:a1655.
9. Sadeghi-Bazargani H, Tabrizi JS, Azami-Aghdash S. Barriers to evidence-based medicine: a systematic review. J Eval Clin Pract. 2014;20:793–802.
10. Hisham R, Liew SM, Ng CJ, Mohd Nor K, Osman IF, Ho GJ, Hamzah N, Glasziou P. Rural doctors' views on and experiences with evidence-based medicine: the FrEEDoM qualitative study. PLoS One. 2016;11:e0152649.
11. Shaneyfelt T, Baum KD, Bell D, Feldstein D, Houston TK, Kaatz S, Whelan C, Green M. Instruments for evaluating education in evidence-based practice: a systematic review. JAMA. 2006;296:1116–27.
12. Ruzafa-Martinez M, Lopez-Iborra L, Moreno-Casbas T, Madrigal-Torres M. Development and validation of the competence in evidence based practice questionnaire (EBP-COQ) among nursing students. BMC Med Educ. 2013;13:19.
13. Adams S, Barron S. Development and testing of an evidence-based practice questionnaire for school nurses. J Nurs Meas. 2010;18:3–25.
14. Johnston JM, Leung GM, Fielding R, Tin KY, Ho LM. The development and validation of a knowledge, attitude and behaviour questionnaire to assess undergraduate evidence-based practice teaching and learning. Med Educ. 2003;37:992–1000.
15. Fritsche L, Greenhalgh T, Falck-Ytter Y, Neumayer H, Kunz R. Do short courses in evidence based medicine improve knowledge and skills? Validation of berlin questionnaire and before and after study of courses in evidence based medicine. BMJ. 2002;325:1338–41.
16. Ramos KD, Schafer S, Tracz SM. Validation of the Fresno test of competence in evidence based medicine. BMJ. 2003;326:319–21.
17. Rice KHJ, Abrefa-Gyan T, Powell K. Evidence-based practice questionnaire: a confirmatory factor analysis in a social work sample. Adv Soc Work. 2010;11:158–73.
18. Iovu MB, Runcan P. Evidence-based practice: knowledge, attitudes, and beliefs of social workers in Romania. Revista de Cercetare si Interventie Sociala. 2012;38:54–70.
19. Upton D, Upton P. Development of an evidence-based practice questionnaire for nurses. J Adv Nurs. 2006;53:454–8.
20. McColl A, Smith H, White P, Field J. General practitioners' perceptions of the route to evidence based medicine: a questionnaire survey. BMJ. 1998;316:361–5.
21. Blenkinsopp A, Paxton P. Symptoms in the pharmacy: a guide to the management of common illness. 3rd ed. Oxford. Blackwell Science; 1998.
22. Gorsuch RL. Factor analysis. 2nd ed. Lawarence Erlbaum Associates: Hillsdale; 1983.
23. Flesch R. A new readability yardstick. J Appl Psychol. 1948;32:221–33.
24. van der Eijk C, Rose J. Risky business: factor analysis of survey data – assessing the probability of incorrect dimensionalisation. PLoS One. 2015;10:e0118900.
25. Kaiser HF. A second generation little jiffy. Psychometrika. 1970;35:401–15.
26. Hidalgo B, Goodman M. Multivariate or multivariable regression? Am J Pub Health. 2013;103:39–40.
27. Cronbach LJ. Coefficient alpha and the internal structure of tests. Psychometrika. 1951;16:297–334.
28. Streiner DN. G. Health measurement scales: a practical guide to their development and use. 2nd ed. Oxford: Oxford University Press; 1995.
29. Terwee CB, Bot SD, de Boer MR, van der Windt DA, Knol DL, Dekker J, Bouter LM, de Vet HC. Quality criteria were proposed for measurement properties of health status questionnaires. J Clin Epidemiol. 2007;60:34–42.
30. Cicchetti DV. Guidelines, criteria, and rules of thumb for evaluating normed and standardized assessment instruments in psychology. Psychol Assess. 1994;6:284–90.
31. Zwolsman S, te Pas E, Hooft L, Wieringa-de Waard M, van Dijk N. Barriers to GPs' use of evidence-based medicine: a systematic review. Br J Gen Pract. 2012;62:e511–21.
32. Dizon JM, Grimmer-Somers K, Kumar S. Effectiveness of the tailored evidence based practice training program for Filipino physical therapists: a randomized controlled trial. BMC Med Educ. 2014;14:147.
33. Chen FC, Lin MC. Effects of a nursing literature reading course on promoting critical thinking in two-year nursing program students. J Nurs Res. 2003; 11:137–47.
34. Bennett S, Hoffmann T, Arkins M. A multi-professional evidence-based practice course improved allied health students' confidence and knowledge. J Eval Clin Pract. 2011;17:635–9.
35. McCluskey A, Lovarini M. Providing education on evidence-based practice improved knowledge but did not change behaviour: a before and after study. BMC Med Educ. 2005;5:40.
36. Levin RF, Fineout-Overholt E, Melnyk BM, Barnes M, Vetter MJ. Fostering evidence-based practice to improve nurse and cost outcomes in a community health setting: a pilot test of the advancing research and clinical practice through close collaboration model. Nurs Adm Q. 2011; 35:21–33.
37. Stevenson K, Lewis M, Hay E. Do physiotherapists' attitudes towards evidence-based practice change as a result of an evidence-based educational programme? J Eval Clin Pract. 2004;10:207–17.

16

Coordinating care for older adults in primary care settings: understanding the current context

Jacobi Elliott[1*], Paul Stolee[1], Veronique Boscart[2], Lora Giangregorio[1] and George Heckman[1]

Abstract

Background: It is well known that older adults are high users of the health care system. Older adults with chronic conditions receive care from multiple providers, across multiple settings, and this care is often unorganized and confusing. In 2005, Ontario established a model of inter-professional primary care (family health teams) with the aim of providing enhanced interdisciplinary primary care to patients. Primary care requires an in-depth understanding of the operations of primary care teams and their relationships with other community services. The aim of this study was to develop a deeper understanding of the current operations of two family health teams in Ontario, including their current processes for referrals, information sharing, and engagement of patients in decision-making.

Methods: Focus group and individual semi-structured interviews with health care providers were conducted. Purposeful sampling was used to ensure information was obtained from different professional perspectives. Interviews were audio-recorded and transcribed verbatim. Using NVivo 10, data were analyzed using line by line thematic analysis techniques. A cluster technique was then applied to group similar codes into themes.

Results: Three focus group interviews (involving 4–6 health care providers/focus group) and six individual interviews were conducted with health care providers from two primary care teams and surrounding community care organizations. Six key themes were identified: 1) challenges engaging older adults in decisions about their care; 2) who is responsible for coordinating the care? 3) fragmented information sharing between health care providers; 4) lack of standardized referral processes and follow-up; 5) identifying services in the community for older adults; and 6) caring for older adults in rural communities.

Conclusions: The results of this study provide an in-depth understanding of the current context in which the primary care teams are currently operating. Improved primary care will require stronger processes of coordination, greater knowledge of and connections with other community services, and enhanced patient engagement processes. This information provides a helpful basis for implementing interventions in primary care.

Keywords: Older adults, Primary care, Qualitative methods, Health care providers, Care coordination

* Correspondence: jacobi.elliott@uwaterloo.ca
[1]University of Waterloo, 200 University Avenue West, Waterloo, ON N2L 3G1, Canada
Full list of author information is available at the end of the article

Background

Older adults use a large amount of health care services, however the current health care system is not well designed to meet their needs. Primary health care is seen as being the health care system "first point of contact" and as the patient's medical "home", helping patients navigate and coordinate their care journey [1, 2]. Effective primary health care also provides continuing care for chronic conditions and involves a wide range of health care providers in the care provided to patients [3].

Although primary health care would seem to be the best place within the system to provide and coordinate care for older adults, it is poorly positioned to do so. Through the development of both structural and funding-based barriers between primary and community care, the delivery of healthcare has become fragmented in many countries [4, 5]. Many patients, particularly those individuals who are older and who experience one or more chronic conditions, may require long-term, often complex care from multiple providers working in a variety of settings [6, 7]. There is a recognition that primary care needs to move away from a focus on episodic care in which the majority of patients seek attention for specific, acute complaints and leave care when treatment has been received [8]. Increasingly, health care providers are acknowledging the need to work together with patients, their families, and informal caregivers, and to collaborate with other health care providers to tailor healthcare to better fit the individual patient context [8].

Furthermore, family physicians are often considered to be the structural link for coordination between primary, community and hospital care for the patient [6]. Family physicians are viewed as the central medical professional in the care and management of chronic disease, in particular; in part, this is due to their longstanding relationship with the patient which allows them to take into account a longer term medical history and greater knowledge of the individual patient context [9]. However, most family physicians are not in a position to take on the duties of a full-time care coordinator. The demands of caring for patients with chronic conditions represents a substantial increase to physician workload [8]. Some primary health care practices have added or reorganized staff and delegated the work of coordination, creating a "care team", who all participate actively in meeting the needs of an individual patient [8]. The idea of primary care "teams" was established in the Ontario, Canada health care context through the launch of Family Health Teams (FHTs) in 2005. FHTs are comprised of physicians, nurses and interdisciplinary care providers such as; social workers, dieticians, or occupational therapists, who provide services such as chronic disease management, counseling, education, and palliative care [10]. The use of care teams is said to improve efficiency, staff satisfaction, and the patient experience of care [8]. Although FHTs were established almost a decade ago, care is still disjointed between primary and community care in Ontario [10].

This study aimed to understand the current context and operation of primary health care teams, focusing on the current process for referring older adults to community care services from primary care; the current state of information sharing; and identification of services available to older adults in the community. This study is the first step of a larger research project where findings from this work will be used to guide implementation and evaluation of a model of care coordination for older adults in primary care. Specifically, this study aimed to answer the following question, what is the local context in which primary care teams were operating, including the available health and support services?

Methods

Through a social constructivist perspective, this study used qualitative methods (focus group and individual interviews) and thematic analysis of the data to understand the current referral and care coordination process between primary care and community care in two primary care locations, a rural and an urban site.

Ethics clearance for this study was obtained from the University of Waterloo's Office of Research Ethics (ORE #20452).

Sampling and recruitment

Purposeful sampling was used to gather the perspectives of persons who might play a role in coordinating care for older persons (e.g. nurse, social worker, care coordinator). Two primary care sites were chosen and the community care organization that served seniors, working around that site were noted. It was also important to involve community care providers - those individuals who work outside of the primary care centre but receive referrals from the primary care centre. These could include community care coordinators, Alzheimer Society program directors, and care providers for community services such as nutrition services or transportation. Individuals were recruited through standardized email communication and participants were asked if they felt anyone else should be involved and contacted.

The target sample size for this phase of the study was approximately 6–8 individuals for each focus group, following common qualitative procedures [11]. Primary care provider and community care provider focus groups were kept homogenous as per common focus group approaches [11].

Data collection

Focus group and individual interviews were conducted with primary care and community care providers. Interviews were conducted at two study sites, one representing a rural community and one an urban community. Focus group interviews were conducted with three groups: urban primary care team, urban community care representatives, rural community care representatives. Individual interviews were conducted with participants who could not attend focus group interviews, including rural primary care team providers. Focus group and individual interviews were conducted face-to-face or by telephone and lasted 60–90 min in length. These were audio-recorded and transcribed verbatim. In order to guide and assist the interviewer, an interview guide (Additional File 1) was created with questions that would enable the researcher to gain a better understanding of the current referral process, communication mechanisms, and information on how providers currently engage patients in care planning.

Data Analysis

Data collected during the interviews consisted of verbatim transcripts for each focus group and individual interview. Using NVivo 10 software [12], all interview data were analyzed using line by line emergent coding as outlined by Lofland and colleagues [13]. Following a process outlined by Lofland and colleagues [13], initial coding was completed followed by focused coding where patterns, themes, and interesting concepts were identified. A clustering technique was completed, where similar codes were grouped into themes [13]. Each cluster was given a name and brief description, with quotations from the data to support the theme.

Ensuring Methodological Rigour

The use of member checking (i.e. sharing categories and interpretations with participants to determine if their realities are adequately represented) and development of an audit trail was used to promote trustworthiness of findings [14]. A process of reflexivity was also completed which allowed the researcher to be aware of their role throughout the project. Specifically, in this project, the researcher collected information from study participants, removing their own biases and allowed the experiences of the participants to be reflected in the results.

Results are presented in detail below, however some findings from this work are also presented in a local public document [15].

Results

Three focus group interviews were completed with 4–8 participants in each group and six participants were interviewed individually ($n = 30$ participants in total). In total, representation from the rural community included six participants from primary care, six from community care, and two hospital representatives. Representation from the urban area included nine participants from primary care, six from community care, and one hospital representative. Community care providers represented organizations providing care including both community support services and home care services.

The findings revealed a number of themes related to the current primary and community care contexts. After reviewing the data and performing appropriate thematic analysis, six key themes emerged. Table 1 outlines the themes and subthemes.

Challenges in engaging older adults in decisions about their care

Evident throughout many of the discussions was the fact that although healthcare providers felt that engagement of patients was important in health care decision-making, however either it was not done as well, or as often, as it should be, or some providers didn't know how to engage patients in a meaningful way. During the interview, health care providers discussed how they currently involve older adults and their family caregivers in healthcare planning; the quotes below illustrate the various responses: quotes.

Yes, we use surveys if that's what you're getting at ... there's really no participatory involvement in the care pathway or planning – Primary Care Provider Urban.

Not as much as they could or should be. I think that many feel powerless – not knowing what is available to them or how to 'work the system'. – Urban Community Care Provider.

Community providers felt that they offered their patients' options but it was up to the patient to decide whether to accept the service. Providers felt that they couldn't do anything if the patients declined services.

We may present all of the options and make our suggestion about what would be most helpful, but ultimately if our client does not want that service then that's up to them. – Community Care Representative (Urban).

Providers recognized that as they get to know their patients better and build a relationship, discussions are open and patients may opt to participate in services.

...as you build trust in the relationship, you can get people engaged in other services – Community Care Provider (Urban).

Community care providers also identified issues when goals and preferences are not discussed with the patient. In the case below, the physician made a referral, however when the community care provider offered the service, the patient was not willing to accept the service. This could also point to limited engagement and education for the patient.

We also want to have a better idea of what their goals are, because what the goal is, let's say, for example, the goal for the family physician might be a med review by psychiatry. When we get in there we might have to do

Table 1 Themes and Subthemes

THEMES	Subthemes
1) *Challenges in Engaging Older adults in Decisions about their Care*	• *Older adults should be engaged more in decision-making than they are currently* • *Understanding why older adults decline services* • *"Time" is needed for meaningful conversations* • *Caregivers are an important part of the circle of care*
2) *Who is Responsible for Coordinating the care?*	• *The role of a coordinator* • *Role clarity needed among patients and providers* • *Primary health care as a hub for coordinating care*
3) *Fragmented Information Sharing between Health Care Providers*	• *Communication between primary care and community care is fragmented* • *Providers going beyond what is expected of them to get information about a client* • *Multiple documentation systems make it hard to access patient information*
4) *Lack of Standardized Referral Processes and Follow Up*	• *Types of referrals to community services* • *Issues with referring patients to external services*
5) *Identifying Services in the Community for Older Adults is challenging*	• *Many organizations offer a variety of services for older complex patients*
6) *Caring for Older Adults in a Rural Communities*	• *Cultural boundaries* • *Coordinating care in large geographical location*

some work arounds, massaging that...and they [patient] may not be ready to say yes... So that sometimes, I think is a challenge.... – Community Care Provider (Rural).

Many providers acknowledged the benefits of engaging patients and families in health care decision-making but identified the challenges that go along with those discussions. In order to engage patients in a meaningful way, there is a level of education that needs to occur for both the providers and the patients. If the patients are not aware of the services that are being offered to them, they may not see the value and therefore may decline the service.

I think it's just a hard thing to have a menu and say what would you like, when they don't really understand maybe fully what each service might bring them, so that needs to be explained when you're offering this service or getting consent for a service – Community Care Provider Rural.

Above all, a strong and trusting relationship is central to involving older adults in healthcare decision-making. However, the current Canadian healthcare system is not designed to support the time it takes to build a trusting relationship. As illustrated in the quote below, the health system also does not support the community care provider being the one touch point for the patient.

It becomes challenging ... it's not efficient for me to drive every day to buy a coffee to drive over to [Bob] to sit for an hour talking about his cat. It's not efficient, it's not productive per se. *So for those 15 to 20 times I have to drive to sit and talk about [Bob's] cat, nothing comes out of that. But on the 21st time, I get buy-in. And then I get support for him. The other kind of caveat to that is because I try so hard and I go out of my way and I kind of bend over backwards to really focus on providing the client with that compassion and empathy that they really not ever experienced in their life, I become the person that they call for everything, which is also not efficient.* – Community Care Provider (Rural).

Overall, patient engagement was recognized as important, however providers stated that a) the system does not support meaningful engagement (e.g. time with patients); b) both providers and patients need to have more time and education around the services available to older adults in the community; and c) providers need more support for relationship building. This will allow for patients to express their goals and preferences and ultimately create a care plan that suits their individualized needs.

Who is responsible for coordinating care?

During the focus group interviews, care coordination was discussed, including who providers felt was most responsible for coordinating care for older adults. Many participants agreed that care coordination should occur in the primary care setting where patients may have longer standing relationships with physicians and nurses. The following excerpts illustrate these views:

Primary care should be the hub of care – and this requires coordination. I don't think this is a new role, however. We have too many ineffective care coordinators throughout the system that are 'system-centred' rather than 'client-centred' – by that I mean that they coordinate the services that they are responsible for and connected to but no more. – Community Care Provider (Urban).

The second quote also demonstrates the feelings expressed by some providers that there are already care coordinators in the system however, they work for an organization rather than working across the system to ensure a patient is connected to the right services.

Regardless of where the coordination happens, having one person to communicate with is important for the patient:

I think having one point of contact that people feel comfortable calling in to is essential. Like, you've got all of these other organizations out there, but especially our community here, being such a rural older population... they don't like having to answer to an answering machine, they like a real voice. So I think having that real voice available to them is important for that system navigation piece. You know, have someone who's going to say "Okay, this is where we need to go, and let's make it happen." – Primary Care Provider (Rural).

Participants in each of the focus group discussions mentioned the important role of a system navigator. Participants debated whether there was a need for a specific navigator role. Others optimistically commented that the system could work collaboratively to coordinate care for an individual without a designated role.

I would expect to see is that system navigation is part of a process or function of primary care and the home team. – Community Care Provider (Urban).

I think that people are not knowledgeable about programs and services until they need them, and then they're in a crisis situation, and then it's not a good time to be searching for information. So if there was someone they could contact then they're not taking up primary healthcare time with a physician or nurse practitioner, over something that could be dealt with by the most appropriate service provider... I think by having a system navigator, that person could be followed and the right services put into place to prevent a serious fall or some other situation that people are picking up on – Primary Care Provider (Urban).

It is also important to recognize that those patients who are familiar with the system and feel empowered to be close involved in their care may desire to take on the role as their own navigator. Having patients engaged in discussions would allow for the best decisions to be made for individual situations, as indicated.

Trying to identify who is the most responsible person for coordinating care and that role may end up in all different places, depending upon the individual. So in some cases it might be someone in the community who has a long standing relationship with that person, in other cases it might be the CCAC[1] care coordinator or perhaps if neither of those, it could be someone in primary care, but instead of having multiple people taking on, like ultimately someone has to take accountability, and it may not always be the same person – Community Care Provider (Rural).

Many providers in the community felt that they were already coordinating care for older adults. However, even these individuals saw the importance of engaging primary care in discussions around patients.

Well, I guess that, see that depends on what you're asking for. Because if they have a requirement for the services that CCAC does, then we're doing that kind of coordination of care piece, but having the primary care physician more engaged in those care plans would be ideal, and I don't know if that happens all the time. – Community Care Provider (Rural).

Although many agree that regardless of where the coordination role occurs, a dedicated individual should care for the patient and take on the responsibility of linking the individual to appropriate services. This raises the question of how feasible it is to dedicate one person to take on responsibility or have a role across the entire system.

We've thought about that... It's just whether the ministry agrees with it, right? So that's the biggest thing... It's a very important role for system navigation. I think some of the things we've put in place here... even though we don't have a dedicated person doing that, we have a few people who do that role. – Primary Care Provider (Rural).

Fragmented information sharing among health care providers

When the topic of *information sharing among health care providers* arose during the focus group and individual interviews, many providers had much to say. Information sharing continues to cause challenges for providers across the entire health care system due in part to the many different electronic medical records (EMRs) being used. In the local health region in which this study was conducted, there are 13 different EMR systems used across the health care system (primary care, community care, hospitals, etc.). Many providers acknowledged this challenge,

At this point what I think our biggest challenge is the whole lack of a common documentation system. Because I don't have access to the client's EMR, which is what doctors rely on for communication between their allied staff. So it's very difficult to have a true sense of good collaboration because...the doctors especially really just don't have the time to step away from the client to come and find me. And I may or may not be in the building. – Primary Care (Rural).

Further to that, there are no standardized forms in place for communication between primary care and community care, creating fragmented, or often non-existent, communication between the two health sectors. Some health care providers have taken it upon themselves to come up with solutions to ensure the information is easily accessible for the physicians who do not have a lot of time to read multiple pages of a report. However, if every community care provider had their own method of reporting, this could cause more complication for a physician who may be trying to quickly review the document, as indicated in the excerpt below from the community care provider who recognizes her method for documenting may be more "detrimental" than helpful.

Three of those four pages are information about a client's name, marital status, and disease diagnosis. So the demographic information that occupies page one is really of no use to the doctor and after looking at page one think this is bananas and skip it. You know. They don't have time. So what I try to do is send my note, I'll do my home visit with the client and do my assessment and be very thorough in putting as much detail as I can about what happened when I was in the home. I really want the doctor to be able to read the note and feel like they were there. Sometimes that's detrimental because sometimes doctors want a one sentence snapshot: Client is good, services are started, check, carry on. And when I send them this mass note that's quite thorough, I'm not sure how many like or dislike that. – Community Care Provider (Urban).

As demonstrated in the following participant quotations, many health care providers identified the need to improve information sharing among providers across the health care system.

We um don't have a lot of conversation going back and forth between primary care. What does happen sometimes ... we would check on Clinical Connect[2] to try and get more information about it which isn't always helpful...sometimes they don't give you all the information. Again, that's limited too because Clinical Connect – not everybody is connected – Community Care Provider (Urban).

I think that's an area that there's a lot of room for growth and improvement on. It is, for us, it's been more individualized, so as an example, if we know, if we've had a referral come from primary care locally and we're working very closely around the care for an individual, there's some natural systems in place to share and to communicate that back, but it really, really depends, we don't have a standard, formal process for that, we talk about how that might happen...but it's a bigger system to try to figure out how we communicate back. – Community Care Provider (Urban).

Ultimately, these issues affect the patient as they are required to repeat their stories multiple times to multiple health care providers. Patients may lose trust in the system because they have already answered questions and don't understand why the new health care provider hasn't received that information.

I agree. I agree. Yeah, no. Because they don't like having to tell their story over and over and over again. The nice thing about here, with me doing kind of that role, is that I know everybody. And I have access to the EMR. So if they've told the story once, I can read through it, and I don't need to ask them again. Right? So just having that peace of being able to tell it that once and that's it. – Primary Care Provider (Rural).

For providers that work within the same organization (or in rural settings), it may be more feasible to have a "quick hallway conversation" to discuss a patient. However, participants acknowledged the privacy issues surrounding those conversations. Participants also suggested that phone conversations should occur more often when a provider needs to get information about a patient.

Call anybody, it's okay to call...I've got this client right, and basically – just like what happened today... our hallway conversation: had a nurse come and say '[Provider Name], come here, I need to bounce something!' so just having that and being able to do it... I know privacy is out there and I know there's a lot of issues, but...

The interview results indicate that information sharing is an issue across the entire health care system.

Lack of standardized referral processes and follow-up

During the focus group and individual interview process, another theme emerged around the current process of appropriately referring patients to services in the community. Interviews with care providers made clear that presently, there is no standardized process for identifying which primary care patients would benefit from additional services.

Interviewer: Do you currently use any standardized assessments on your older adults?

Primary Care Provider (Urban): No, definitely not on every older adult. Sometimes the Montreal Cognitive Health Assessment (MoCA) or screening for diabetes and hypertension. We go for the most commonly used ones.

Interviewer: And what about referral pathways for those patients, would most of your assessments have a referral piece to them as well?

Primary Care Provider (Urban): Not always, no.

Care providers did discuss however, that when a patient was referred to a service, multiple modes of communication are used to make the referral including phone calls, fax, e-referrals, self-referral or referrals from friends and family,

We do get referrals over the phone on our secure voicemail and by fax from various providers, generally they're physicians, who do it that way, we also get referrals through the e-referral aspect as well – Community Care Provider.

Health care organizations on the receiving end of the referral then need to keep track of the different referrals coming in through the various modes of communication. Multiple modes of communication make it challenging to track referrals and ensure patients are receiving the services they need.

In this particular health region, there is a centralized intake process for referring to specialized geriatric services. This allows a nurse who works for centralized intake to review the referral, access multiple databases of patient health information and put together a package that is sent on to the specialist. This helps to prioritize patient urgency as well provide information to the next health care provider who may not have access to all of the different EMR systems.

For some programs, there are a number of referrals made by friends and family on behalf of the patients, *"Phone calls, a majority of them are clients or family members" (Community Care Provider).* Sometimes health care providers discuss a service with the patient and then leave it up to the patient to access the service. One Family Health Team in the rural community indicated that they generally ask patients *"how confident are you feeling that you can make that call?"* and depending on the answer, providers may help make connections for that patient. Participants noted that patients can be informed about a service, but if they do not have someone helping to make the connection or attend with them, the referral may not follow through.

Another major issue discussed by multiple health care providers (participants) was the concern around offering programs or services to patients who needed the service but did not want to accept it.

We'll go out and visit people and a referral has been made, but really they don't want the service and they don't want any involvement.... but I also think, I mean the other part that I just also want to raise, is there are some people where the referrals don't get made, and that to me is also an equally important issue. – Community Care Provider (Urban).

Participants acknowledged these issues of patients declining services or people not being referred in the first place. Community care providers spoke about how important it was to educate primary care providers on the services that are offered in the community. Primary care providers tended to know about the few services that they referred to often.

Identifying services in the community for older adults is challenging

During the focus group discussions with primary care providers at both study sites, it was evident that more education was needed in terms of what services were available in the community for older adults. Providers seemed to be familiar with the common services such as those offered by the Alzheimer Society or the Community Care Access Centre (CCAC) but they were not familiar with programs or services that could help older adults who were not yet considered frail. One provider summarized the issue well in the following comment,

I think whoever is doing the referral or suggesting the referral, needs to be educated on services and resources and understand the system enough to say "here's some of the options available to you" and "where would you like to start?" Because I think, you know, a care coordinator, for example, in the community, might see that there is a dementia that is starting with a client and feels that going to memory clinic might be a good option for the client, but says "but you can also see a specialist, that might be a good option too" knowing that the client is not able to access community very well, or there's lots of other issues with the client, they may say "let's start with outreach team, it's a team of a care coordinator and specialized nurses that will look at your situation, do an assessment, talk to your physician about that assessment", then maybe determine next steps, whether it's seeing a geriatrician, so there's always next steps. And it's very individualized based on the client situation, so I think the person who is doing that assessment, be it the nurse, care coordinator, or family physician, is individuals deciding what might be the next steps based on what they know about the client – Community Care Provider (Rural).

In order to create care plans that are appropriate for the patient, it would be important to be familiar with a wide range of services in the community that could be of benefit to older adults. Participants were asked to list the services to which they commonly referred, these included internal programs within the Family Health Teams such as diabetes management or nutrition classes, or external programs such as memory clinics, specialists' referrals, or the CCAC. Subsequently, during the focus group discussions with community care providers, participants were asked to discuss services that their organizations offered that would be appropriate for older adults. The list generated from these discussions include transportation services, in home and community exercise programs, hearing clinics, arthritis education, meals on wheels, cooking class, friendship programs, support groups, and many more. Community care providers also identified that many of these services would be beneficial for older adults who are looking to maintain their health and independence in the community.

Caring for older adults in a rural community

The last theme that emerged through the interviews was one related to caring for older adults in rural communities. Community care and primary care providers in the rural community discussed facilitators and challenges that they encounter when working with older adults. Within a rural community, providers talked about how "everyone knows everyone" both in terms of the patient knowing the care provider and care providers knowing each other. Both of these examples are illustrated in the excerpts below:

I'm from this community and have been here for a number of years. So it makes it easier when I'm talking to these people, because they usually know me or my family. So that's a big plus...they feel comfortable that way. – Rural Primary Care Provider.

One community provider also discussed the importance of building a trusting relationship with patients. It is difficult to have patient buy-in without a long-standing relationship. New providers (within the rural community or from an urban organization) may be able to develop relationships with patients if they are connected through a provider with whom the patient already has an established relationship. This idea is further described in the two quotes below:

The only other thing I would like to add is I think rural is unique, and I think that you know that the organizations in this community work very well together, and have trusting relationships with seniors, so often it's someone from one of the core organizations in the rural townships that will then make the introduction to someone else and then the service will be accepted. – Community Care Provider (Rural).

As illustrated above, older adults are concerned with their privacy and developing trust between the patient and provider is important.

One challenge encountered by rural community care providers is the large geographical area that they have to cover to provide services to older adults. Within one day, the community care provider could be driving long distances across the rural region to see different patients.

It has been a real challenge, especially when I am one person who is working out of such a massive geography. – Community Care Provider (Rural).

There are also limited care providers working in the region, so it may be that there is only one provider for the specific organization across the entire rural area.

Providing care for older adults in the rural community presents some unique challenges or differences. As discussed by the participants, relationships are key to the success of providing care to older adults, especially in rural communities where trust and privacy are a concern. Relationships between the patient and provider allow for greater buy-in by the patient to accept services, and relationships between providers allow for knowing who to contact when looking for specific services or information. The strengths and challenges identified above were not present in the urban setting. Although care providers in an urban setting may build a long-standing relationship with a patient, this is not the same as "everyone knows everyone" and therefore building the relationship takes time. Furthermore, community care providers are not working across large geographical regions, rather, they are responsible for small sub-sections of the urban region.

Discussion

The aim of this paper was to understand the current state of primary care and the environment in which it operates, in relation to engaging patients in decision-making, referral processes and information sharing. Data were gathered from in-depth focus group and individual interviews with 30 health care providers in rural and urban centres. Data analysis yielded six key themes that allow for better understanding of the current context of primary care teams. Although many of the findings identified through this project were not entirely unfamiliar in health care system research, these results provide greater awareness of the current issues faced by the primary health care sector [2, 16–19]. Furthermore, the issues were echoed by multiple participants across different professions (nurse, physician, manager, etc.) and across different health care sectors (primary care and community care).

The first theme, *challenges in engaging older adults in health care decision making*, highlighted the importance of engaging older adults in care planning, however it was strongly identified that this is not what currently happens in daily practice. Previous studies have identified that caring for older adults is most effective in improving outcomes when it includes active in-person contact with patients and families [20]. Specifically, older adults living with multiple chronic conditions emphasize the need for convenient and flexible access to their healthcare providers, clear communication of plans for their care that are specific to their individual circumstances, and support from a care coordinator who is able to help in prioritizing their needs and who can also promote continuity in their care relationships [9, 20]. This is an area for improvement in primary care where long-standing relationships are already developed between patients and health care providers.

The second theme, *who is responsible for coordinating care?* and the third theme, fragmented *information sharing between health care providers*, both highlighted the current challenges experienced by health care providers when coordinating care for older adults. Participants felt that a specific coordinator role could be valuable however this role would not be of benefit to patients and providers unless it was supported by better engagement of patients and families in decision-making, as well continuity of care across the health system. Literature suggests that caring for and supporting patients and families includes utilizing the right services, at the right time, determined by level of complexity [18].

The fourth and fifth themes, *lack of standardized referral processes and follow-up, and identifying services in the community for older adults*, touched on current processes that occur when trying to organize services for older adults. Data indicated that multiple communication methods are used to make referrals. Furthermore, providers acknowledged they are unfamiliar with all of the services available in the community, and sometimes referrals to services are not made on behalf of the patients when they should be. These are areas for significant improvement to primary care for older adults. Literature demonstrates the need for multidisciplinary care for older frail adults because it significantly reduces fall risk, hospital use and nursing home admissions [21].

The final theme, *caring for older adults in rural communities*, identified some of the unique challenges and facilitators when providing care for older adults in rural communities including, community care providers working across large geographical regions, "everybody knowing everyone", and the importance of building trusting relationships. Although there were some strengths of rural communities identified, such as providers knowing who to contact for services, there are significant challenges. There are not enough health care providers to adequately serve the number of older adults in rural communities [22]. Sometimes rural communities are described as wealthy in terms of social networks that can support older adults, however there is a lack of available community resources to support older adults who wish to age in their own home [22, 23]. The lack of access to specialists also poses a significant challenge for individuals who need geriatric support for complex health conditions.

Limitations

There are two limitations of the study. First is the study recruitment process. The researcher used networks in the community to make connections with community care providers who might be interested in participating, limiting access to the smaller organizations who may not be as well known in the community. Secondly, the study is limited to only two sites within one Canadian province and therefore the results may not be representative of other primary care teams across Ontario or Canada. However, a rural and urban location were selected to illustrate two different contexts.

Conclusions

This study has provided information that will be useful for the next phases of this larger research focus. This research identified issues experienced by providers when providing care to older adults and areas that future work should focus on to improve care coordination for older adults. This study resulted in more detailed understanding of the primary care environment as it relates to providing care to older adults. Specific issues related to caring for older adults were identified including: lack of involvement of older adults in care planning; trouble coordinating care across the system, including challenges with sharing and receiving information; and limited knowledge by primary care providers of appropriate services for individuals in the community. Based on these findings, further education is necessary for both providers and patients in terms of service availability as well as the importance of engagement in decision-making and how this can be achieved.

Endnotes

[1]Community Care Access Centre (CCAC): There are 14 CCACs across Ontario funded through the Ontario Ministry of Health and Long-Term Care, CCACs coordinate home care services and long-term care placements.

[2]Clinical Connect is a secure, web-based portal that provides physicians and other health care providers with access to patients' EMR from hospitals and CCACs.

Abbreviations

CCAC: Community Care Access Centre; EMR: Electronic Medical Record; FHT: Family Health Team; MoCA: Montreal Cognitive Health Assessment

Acknowledgements

We wish to thank all of the individuals who participated in our study.

Funding

Jacobi Elliott was funded by a fellowship award from the Canadian Frailty Network (IFP2015W-07). Further support for this project was received from St. Joseph's Health Centre Guelph. These organizations provided financial support but did not have direct involvement in carrying out the research protocol or writing of the manuscript.

Authors' contributions

JE, PS, VB, LG and GH designed the study. JE collected data. JE carried out data analysis with support from PS. JE wrote the first draft of the article, which was then revised by all of the authors. All authors approved the final version of the article.

Consent for publication

The information participants received about the study included an explanation that results would be published. Thus, their written consent covered publication as well as participation.

Competing interests

The authors declare that they have no competing interests.

Author details

[1]University of Waterloo, 200 University Avenue West, Waterloo, ON N2L 3G1, Canada. [2]Conestoga College, 299 Doon Valley Dr, Kitchener, ON N2G 4M4, Canada.

References

1. Starfield B, Shi L, Mackino J. Contribution of primary care to health systems and health. Milbank Q. 2005;8:457–502.
2. Bodenheimer T. Coordinating care--a perilous journey through the health care system. N Engl J Med. 2008;358(10):1064.

3. Health Council of Canada. Primary health care: background paper. 2005. Retrieved on May 20, 2015 from https://healthcouncilcanada.ca/files/2.44-BkgrdPrimaryCareENG.pdf.
4. Glasby J, Dickinson H, Peck E. Guest editorial: partnership working in health and social care. Health Soc Care Community. 2006;14(5):373–4.
5. Banfield M, Gardner K, McRae I, Gillespie J, Wells R, Yen L. Unlocking information for coordination of care in Australia: a qualitative study of information continuity in four primary health care models. BMC Fam Pract. 2013;14(34). https://doi.org/10.1186/1471-2296-14-34.
6. Van Houdt S, Heyrman J, Vanhaecht K, Sermeus W, De Lepeleire J. (2013). Care pathways across the primary-hospital care continuum: using the multi-level framework in explaining care coordination. Bmc Health Services Research,13.
7. Robben SH, Huisjes M, van Achterberg T, Zuidema SU, Olde Rikkert MG, Schers HJ, Melis RJ. Filling the gaps in a fragmented health care system: development of the health and welfare information portal (ZWIP). JMIR Res Protoc. 2012;1(2):e10. https://doi.org/10.2196/resprot.1945.
8. Sevin C, Moore G, Shepherd J, Jacobs T, Hupke C. Transforming care teams to provide the best possible patient-centered, ollaborative care. Journal of Ambulatory Care Management. 2009;32(1):24–31.
9. Boeckxstaens P, De Graaf P. Primary care and care for older persons: position paper of the European forum for primary care. Qual Prim Care. 2011;19(6):369–89.
10. Sweetman A, Buckley G. Ontario's experiment with primary care reform. SPP Research Papers. 2014;7(11). https://doi.org/10.2139/ssrn.2434658.
11. Krueger R, Casey M. Focus groups. 3rd ed. Thousand Oaks: Sage Publications; 2000.
12. QSR International. NVIVO 10. 2012. Retrieved April, 2015. from https://www.qsrinternational.com/.
13. Lofland J, Snow DA, Anderson L, Lofland LH. Analyzing social settings: a guide to qualitative observation and analysis. 4th ed. Belmont: Wadsworth Publishing; 2006.
14. Shenton AK. Strategies for ensuring trustworthiness in qualitative research projects. Educ Inf. 2004;22:63–75.
15. Elliott J, Gregg S, Stolee P. Implementing and evaluating the assessment urgency algorithm in primary care and an emergency department. Waterloo: University of Waterloo; 2016.
16. Elliott J, Forbes D, Chesworth BM, Ceci C, Stolee P. Information sharing with rural family caregivers during care transitions of hip fracture patients. International Journal of Integrated Care. 2014;14(16). https://doi.org/10.5334/ijic.1195.
17. Sinha, S. (2012). Living longer, living well: recommendations to inform a seniors strategy for Ontario. Government of Ontario. Retrieved from http://www.longwoods.com/blog/wp-content/uploads/2013/01/seniors_strategy.pdf
18. Rothman AA, Wagner EH. Chronic illness Management : what is the role of primary Care ? Ann Intern Med. 2003;138(3):256–62.
19. McMurray J, Hicks E, Johnston H, Elliott J, Byrne K, Stolee P. "Trying to find information is like hating yourself every day" the collision of electronic information systems in transition with patients in transition. Health Informatics J. 2013;19(3):218–32. https://doi.org/10.1177/1460458212467547.
20. Bayliss EA, Balasubramianian BA, Gill JM, Stange KC. Perspectives in primary care: implementing patient-centered care coordination for individuals with multiple chronic medical conditions. The Annals of Family Medicine. 2014; 12(6):500–3.
21. Beswick AD, Rees K, Dieppe P, Ayis S, Gooberman-Hill R, Horwood J, Ebrahim S. Complex interventions to improve physical function and maintain independent living in elderly people: a systematic review and meta-analysis. Lancet. 2008;371(9614):725–35.
22. Keating N, Eales J. Diversity among older adults in rural Canada: health in context. In: Health in rural Canada. Vancouver, BC: UBC Press; 2012. p. 427–46.
23. Sims-Gould J, Martin-Mathews A. Distance, privacy and independence: rural homecare. In: Rural ageing: a good place to group old? 2008. p. 43–51.

17

Stroke follow-up in primary care: a prospective cohort study on guideline adherence

Rune Aakvik Pedersen*, Halfdan Petursson and Irene Hetlevik

Abstract

Background: After a stroke, a person has an increased risk of recurrent strokes. Effective secondary prevention can provide significant gains in the form of reduced disability and mortality. While considerable efforts have been made to provide high quality acute treatment of stroke, there has been less focus on the follow-up in general practice after the stroke. One strategy for the implementation of high quality, evidence-based treatment is the development and distribution of clinical guidelines. However, from similar fields of practice, we know that guidelines are often not adhered to. The purpose of this study was to investigate to what degree patients who have suffered a stroke are followed up in general practice, if recommendations in the national guidelines are followed, and if patients achieve the treatment goals recommended in the guidelines.

Methods: The study included patients with cerebral infarction identified by the ICD-10 discharge diagnoses I63.0 trough I63.9 in two Norwegian local hospitals. In total 51 patients participated. They were listed with general practitioners in 18 different clinics. The material consists of the general practitioners' (GPs') medical records for these patients in the first year of follow-up; in total 381 consultations.

Results: Of the 381 consultations during the first year of follow-up, 71 (19%) had stroke as the main topic. The blood pressure (BP) target value < 140/90 mmHg was reached by 24 patients (47%). The low density lipoprotein (LDL) cholesterol target value < 2.0 mmol/L was reached by 14 (27%) of the 51 patients. In total six patients (12%) got advice on physical activity and three (6%) received dietary advice. No advice about alcohol consumption was recorded.

Conclusions: The findings support earlier claims that the development and distribution of guidelines alone is not enough to implement a certain practice. Despite being a serious condition, stroke gets limited attention in the first year of follow-up in general practice. This can be explained by the complexity of general practice, where even a serious condition loses the competition for attention to other apparently equally important issues.

Keywords: Stroke, Practice guidelines, General practice, Secondary prevention

Background

Stroke

Ischemic stroke is a frequent disorder with extensive personal and social consequences. In the Western world, stroke is regarded the third most common cause of death [1]. In Norway, about 15,000 persons suffer a stroke each year, and a 50% increase is expected in the period 2010–2030 [2]. The average cost of an acute ischemic stroke hospitalization in Europe has been estimated to $11,900 (2013) and one-year follow-up is estimated to an average of $3720 [3]. Patients with recurrent strokes have more adverse clinical outcomes and costs are higher compared with patients suffering first-ever strokes [4].

Recurrent stroke and secondary prevention

Having had a first stroke, a person has an increased risk of recurrent strokes; 11% within 1 year, 26% within 5

* Correspondence: rune.pedersen@ntnu.no
General Practice Research Unit, Department of Public Health and Nursing, NTNU, Norwegian University of Science and Technology, PO Box 8905 MTFS, N-7491 Trondheim, Norway

years and 39% within 10 years. The numbers refer to all strokes [5]. The mortality after a recurrent stroke is particularly high [6, 7].

Risk factors for recurrent cerebrovascular events are well known. Handling these with effective individualized secondary prevention can provide substantial gains in preventing cerebrovascular disease and death [8]. Based on estimates of the benefits from preventive measures for heart attack, it has been suggested that the various secondary preventive measures in combination can reduce the risk of recurrent stroke with up to 70% [1].

Adherence to recommendations for such secondary prevention and to offer the patients the necessary follow-up is a challenge for the health services [8]. Although management of secondary prevention for stroke and transient ischemic attack (TIA) may differ [9], reports on follow-up of TIA may indicate that many patients do not receive secondary prevention at all [10]. Considerable under-treatment with statins in patients with prior cardiovascular disease is documented [11] as is diminishing compliance over time [11, 12]. One answer to such challenges has been development and implementation of clinical guidelines.

Follow-up in primary care

General practice is well placed to provide follow-up of stroke patients, but this potential is not necessarily fulfilled [13]. Norwegian National guidelines for treatment and rehabilitation of stroke patients [2] were issued in 2010. According to these guidelines, the general practitioner (GP) is supposed to play a key role in the follow-up of patients who have suffered a stroke. Furthermore, the guidelines provide specific advice on the content of the follow-up. It is recommended that patients with stroke should usually be treated with lipid-lowering medication in the form of statins, and that creatine kinase (CK) and transaminase blood samples are taken to control possible side-effects of this treatment. The recommended target value for low-density lipoprotein (LDL) is < 2.0 mmol/L. For blood pressure (BP), the recommended target value is < 140/90 mmHg. Diet, body mass index (BMI), physical activity, alcohol consumption and smoking affect the risk for stroke and recurrent stroke. These lifestyle factors should therefore also be part of the post-stroke follow-up. In the Netherlands, it was found that advice in a protocol corresponding to the Norwegian guidelines is followed only to some extent. As an example, lifestyle advice was offered to only one in four patients [14]. After the introduction of the Dutch protocol, only minimal impact was noted on clinical practice and no major changes in survival or secondary outcomes were found [15].

However, it is still not known to what degree the patients are followed up in general practice in Norway, nor is it known if the follow-up is in accordance with the guidelines. It is known that development and distribution of guidelines alone is not sufficient for implementation in general practice [16]. It is therefore recommended to make use of more active methods for implementation [16], but even comprehensive active implementation does not necessarily lead to adherence to the clinical guidelines [17, 18].

In this study, the aim was to investigate the extent to which patients who have had a stroke are being followed up in general practice, if the recommended procedures have been applied and whether or not patients achieve the treatment goals recommended in the national guidelines.

Methods

Design and setting

The study took place in Møre og Romsdal County in Western Norway. This is an affluent area with good access to primary and secondary health care. In 2016 the county had the highest life expectancy for boys and the second highest for girls among all 19 Norwegian counties [19]. In Norway, all residents are entitled to a regular general practitioner (RGP). When a resident is registered on a GP's list of patients, the GP has the medical responsibility for this person. At the time of this study, about 99% of the Norwegian population was registered on GPs' patient lists [20]. When a person registered on a GP's list is discharged from hospital, the GP normally receives a discharge summary. The discharge summary is a transfer of information from the hospital to the GP, not a formal referral. The guidelines [2] state that discharge summaries of good quality sent to the RGP is a prerequisite for the follow-up of stroke patients.

The study included patients treated for ischemic stroke in two Norwegian local hospitals in 2011 and 2012. Patients with hemorrhagic stroke were not included. The reason for this was that the guidelines do not apply to all forms of hemorrhagic stroke. A search for the ICD-10 discharge diagnosis I63.0 trough I63.9 identified patients with cerebral infarction in the hospital files. The patients' RGPs were identified by The Norwegian Health Economics Administration (Helfo). All patients identified in the hospital files were registered with an RGP, and all patients included had active practicing RGPs in clinics with regular office hours and availability. All clinics were available for wheelchair users, and all clinics had secretaries available by phone. All clinics also had laboratory services including availability of blood investigations such as CK, transaminases and cholesterol. The costs of laboratory services are covered by the National Insurance Scheme. Residents in Norway have compulsory membership in this scheme. None of the clinics had dietitians or rehabilitation therapists as part of their staff.

Invitation to participate in the study was sent to each of the GPs identified as described above. Only patients living in their own home and registered with an RGP who accepted participation, were subsequently invited to participate in the study. Patients in nursing homes were excluded.

One of the authors (RAaP) visited each clinic personally. All clinics kept electronic medical records, and each clinic provided access for the researcher. The GPs used three different electronic medical record systems. We evaluated the records of each consultation (n = 381) in the RGPs' clinic the first year after the hospital stay or the last outpatient hospital consultation. The record's laboratory results, prescribing registries and diagnosis registries were all used to support the evaluation of the written text record of each individual consultation. An operational definitions list was used to standardize the coding of data (Additional file 1).

We noted the number of consultations with any content relevant for stroke follow-up, as was the number of consultations mainly concerning stroke. A note was made where we found that any of the lifestyle factors diet, BMI, physical activity, alcohol consumption or smoking had been addressed in the consultation. We chose to include those who had a recorded BMI, also when recorded before the specific follow-up year. Furthermore, we recorded whether or not the recommended blood tests were taken and the results of blood pressure measurements and LDL laboratory results, as these tests have specified targets in the guideline, expected to be reached.

Results

Among 100 invited GPs, 37 agreed to participate. These 37 GPs had a total of 138 stroke patients from 2011 and 2012 on their lists. We invited all these 138 patients to participate in the study, and 51 gave their written consent. Age varied from 38 to 90 years (mean 68.5 years). Thirty (59%) were male and 21 (41%) female. These 51 patients had RGPs in 18 different clinics.

In total 46 patients (90%) had suffered from an acute stroke. Among these, 40 had their first-ever stroke, and 6 had a recurrent stroke. The rest of the patients in the total group of 51 patients had TIA following a previous stroke or previous stroke with new symptoms not classified as TIA, and where new stroke could not be detected. In one patient, we found that the stroke diagnosis was used, but not further discussed in the discharge summary. Five patients got acute thrombolytic treatment and 19 of the patients were discharged with an outpatient control appointment.

Consultations

These 51 patients had 381 consultations with their RGP the first year after discharge from hospital, an average of 7.5 (0–24) consultations.

Stroke follow-up

In 148 consultations (39%), stroke was documented as a topic. We found that 71 (19%) of the consultations had stroke as the main topic. The medical record in these cases was primarily concerned with stroke, although other issues also were discussed. On average, each patient had 1.4 (0–7) consultations mainly concerning stroke during the first year of follow up in general practice.

Adherence to the most central advice for the follow-up

Table 1 gives information about the number (percentage) of relevant lifestyle information registered in the patient records, as well as procedures performed (BP and LDL-cholesterol) in addition to the number of patients where the recommended goals were reached.

Other recommendations

On discharge from hospital, 45 of the 51 patients were treated with statins. In the GPs' medical records, we found confirmation of ongoing statin treatment in 39 patients. In our material, CK and transaminase blood samples were taken in 8 (16%) of the 51 patients, and in 7 of the 39 patients where we could find confirming

Table 1 Variables registered and goals reached

	Women (n = 21)		Men (n = 30)		Total (n = 51)	
	N	%	n	%	n	%
Variables registered						
Lifestyle[a]	7	33	9	30	16	31
BMI[b]	6	29	6	20	12	24
Diet[c]	2	10	1	3	3	6
Physical activity[d]	4	19	2	7	6	12
Smoking[e]	1	5	3	10	4	8
Alcohol[f]	0	0	0	0	0	0
BP[j]	20	95	26	87	46	90
LDL[h]	13	62	15	50	28	55
Goals reached						
BP[i]	11	52	13	43	24	47
LDL[j]	7	33	7	23	14	27

[a]Patients with any notes on lifestyle made the first year of follow-up. [b]Patients with a BMI measure made before or the first year after the stroke. [c]Any notes on diet during the first year of follow-up. [d]Any notes on physical activity the first year of follow-up. [e]Any notes on smoking the first year of follow-up. [f]Any notes on alcohol consumption the first year of follow-up. [j]Blood pressure measured the first year of follow-up. [h]LDL measured the first year of follow up. [i]BP < 140/90 mmHg in the last registration in the study period. [j]LDL < 2.0 mmol/L

information about ongoing statin treatment in the GPs' medical records.

Discussion

Main findings

In this study we examined the follow-up of patients with stroke in general practice. We compared the recommendations in the national guidelines with clinical practice in real life. Nearly all patients had their blood pressure measured within the first year of follow-up in general practice. Despite this, only about half of the patients had reached the blood pressure target value. Fewer patients had their LDL-cholesterol level measured, and the LDL-cholesterol target value was reached by less than one third of the patients. We found limited information on diet and physical activity and none about alcohol consumption in the medical records.

Patients residing in the community had on average consulted their GP more than seven times the first year after being discharged from hospital with a stroke diagnosis. In 2012, Norwegians on average consulted their RGP 2.6 times [21]. However, in our material we also found that stroke was not necessarily the foremost concern in the consultations with the GP in this period. In fact, stroke was not documented as an issue at all in most of these consultations. The findings reveal that the median number of consultations mainly concerning stroke was one in the first year of follow up. Stroke got limited attention in the consultations with the GP the first year after the incident, even though it is a serious condition. This may be because the stroke diagnosis faced competition from other issues that were perceived as equally important by the patient or by the GP at the moment of consultation.

The guidelines give evidence-based advice on the follow-up of stroke survivors. They are based on a thorough review of an extensive amount of research and are intended to ensure good clinical practice. They can be regarded as a map that gives direction and guides the most important clinical decisions for the treatment of patients who have experienced stroke. Our study, however, shows that this map is not in accordance with the terrain in general practice.

Strengths and weaknesses

Based on the GPs' medical records, this study investigates how the follow-ups of the patients have been recorded. It does not involve any form of possible biased self-reporting. The inclusion of patients started out wide, and although the participation rate was low, the researchers did not make any selections. All data collection was done by the same person. In this way, there were no different practices in the review of the medical records or data registration. The possibility of intra-observer variations is nevertheless still present.

We found a low degree of adherence to the guideline. We have no reason to believe that the GPs who accepted participation in this study have a less optimal practice than those who rejected the request. On the other hand, we have some indication of the opposite. When we made reminding telephone calls to all the invited GPs that did not respond to our invitation letters one GP admitted that it was scary to have her practice investigated by researchers.

Still, there are several limitations to this study. There were relatively few patients included, and although the GPs are practicing in 18 different clinics, the clinics are all in the same county. In addition to a low rate of participation among of GPs, there was also a low degree of participation among patients. Possible explanations for this could be poor health, high age and impaired physical and mental functioning in the patients. We needed, for example, to exclude a patient because this persons' partner had signed a declaration of consent, without documentable transfer of authority for consent. The experienced treatment burden among those with stroke is shown to be considerable [22] and combined with the reduced patient capacity, this may also be the reason for the low degree of participation among the invited patients. While the chosen method of reading medical records has its strengths, it also carries with it some weaknesses. There is a possibility of making incorrect recordings. To check this, one would have to visit the clinics again to read the records once more. Given the geographical spread, this would be very resource-demanding.

Furthermore, physicians do not necessarily document every topic of the consultation. Therefore, it is possible that the GP or the patient have addressed topics without it being included in our counts. Despite these weaknesses, we claim the findings to be valid for the performance of secondary stroke-prevention in general practice.

Findings in the light of current knowledge

We have found that the patients often consult their GPs in the period after having had a stroke. In this way, our study is consistent with previous claims that general practice is well placed for the follow-up of patients who have had a stroke [12]. The reasons for lack of guideline adherence are largely unknown. It could be that the GPs do not know the recommendations for secondary prevention after stroke [16], that the guidelines do not fit in with the patients` complexity [23] or that the guidelines are poorly adapted to general practice in other ways [24]. There are also critical questions as to whether the theoretical basis for clinical guidelines is good enough as guidelines are mostly organ-specific. This results in a high degree of complexity in general practice where patients often have many diseases at the same time [25]. International expert guidelines are also documented to be non-implementable in Norwegian general practice because of the resource utilization recommended is not compatible with the resources available. For example, international guidelines on high blood pressure alone have been estimated to impose a workload that exceeds the total working capacity of Norwegian GPs [26]. To the extent that the guidelines are followed with respect to recommended procedures being carried out, it is nevertheless a recognized problem that this does not have to significantly affect health goals for patients [17, 18].

It is known that the risk of stroke can be reduced by adjustments in lifestyle and that lack of knowledge is a main obstacle for patients in achieving this benefit [27]. The guidelines [2] are explicit on lifestyle advice; they give recommendations on physical activity, diet and alcohol consumption in addition to BMI. One prominent finding in this study is the absence of such lifestyle advice, and especially advice on diet and alcohol consumption. This corresponds to previous findings, pointing out that patients report having received little or no information about lifestyle following a stroke [28].

We recommend future research to explore reasons for non- adherence to guidelines. Other studies point out that the majority of patients with a chronic disease in primary care, also have other chronic diseases; multimorbidity [29]. Also, most persons aged 65 and older are multimorbid [30, 31]. In our research group, we will therefore conduct further research on stroke follow-up in the presence of multimorbidity. General practice is not meant to focus on one single disease, but practices an integrated approach. An understanding of this complexity might give answers to why the follow-up of patients who have had a stroke seems to be so limited in general practice.

Conclusions

Although patients frequently consulted their GPs in the first year after a stroke, most consultations were concerned with issues other than the stroke. When stroke was an issue, the recommendations in the guidelines were often not adhered to. This means that even a medical condition considered to be serious, may receive only limited attention in general practice. As the access to the GP did not seem to be limited, the results may rather be caused by the complexity of general practice. Other complaints may be regarded as equally important by the patient or by the GP. This complexity should be considered in the development of clinical guidelines.

Abbreviations

BMI: Body mass index; BP: Blood pressure; CK: Creatine kinase; GP: General practitioner; Helfo: The Norwegian Health Economics Administration; LDL: Low-density lipoprotein; REK: Regional committees for medical and health research ethics; RGP: Regular general practitioner; TIA: Transient ischemic attack

Acknowledgements

The authors of this study would like to thank all the participating GPs for taking their time to facilitate the data collection. We would also like to thank Helse Møre og Romsdal HF for help in identifying the patients and Helfo for identifying the GPs.

Funding

This study was funded by the Norwegian Research Fund for General Practice, The Norwegian Committee on Research in General Practice and The Norwegian Centre of Rural Medicine.

Authors' contributions

RAaP, HP and IH took part in the planning of the study. RAaP registered data from the medical records and wrote the first draft of the manuscript. HP and IH read the paper and made improvements of the content and wording. RAaP, HP and IH have read and approved the final manuscript.

Authors' information

RAaP is a neurologist, a former family doctor and holds a masters' degree in social studies. HP is a family doctor and PhD. IH is a Professor of General practice at NTNU.

Consent for publication

Not applicable.

Competing interests

The authors declare that they have no competing interests.

References

1. Lo EH, Dalkara T, Moskowitz MA. Mechanisms, challenges and opportunities in stroke. Nat Rev Neurosci. 2003;4(5):399–415.
2. The Norwegian Directorate of Health. Nasjonal faglig retningslinje for behandling og rehabilitering ved hjerneslag [National guideline for treatment and rehabilitation in stroke] (In Norwegian). Oslo: The Norwegian Directorate of Health (Helsedirektoratet); 2010.
3. Nicholson G, Gandra SR, Halbert RJ, Richhariya A, Nordyke RJ. Patient-level costs of major cardiovascular conditions: a review of the international literature. Clinicoecon Outcomes Res. 2016;8:495-506.
4. Engel-Nitz NM, Sander SD, Harley C, Rey GG, Shah H. Costs and outcomes of noncardioembolic ischemic stroke in a managed care population. Vasc Health Risk Manag. 2010;6:905–13.
5. Mohan KM, Wolfe CD, Rudd AG, Heuschmann PU, Kolominsky-Rabas PL, Grieve AP. Risk and cumulative risk of stroke recurrence: a systematic review and meta-analysis. Stroke. 2011;42(5):1489–94.
6. Ellekjaer H, Holmen J, Indredavik B, Terent A. Epidemiology of stroke in Innherred, Norway, 1994 to 1996. Incidence and 30-day case-fatality rate. Stroke. 1997;28(11):2180–4.
7. Aarnio K, Haapaniemi E, Melkas S, Kaste M, Tatlisumak T, Putaala J. Long-term mortality after first-ever and recurrent stroke in young adults. Stroke. 2014;45(9):2670–6.
8. Russell D, Lund C, Dahl A. Sekundærprofylakse etter hjerneinfarkt og transitorisk iskemisk anfall [secondary prophylaxis after ischemic stroke and transitoric ischemic attack] (in Norwegian). Tidsskr Nor Legeforen. 2007; 127(10):1379–82.
9. Gladstone DJ, Kapral MK, Fang J, Laupacis A, Tu JV. Management and outcomes of transient ischemic attacks in Ontario. CMAJ. 2004;170(7): 1099–104.

10. Corrao G, Rea F, Merlino L, Mazzola P, Annoni F, Annoni G. Management, prognosis and predictors of unfavourable outcomes in patients newly hospitalized for transient ischemic attack: a real-world investigation from Italy. BMC Neurol. 2017;17(1):12.
11. Nilsson G, Samuelsson E, Soderstrom L, Mooe T. Low use of statins for secondary prevention in primary care: a survey in a northern Swedish population. BMC Fam Pract. 2016;17(1):110.
12. Ho PM, Bryson CL, Rumsfeld JS. Medication adherence: its importance in cardiovascular outcomes. Circulation. 2009;119(23):3028–35.
13. Whitford DL, Hickey A, Horgan F, O'Sullivan B, McGee H, O'Neill D. Is primary care a neglected piece of the jigsaw in ensuring optimal stroke care? Results of a national study. BMC Fam Practice 2009;10:27.
14. de Weerd L, Rutgers AW, Groenier KH, van der Meer K. Health care in patients 1 year post-stroke in general practice: research on the utilisation of the Dutch transmural protocol transient ischaemic attack/cerebrovascular accident. Aust J Prim Health. 2012:18(1):42–9.
15. de Weerd L, Groenhof F, Kollen BJ, van der Meer K. Survival of stroke patients after introduction of the 'Dutch transmural protocol TIA/CVA. BMC Fam Pract. 2013;14:74.
16. Treweek S, Flottorp S, Fretheim A, Havelsrud K, Kristoffersen DT, Oxman A, Aasland OG. Retningslinjer for allmennpraksis - blir de lest og blir de brukt? [guidelines in general practice--are they read and are they used?]. Tidsskr Nor Legeforen 2005;125(3):300–3.
17. Hetlevik I. The role of clinical guidelines in cardiovascular risk intervention in general practice. Trondheim, Norway: NTNU; 1999.
18. Fretheim A, Oxman AD, Havelsrud K, Treweek S, Kristoffersen DT, Bjorndal A. Rational prescribing in primary care (RaPP): a cluster randomized trial of a tailored intervention. PLoS Med. 2006;3(6):e134.
19. Statistics Norway: Deaths 2015. https://www.ssb.no/en/befolkning/statistikker/dode/aar/2016-03-09. Accessed 27 Apr 2018.
20. The Norwegian Directorate of Health: Fastlegestatisitkken. https://helsedirektoratet.no/statistikk-og-analyse/fastlegestatistikk#fastlegestatistikk-2012 (2018). Accessed 27 Apr 2018.
21. Statistics Norway: General practitioners consultations, by age and sex (C) 2010–2016 [https://www.ssb.no/statbank/table/09535/?rxid=a9a876f4-ce50-4c95-b371-9f86d663c25b] Accessed 27 Apr 2018.
22. Gallacher KI, May CR, Langhorne P, Mair FS. A conceptual model of treatment burden and patient capacity in stroke. BMC Fam Pract. 2018;19(1):9.
23. Austad B, Hetlevik I, Mjolstad BP, Helvik AS. Applying clinical guidelines in general practice: a qualitative study of potential complications. BMC Fam Pract. 2016;17:92.
24. Bloy G, Rigal L. General practitioners' relationship with preventive knowledge: a qualitative study. Aust J Prim Health. 2016;22(5):394–402.
25. Hetlevik I, Getz L, Kirkengen AL. General practitioners who do not adhere to practice guidelines- do they have valid reasons? Tidsskr Norske Legeforen. 2008;128(19):2218–20.
26. Petursson H, Getz L, Sigurdsson JA, Hetlevik I. Current European guidelines for management of arterial hypertension: are they adequate for use in primary care? Modelling study based on the Norwegian HUNT 2 population. BMC Fam Pract. 2009;10:70.
27. Galimanis A, Mono ML, Arnold M, Nedeltchev K, Mattle HP. Lifestyle and stroke risk: a review. Curr Opin Neurol. 2009;22(1):60–8.
28. Lawrence M, Kerr S, Watson H, Paton G, Ellis G. An exploration of lifestyle beliefs and lifestyle behaviour following stroke: findings from a focus group study of patients and family members. BMC Fam Pract. 2010;11:97.
29. Sinnige J, Korevaar JC, Westert GP, Spreeuwenberg P, Schellevis FG, Braspenning JC. Multimorbidity patterns in a primary care population aged 55 years and over. Fam Pract2015;32(5):505–13.
30. Barnett K, Mercer SW, Norbury M, Watt G, Wyke S, Guthrie B. Epidemiology of multimorbidity and implications for health care, research, and medical education: a cross-sectional study. Lancet (London, England). 2012; 380(9836):37–43.
31. Tomasdottir M, Getz L, Sigurdsson J, Petursson H, Kirkengen A, Krokstad S, McEwen B, Hetlevik I. Co- and multi-morbidity patterns in an unselected Norwegian population: cross-sectional analysis based on the HUNT study and theoretical reflections concerning basic medical models. Europ J Pers Cent Healthc. 2014:2(3):335–45.

Internists' career choice towards primary care

Nathalie Scherz[1,2*], Stefan Markun[1], Vera Aemissegger[1], Thomas Rosemann[1] and Ryan Tandjung[1,3]

Abstract

Background: Swiss primary care (PC) is facing workforce shortage. Up to 2011 this workforce was supplied by two board certifications: general medicine and internal medicine. To strengthen them against subspecialties, they were unified into one: general internal medicine. However, since unification general practitioners' career options are no longer restrained by early commitment to PC. This may lead to a decrease of future primary care physicians (PCPs).

Methods: To gain insights in timing and factors influencing career choice of internists, we addressed a cross sectional survey to all board certified internists in the years 2000–2010 ($n = 1462$). Main measures were: final career choice (PCPs, hospital internists or subspecialists), timing and factors influencing career choice, and attractiveness of PCP career during medical school and residency.

Results: Response rate was 53.2%, 44.8% were female and median age was 45 years old. Final career choice was PCP for 39.1% of participants, 15.0% chose to become hospital internists, 41.8% became subspecialists and 4.0% other. Timing of career choice significantly differed between groups. Most of the subspecialists have chosen their career during residency (65.3%), while only 21.9% of the PCPs chose during residency. Work experience in an academic hospital was negatively associated with becoming PCP ($P < 0.001$). Family influence on career choice was more frequently reported among PCPs and chiefs' influence more reported among non-PCPs ($P < 0.001$). Fifty-nine percent of the participants considered a career as PCP to be attractive during medical school, this proportion decreased over time.

Conclusions: Timing of career choice of PCPs and subspecialists strongly differed. PCPs opted late for their career and potentially modifiable external factors seem to contribute to their decision. This stresses the importance of fostering attractiveness of PC during medical school as well as during and after residency and of tailored residency positions for future PCPs in the hospital-dominated new general internal medicine training.

Keywords: Medical education, career choice, Primary care, Survey research, Workforce

Background

As in many countries, primary care in Switzerland is challenged by a shortage of workforce and several negative prognostic factors are found when evidence across different biographical stages of physicians is looked at: during medical school, primary care has low attractiveness as a career choice [1–4]. For career choice, however, residency was found to be more determining than medical school, but attractiveness of primary care even decreases during residency [5–7]. Ultimately an important proportion of residents initially aiming at a career in primary care changes its goal during residency [1, 8, 9]. Thus, spontaneous amelioration of the workforce shortage in primary care seems unlikely.

In Switzerland, up to 2010 two different board certifications contributed to primary care workforce: the first being internal medicine with a mainly hospital based residency which also served as basis for subspecialties in internal medicine and the second being general medicine.

Both board certifications required 5 years of postgraduate medical training. There was no nationally coordinated structured curriculum, neither for future PCP

* Correspondence: nathalie.scherz@usz.ch
[1]Institute of Primary Care, University Hospital of Zurich, University of Zurich, Pestalozzistrasse 24, 8091 Zurich, Switzerland
[2]Arud Centres for Addiction Medicine, Zurich, Switzerland
Full list of author information is available at the end of the article

nor for hospitalists. The residents designed their curriculum themselves by applying for different residency positions, mainly in hospitals. After 5 years and an examination, they submitted their completed curriculum to the institute for medical postgraduate education [10]. The institute reviewed if the criteria for the board certification were fulfilled. Board certification in general medicine required residency in- and outpatient internal medicine, surgery and different possible rotations like for example pediatrics, gynecology, psychiatry. Those board certified generalists were most likely to join primary care workforce [5, 11].

Conversely board certified internists worked mainly in internal medicine in hospital and performed rotations in internal medicine subspecialties (for example, cardiology, nephrology, angiology, endocrinology etc.) Thus they became versatile physicians qualifying for many different careers: In Switzerland internists are working as hospitalists, subspecialists and also as primary care physicians (PCPs). Therefore, residents in internal medicine are not necessarily committed to a specific career in medicine. While some residents in internal medicine clearly aim at a particular career, others may initially choose internal medicine because they thereby remain open to a broad variety of career opportunities even after board certification. Repeated surveys in Switzerland and in the US have shown that residents in internal medicine increasingly tend to opt for subspecialties and are overall inconstant in their preferences [8, 12–14].

In contrast to regulations in other countries, vocational trainings in Swiss primary care have not been mandatory for future PCPs. Between 2000 and 2010 only 30–60% of the candidates made such a vocational training [11, 15].

Countries like the Netherlands, United Kingdom, and Denmark, could address workforce shortage creating centralized dedicated primary care curricula. Most central European Countries launched similar programs. [16] Australia set incentives and programs for rural primary care workforce [17]. Another pathway was chosen In Switzerland: to counter the trend towards more subspecialization and strengthen general internal medicine against subspecialties, the board certification in general medicine and internal medicine were merged into a single certification of "general internal medicine" in 2011. Residents are still able to design a curriculum including in- an outpatient internal medicine, subspecialties and other specialties such as surgery, pediatrics, gynecology, psychiatry in accordance to their interest and goal. Vocational training in primary care is encouraged for ongoing primary care physicians [18–20]. The effect on this merger of board certifications, however, is unknown and it may even result in a further decline of primary care workforce. Indeed, with the new certification, there will no longer be a group of general medicine practitioners that commit early to a career in primary care. Given the versatility of general internists and their broad opportunities a decrease of future PCPs might occur. We therefore aimed to gain further insights on timing of final career choice of internists and on influencing factors. We retrospectively assessed attractiveness of primary care during medical school and internal medicine residency.

Methods

Study design

The study is a cross-sectional survey. All physicians in the target population were invited to participate by a postal invitation letter containing a paper version of the questionnaire in either French or German language. Additionally, a link was provided leading to an identical online questionnaire. An identification code assured that only a single entry per participant was considered in the analysis. Five weeks after the first postal letter, a second postal letter was sent to non-respondents only. Both preliminary versions of the French as well as the German questionnaire were pre-tested with 15 physicians from the study population.

Study population

All physicians who received a Swiss board certification in internal medicine in the years 2000 to 2010 were eligible. Exclusion criterion was a missing answer to the primary outcome question about final career choice. The addresses were provided by the Swiss Medical Association, FMH.

Questionnaire

To gain insights on factors potentially influencing the career choice of medical students and residents, we conducted a literature search with the scope of general medicine, career planning and specialty choice to compose the questionnaire.

Inclusion criteria were verified with questions about years and types of board certifications.

Baseline characteristics: To characterize the study population, we included questions about demographic characteristics (sex, current age) education (age at end of medical school, place of graduation) and residency (PCP vocational training, residency at academic hospital, months of outpatient work) and current work situation (part-time, leading position, employed vs self-employed, setting, working half-days a week).

Primary outcome: The primary outcome final career choice was defined as the participants' answer to the question "What will be your main lifetime activity". Possible answers were: "PCP", "hospital internist", "subspecialists" and "other". If the box "other" was ticked, we reclassified the participants based on their free-text answer. We reclassified them as PCP if they did not have a second board certification and currently worked in a practice. We reclassified them as "subspecialists" if they indicated a second board certification and as "hospital internist" if they were working in hospital without a second board certification. Those who were not working with patients or who did not fulfill one of the categories were classified as "others". As our focus was PCP as a career choice, we categorized respondents as PCP versus non-PCP to compare the association of influencing factors with final career choice. Non-PCP included respondents with answers: hospital internists, subspecialists, and other career choices.

Secondary outcomes and influencing factors: To compare timing of final career choice over categories we asked "When did you decide about your main lifetime activity?" with a multiple choice answer. To investigate factors associated with the final career choice we asked about perceived influence of participants' peers on final career choice, availability of resident positions and practice moratorium (i.e., a federal law restricting the opening of private practices in Switzerland from 2002 to 2011).

Finally we explored (non-mutually-exclusive) attractiveness of following careers: "being an internist without further subspecialty", "being a specialist", "working in a practice" and "working in a hospital" at different biographical time intervals: "during medical school", "during internal medicine residency" and "final career choice". We categorized a career in primary care to be perceived as attractive if participants rated "working in a practice" and "being an internist without further subspecialty" as attractive within the same biographical time interval.

Statistical analyses

We summarized data using counts and proportions for categorical variables and median and interquartile range for continuous variables as all of them were all not normally distributed. Participants were grouped into PCPs and non-PCPs according to primary outcome response. Group comparisons were performed using chi-squared test defining a $P < 0.05$ as statistically significant between-group difference. Data analysis was performed using R Statistics (version 3.2.0).

Results

Out of 3287 questionnaires 1749 were returned (response rate 53.2%). Although being in the provided address list, 266 were not board certified in internal medicine or not in the years 2000 to 2010 and thus were not included. Missing answer to the primary outcome question led to exclusion of 21 participants. Finally, 1462 answers were considered in the analysis: 1024 German, 390 French and 48 Italian (See Flowchart in Additional file 1). Overall completeness of responses was >95% for all questions. Participants' median age was 45 years (IQR: 42–49), 44.8% of them were female and 17.6% had finished medical school outside of Switzerland. The median number of working days per week was 5 (IQR: 3.5–5) with 47.3% of the participants working part time, 40.0% self-employed and 47.7% having a leading position.

Primary outcome

When asked about their final career choice: 573 (39.2%) responded PCPs, 219 (15.0%) hospital internists, 611(41.8%) subspecialists and 59 (4.0%) mentioned another career choice. The baseline characteristics categorized by final career choice are presented in Table 1.

Timing of career choice

Timing of final career choice significantly differed between different groups (Fig. 1, $P < 0.001$). Most of the subspecialists have chosen their career during residency (65.3%) whereas only 37.0% of the PCPs have chosen it during that time. Conversely, more PCPs than subspecialists chose their career during medical school (21.9% versus 12.1%) and after board certification (41.1% versus 22.6%).

Factors influencing career choice

Significantly more non-PCPs than PCPs felt that former chiefs (62.9% vs 26.9%, $P < 0.001$) and professors (20.0% vs 6.5%, $P < 0.001$) influenced their career choices. On the other hand, more PCPs reported influence from their family on their career choice (56.5% versus 42.0%, $P < 0.001$, Fig. 2).

Overall 25.6% of the PCPs and 24.2% of the hospital internists reported that the availability of residency positions kept them away from a sub-specialization. When asked about the influence of practice moratorium, 8.5% of the participants reported that it influenced their career choice. Among those 3.8% of the PCPs reported that it kept them from becoming a subspecialists; 8.7% of the subspecialists and 10.4% of hospital internists reported that it kept them from becoming a PCP.

Overall, a minority of the participants has completed a vocational training in primary care. More PCP than non-PCP reported having completed such a training (28.1% vs 13.7%, $P < 0.001$) and more non-PCP completed a residency in an academic hospital (38.2% vs 25.8% $P < 0.001$).

Attractiveness of a career as a PCP

The perceived attractiveness of a career as a PCP changed importantly over time: 59.1% of the

Table 1 Baseline characteristics

	PCPs		Hospital internists		Subspecialists		Others	
	n	%	*n*	%	*n*	%	*n*	%
Total	573	100	219	100	611	100	59	100
Female	311	54.3	109	49.8	203	33.2	32	54.2
Education and residency								
Swiss medical diploma	479	83.6	185	84.5	490	80.2	50	84.7
PCP vocational training	161	28.1	34	15.5	79	12.9	9	15.3
residency in an academic hospital	350	61.1	166	75.8	449	73.5	44	74.6
Current work situation								
Part time	372	64.9	85	38.8	196	32.1	26	44.1
Leading position	174	30.4	156	71.2	341	55.8	26	44.1
Employed	156	27.2	210	95.9	448	73.3	47	79.7
Setting								
Practice	527	92.0	6	2.7	189	30.9	16	27.1
Hospital	19	3.3	197	90.0	351	57.4	16	27.1
Outpatient clinic	13	2.3	10	4.6	52	8.5	4	6.8
Nursing home	4	0.7	2	0.9	4	0.7	1	1.7
Other[a]	4	0.7	2	0.9	5	0.7	21	35.6
	Median	IQR	Median	IQR	Median	IQR	Median	IQR
Age	46	42–51	45	42–49	44	41–47	45	43–49
Education and residency								
Age at end of med. school	27	26–28	26	26–28	26	26–27	27	26–28
Months of outpatient work	12	9–24	14	10–24	12	9–18	12	6–17.25
Current work situation								
Working half-days a week	9	6–10	10	7–11	10	8–11	10	6.75–10

[a]Including: administration, research & teaching, insurance, company

participants ($n = 864$) considered a career as a PCP as attractive during medical school. Until residency, there was a net decrease of 98 (52.4%) perceiving PC as attractive: A career as a PCP lost attractiveness for $n = 169$; gained attractiveness for $n = 71$. Later on, of the 766 considering a career as PCP to be attractive during residency, 333 finally chose a non-PCP career (Fig. 3).

Discussion

We aimed at investigating timing of career choice and factors influencing choice of internists and found that those strongly differed between internists choosing to become PCPs compared to those opting for other career choices. While most of the subspecialists took their decision on future career during residency in internal medicine, more PCPs chose their career after residency. Influence of peers' opinions also significantly differed between PCPs and non-PCPs, with non-PCPs reporting more influence of chiefs and professors and PCPs reporting more influence of family on their career choice. Half of physicians perceiving a career in primary care as attractive during residency finally opted for different career choices.

Our results complement a study made on a sample of PCPs with a board certification in general medicine: for general practitioners, residency was shown to be the most important time period for the decision to become PCPs; 53.7% of the general medicine practitioners decided during that time and overall 95.3% of them decided before board certification [5]. These numbers clearly differ from our findings in the group of PCPs with a certification in internal medicine where only 58.9% had committed to their PCP career before board certification. In our study PCPs perceived a higher influence for their career decision of their families than non-PCPs. This confirms similar results in other settings [21–24]. Meanwhile, PCPs reported less influence of chiefs and professors in their career decision. Similarly, lack of role model and "badmouthing" of PC has been shown to reduce attractiveness of PC among medical students [25, 26].

Considering Swiss healthcare's overall shortage of physicians, the pool of residents in general internal medicine

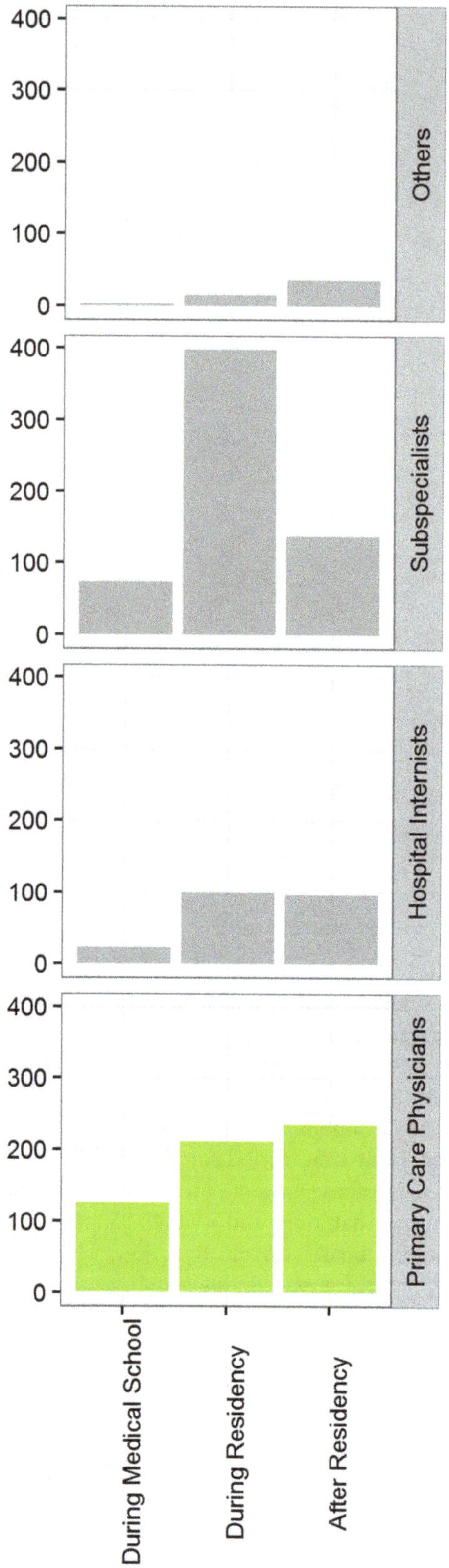

Fig. 1 Timing of career choice

is an attractive source of workforce for almost all non-surgical medical subspecialties. Given the circumstance that general internal medicine board certification requires hospital experience but no experience in primary care, hospital careers or subspecializations simply have substantially higher odds to present themselves attractively to residents. Meanwhile, primary care remains unexperienced and unseen by most internists, even if theoretically considered to be attractive along with other possibilities. This situation might result into increasing number of undecided residents getting offered a subspecialization and to decreasing interest for a career as PCP during residency as shown in our and former studies [8, 9, 12]. The steadier primary care workforce in countries without hospital-based primary care training support this hypothesis as well [15].

We observed that during and after medical school the majority of future internists perceived a career in primary care as an attractive option. Overall the attractiveness of a career as a PCP suffered a net decrease over the career timeline: an important part of them shifts away from a PCP career when simultaneously less shift toward this career choice. For many internists, primary care rather seems to be one option in direct competition with all other career possibilities, than a specific career goal. Therefore, residents interested in primary care are vulnerable to reorientation: to a relevant extent PCPs declared to be influenced by external factors such as the availability of residency positions or the restriction to open new practices. With rising numbers of subspecialty residencies, this might contribute to the overall tendency towards more subspecialization.

Our study further showed that internists finally working as PCPs completed more primary care vocational training than non-PCPs. Still a considerable proportion of subspecialists and hospital internists had a primary care vocational training as well. Studies have shown that residents with a specific primary care residency can also be discouraged from pursuing their career goal when unsatisfying experiences are made [7, 27]. This scenario may have occurred in some of the 15.5% of hospital internists and 12.9% of subspecialists who completed a vocational training in primary care.

Strength and limitations

Our study has potential limitations: First the cross-sectional design based on retrospective career questions is subjected to recall bias considering influencing factors and timing of the career choice. This limitation could be only addressed by prospective cohort studies starting at medical school. However, we showed that the timeline between medical school and final choice is long, so that the follow-up must be planed over more than 10 years in order to capture the late decision concerning a very

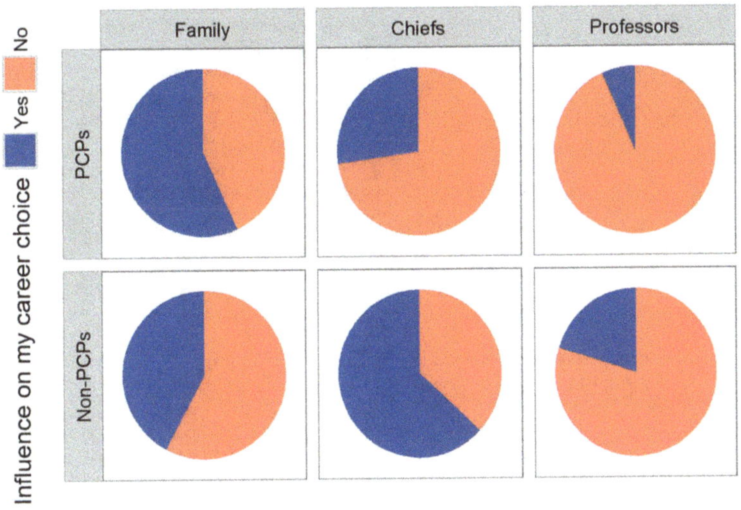

Fig. 2 Influence of peers on career choice

important amount of the physicians. Second our questionnaire contained no comprehensive set of all possible factor influencing the career choice, as those are complex, partly conscious and sometime very individual. Strengths are the successful sampling of the study with a high response rate of the survey and across internists graduating during a broad time interval ranging from 2000 to 2010. The presented spectrum of influencing factors is therefore less likely to be influenced by single events.

Implication for practice

In Switzerland, since the unification of internal and general medicine, all residents aiming to become general internists – independently whether they aim to become PCPs early or not – are qualifying for many different careers. Considering that external factors (including chiefs' opinion, availability of residency positions) are influencing their career choice during residency, the new combined board certification in general internal medicine might even decrease the number of PCPs [8, 14, 21]. Attention must therefore be taken to keep motivation high for future PCPs. Residency has been shown to be crucial concerning career choice leading to primary care. Besides attractive career paths with structured residency programs, role models as well as support by chief and academic staff are important, which can be supported by academic institutes of primary care and mentoring programs. [28–30] If these measures fail, the number of future PCPs might decline even more despite the increasing number of certified general internists [31].

Conclusion

Career choice timing and influence factors of PCPs and subspecialists strongly differ. Internists working as PCPs decide late for a career in primary care and remain vulnerable to external factors, including the availability of residency positions or issues influencing future working conditions. In a very flexible system such as the one in Switzerland, where residents are able to change career orientation at any time of their medical education, continuous investments to keep attractiveness of primary care high during medical school and during and after residency.

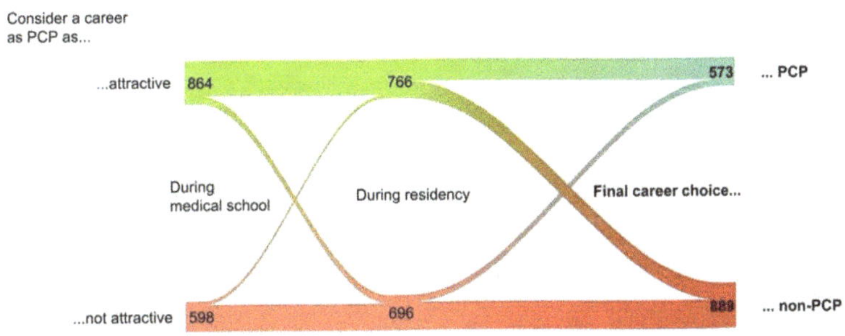

Fig. 3 Attractiveness of a career as PCP during medical school and residency and final career choice

Abbreviations
PC: Primary care; PCP: Primary care physician

Acknowledgment
We thank the Swiss Medical Association FMH for providing the addresses of the participants.

Funding
The study had no funding source.

Authors' contributions
NS designed the questionnaire, performed the data analysis and drafted the manuscript, SM designed the questionnaire, performed the data analysis and drafted the manuscript, VA designed the questionnaire and drafted the manuscript, TR drafted the manuscript, RT designed the questionnaire, performed the data analysis and drafted the manuscript. All authors read and approved the final manuscript.

Competing interests
The authors declare that they have no competing interests.

Consent for publication
Not applicable.

Author details
[1]Institute of Primary Care, University Hospital of Zurich, University of Zurich, Pestalozzistrasse 24, 8091 Zurich, Switzerland. [2]Arud Centres for Addiction Medicine, Zurich, Switzerland. [3]Federal Office of Public Health, Bern, Switzerland.

References
1. Buddeberg-Fischer B, Klaghofer R, Stamm M, Marty F, Dreiding P, Zoller M, et al. Primary care in Switzerland-no longer attractive for young physicians? Swiss Med Wkly. 2006;136:416–24.
2. Tschudi P, Bally K, Zeller A. Wer will heute noch Hausarzt/ärztin werden… ? Umfragen bei Medizinstudierenden und Jungärzten. PRAXIS. 2013;102:335–9.
3. Wright B, Scott I, Woloschuk W, Brenneis F. Career choice of new medical students at three Canadian universities: family medicine versus specialty medicine. Can Med Assoc J. 2004;170:1920–4.
4. Hauer KE, Durning SJ, Kernan WN, Fagan MJ, Mintz M, O'Sullivan PS, et al. Factors associated with medical students' career choices regarding internal medicine. JAMA. 2008;300:1154–64.
5. Tandjung R, Senn O, Marty F, Krauss L, Rosemann T, Badertscher N. Career after successful medical board examination in general practice – a cross-sectional survey. Swiss Med Wkly. 2013;143:w13839.
6. Chaudhuri E, Mason NC, Newbery N, Goddard AF. Career choices of junior doctors: is the physician an endangered species? Clin Med. 2013;13:330–5.
7. Stanley M, O'Brien B, Julian K, Jain S, Cornett P, Hollander H, et al. Is training in a primary care internal medicine residency associated with a career in primary care medicine? J Gen Intern Med. 2015;30:1333–8.
8. West CP, Dupras DM. General medicine vs subspecialty career plans among internal medicine residents. JAMA. 2012;308:2241–7.
9. Garibaldi RA, Popkave C, Bylsma W. Career plans for trainees in internal medicine residency programs. Acad Med. 2005;80:507–12.
10. SIWF Homepage. http://www.fmh.ch/bildung-siwf.html. Accessed 4 Apr 2017.
11. Marty F, Zemp N. Titelverleihungen Fachärztin/Facharzt FMH für Allgemeinmedizin 2009. PrimaryCare. 2010;10:149-150. doi:10.4414/pc-d.2010.08600. Accessed 2 Jan 2017.
12. West CP, Popkave C, Schultz HJ, Weinberger SE, Kolars JC. Changes in career decisions of internal medicine residents during training. Ann Intern Med. 2006;145:774–9.
13. Ratelle JT, Dupras DM, Alguire P, Masters P, Weissman A, West CP. Hospitalist career decisions among internal medicine residents. J Gen Intern Med. 2014;29:1026–30.
14. Jolly P, Erikson C, Garrison G. U.S. Graduate medical education and physician specialty choice. Acad Med. 2013;88:468–74.
15. Djalali S, Frei A, Rosemann T, Tandjung R. Weiterbildung zum Hausarzt – ein europäischer Vergleich. PRAXIS. 2013;102:327–33.
16. Krztoń-Królewiecka A, Švab I, Oleszczyk M, Seifert B, Smithson WH, Windak A. The development of academic family medicine in central and eastern Europe since 1990. BMC Fam Pract. 2013;14:37.
17. Joyce CM, Scott A, Jeon S-H, Humphreys J, Kalb G, Witt J, et al. The "Medicine in Australia: Balancing Employment and Life (MABEL)" longitudinal survey - Protocol and baseline data for a prospective cohort study of Australian doctors' workforce participation. BMC Health Serv Res. 2010;10:50.
18. Bauer W, Hänggeli C. Eine neue Epoche: das neue Weiterbildungsprogramm Allgemeine Innere Medizin. Schweiz Ärzteztg. 2010;91:1929–32.
19. Ghali WA, Greenberg PB, Mejia R, Otaki J, Cornuz J. International perspectives on general internal medicine and the case for "globalization" of a discipline. J Gen Intern Med. 2006;21:197–200.
20. Cassel CK, Reuben DB. Specialization, subspecialization, and subsubspecialization in internal medicine. N Engl J Med. 2011;364:1169–73.
21. Lambert T, Goldacre R, Smith F, Goldacre MJ. Reasons why doctors choose or reject careers in general practice: national surveys. Br J Gen Pract. 2012; 62:851–8.
22. Macdonald C, Cawood T. Factors influencing career decisions in internal medicine: career decisions in internal medicine. Intern Med J. 2012;42:918–23.
23. West CP, Drefahl MM, Popkave C, Kolars JC. Internal medicine resident self-report of factors associated with career decisions. J Gen Intern Med. 2009; 24:946–9.
24. Smith F, Lambert TW, Goldacre MJ. Factors influencing junior doctors' choices of future specialty: trends over time and demographics based on results from UK national surveys. J R Soc Med. 2015;108:396–405.
25. Erikson CE, Danish S, Jones KC, Sandberg SF, Carle AC. The role of medical school culture in primary care career choice. Acad Med. 2013;88:1919–26.
26. Puertas EB, Arósquipa C, Gutiérrez D. Factors that influence a career choice in primary care among medical students from high-, middle-, and low-income countries: a systematic review. Rev Panam Salud Publica. 2013;34:351–8.
27. Peccoralo LA, Tackett S, Ward L, Federman A, Helenius I, Christmas C, et al. Resident satisfaction with continuity clinic and career choice in general internal medicine. J Gen Intern Med. 2013;28:1020–7.
28. Buddeberg-Fischer B, Stamm M, Marty F. Family medicine in Switzerland: training experiences in medical school and residency. Fam Med. 2007;39:651–5.
29. Buddeberg-Fischer B, Klaghofer R, Stamm M. Family physicians in Switzerland: transition from residency to family practice. Fam Med. 2011;43:29.
30. Tandjung R, Ritter C, Haller DM, Tschudi P, Schaufelberger M, Bischoff T, et al. Primary care at Swiss universities-current state and perspective. BMC Res Notes. 2014;7:308.
31. Hanhart A, Rosemann T, Marty F, Tandjung R. Weiterbildung zum Facharzt für Allgemeinmedizin in der Schweiz – welche Fächer werden gewählt? Z Allg Med. 2014;90:234–9.
32. Federal Act on Research involving Human Beings (Human Research Act, HRA) of 30 September 2011, SR810.30, Swiss Federal Law. https://www.admin.ch/gov/en/start/federal-law/classified-compilation.html. Accessed 4 Apr 2017.

19

Medical appropriateness of adult calls to Danish out-of-hours primary care

Karen Busk Nørøxe*, Linda Huibers, Grete Moth and Peter Vedsted

Abstract

Background: Optimal utilisation of the out-of-hours primary care (OOH-PC) services remains a concern in public health policy. We need more knowledge on potentially avoidable contacts. This study examines the frequency of medically assessed inappropriate OOH-PC calls from adults, explores factors associated with such assessment, and examines the relation to patient-assessed severity of health problem and fulfilment of expectations.

Methods: We performed secondary analyses of data from a large cross-sectional survey on contacts to Danish OOH-PC. As access to Danish OOH-PC is provided through telephone triage delivered by a general practitioner (GP), we included only telephone contacts. A contact was characterised as medically inappropriate when the triage GP assessed that the request from a medical perspective should have been directed to daytime primary care. Appropriateness was examined in relation to patient characteristics, reason for encounter, time of contact, and whether the contact was triaged to a face-to-face consultation, and in relation to patient-assessed severity of the health problem and fulfilment of expectations. Associations were estimated with odds ratios (ORs) using multivariate analysis.

Results: Of all contacts, 23.7% were assessed as medically inappropriate. Such assessment was associated with: younger age, longer symptom duration, exacerbation of chronic condition, and contact only few hours away from own GP's office hours. Of medically inappropriate contacts, 31.3% were from patients aged 18–30 years, 41.5% concerned symptoms of > 24 h, 19.4% concerned exacerbation of chronic condition, and 21.3% were calls < 3 h away from own GP's regular office hours. Medicine request was the most frequent reason for an inappropriate contact (14.3% of medically inappropriate contacts). In 53.4% of contacts assessed as inappropriate, the health problem was considered as severe by patients and medical assessed inappropriateness was significantly associated with unfulfilled patient expectations.

Conclusions: One in four OOH-PC calls was considered medically inappropriate. Future efforts to reduce suboptimal use of OOH-PC should focus on the types of contacts with the highest optimisation potential, e.g., medication requests, long-lasting symptoms, and exacerbations. Such interventions should aim at bridging the gap between the GP's medical assessment and the patient's expectations to appropriate OOH-PC use.

Keywords: Denmark, After-hours care, Primary health care, Health care seeking behaviors, Delivery of health care, Health care utilisation

* Correspondence: karen.bn@ph.au.dk
Department of Public Health, Research Unit for General Practice, Aarhus University, Bartholins Alle 2, 8000 Aarhus C, Denmark

Background

Patient contacts to out-of-hours primary care (OOH-PC) are sometimes perceived as medically inappropriate by health care professionals [1–3]. A few contacts should have been directed to an emergency department (ED), some are considered manageable by self-care, and others should have been presented within the regular office hours in primary care [4, 5]. As the demands for OOH-PC are high, a major health policy concern is to reduce the sub-optimal use of these services [6]. It is frequently debated how to lower the number of inappropriate contacts without endangering the health and safety of the patient. However, 'inappropriate' use of acute health-care services is a complex issue, and the concept is poorly defined [7, 8]. In this study, we focus on contacts that according to a medical assessment made by the triage GP should have been directed to primary care within the regular office hours.

The organization of day-time and out-of-hours primary care affects the patients' use of OOH-PC. Lower availability and accessibility of primary health care during daytime has been shown to cause increased use of acute care; this also includes OOH-PC services [9–12]. The direct access in Danish OOH-PC to a general practitioner (GP) who promptly performs telephone triage may stimulate patients' use of OOH-PC as this direct access to medical care may be preferred over their own GP. In addition to the organisation of health care, the help-seeking behaviour among the patients depends on many other determinants, such as sociodemographic and cultural factors, previous experience, attitude to health-service use, and perception of symptoms [8, 13–16]. Patients often perceive their symptoms as more severe and urgent than health-care professionals [3, 8, 17–19].

Discrepancies between patients' and GPs' assessment of severity of symptoms and appropriateness of requests for OOH-PC may limit the potential of reducing the OOH-PC contacts that are considered inappropriate by GPs. The different views may also lead to poor fulfilment of the patients' expectations for care. Development of interventions that may target medically inappropriate (and potentially avoidable) use of OOH-PC requires a deep understanding of the requests for OOH-PC services that are put forward by patients [6]. In particular, we need to study the medical assessment of inappropriateness in relation to the patient-assessed severity of the problem presented. However, to our knowledge, the existing information about medical appropriateness of patient use of acute care is sparse and mainly concerns ED [3, 9, 20].

The aims of this study were (1) to describe the frequency and the characteristics of "medically inappropriate" OOH-PC calls performed by adult patients, (2) to identify factors associated with contacts assessed by GPs as medically inappropriate, and (3) to examine the patient-assessed problem severity and the fulfilment of expectations in relation to the GP-assessed medical inappropriateness of the contact.

Methods

Study design and setting

The study was based on a large cross-sectional survey on patient contacts to OOH-PC in the Central Denmark Region (CDR) over a period of 12 months in 2010–2011 (LV-KOS 2011) [21]. Data was collected using questionnaires completed by GPs and patients and from the OOH electronic registration system.

Denmark is divided into five regions, and each is responsible for organising its own OOH-PC. In four of the regions, OOH-PC is organized by GPs in large-scale co-operatives; this also includes the CDR with 1.2 million inhabitants. Patients access OOH-PC by telephone, and GPs answer all patient calls and perform triage. Only fully licensed GPs perform triage. The triage GPs can manage the patient's health problem by telephone (telephone consultation) or refer to a subsequent face-to-face contact (clinic consultation or home visit) or to hospital (ED or admission). The OOH-PC service is tax-paid and free for patients. The GPs are paid a fee-for-service. The service is available from 4 pm to 8 am on weekdays plus weekends and national holidays; it is intended to deal with requests for urgent medical assistance that cannot wait until regular office hours [22–24].

Data collection

GP pop-up questionnaire

GPs were electronically invited to participate in the study when logging onto the OOH computer system at the start of a shift. Of all GPs doing telephone shifts, one GP per 8-h shift could participate. A short pop-up questionnaire integrated into the existing electronic patient administration system appeared after every 10th telephone contact. The registered contacts have been shown to be highly representative for all OOH-PC contacts in the CDR as patients included in the study varied less than three per cent compared with all patients in the study period regarding the distribution of age and gender [21].

The GP questionnaire included the question: 'Should the patient from a medical perspective have contacted his/her own GP during daytime?' The response categories were: 'Yes', 'No' and 'Don't know'. We defined 'Yes' as a contact assessed by GPs as medically inappropriate for OOH-PC. The GPs also stated triage outcome (telephone consultation or subsequent face-to-face contact in OOH-PC or at hospital), symptom duration, and estimated severity of the health problem by answering additional questions (as seen in Table 1). Finally, the GPs stated whether the contact concerned exacerbation of known chronic disease, new event

Table 1 Characteristics of all OOH-PC telephone contacts and frequency of contacts assessed as medically inappropriate

	All OOH-PC contacts	Contacts assessed by triage GP as medically inappropriate	
	N (%)	n (%)	n/100 contacts (95% CI)
All contacts	5333 (100)	1266 (100)	23.7 (22.6–24.9)
Level of care			
Telephone consultation only	2884 (54.1)	993 (78.4)	34.4 (32.7–36.2)
Triaged to face-to-face contact in OOH-PC	2188 (41.0)	258 (20.4)	11.8 (10.5–13.2)
Triaged to ED or hospital admission	261 (4.9)	15 (1.2)	5.7 (3.3–9.3)
Patient characteristics			
Sex			
Male	2336 (43.8)	539 (42.6)	23.1 (21.4–24.8)
Female	2997 (56.2)	727 (57.4)	24.3 (22.7–25.8)
Age groups (years)			
18–30	1410 (26.4)	396 (31.3)	28.1 (25.8–30.5)
31–40	1010 (18.9)	251 (19.8)	24.9 (22.2–27.6)
41–60	1368 (25.7)	350 (27.6)	25.6 (23.3–28.0)
61–75	786 (14.7)	168 (13.3)	21.4 (18.6–24.4)
> 75	759 (14.2)	101 (8.0)	13.3 (11.0–15.9)
Symptom characteristics (medical perspective)			
Top 10 RFE for medically assessed inappropriate contacts[a]			
1. Request for medication (-50)[b]	334 (6.3)	181 (14.3)	54.2 (48.7–59.6)
2. Fever (A03)	440 (8.3)	75 (5.9)	17.0 (13.6–20.9)
3. Cough (R05)	257 (4.8)	71 (5.6)	27.6 (22.3–33.5)
4. Abdominal pain/cramps general (D01)	302 (5.7)	58 (4.6)	19.2 (14.9–24.1)
5. Throat symptom/complaints (R21)	193 (3.6)	47 (3.7)	24.4 (18.5–31.0)
6. Headache (N01)	189 (3.5)	45 (3.6)	23.8 (17.9–30.5)
7. Back symptom/complaint (L02)	137 (2.6)	37 (2.9)	27.0 (19.8–35.2)
8. Vertigo/dizziness (N17)	145 (2.7)	35 (2.8)	24.1 (17.4–31.9)
9. Nausea (D09)	155 (2.9)	33 (2.6)	21.3 (15.1–28.6)
10. Ear pain (H01)	100 (1.9)	33 (2.6)	33.0 (23.9–43.1)
Other RFE(s) (includes 276 different RFEs)	3532 (66.2)	754 (59.6)	21.3 (20.0–22.7)
Reason for contact			
New episode (including symptoms of long duration)	4120 (77.3)	860 (67.9)	20.9 (19.6–22.1)
Exacerbation of chronic disease	868 (16.3)	246 (19.4)	28.3 (25.4–31.5)
Other	345 (6.5)	160 (12.6)	46.4 (41.0–51.8)
Duration of symptoms			
< 5 h	1712 (32.1)	215 (17.0)	12.6 (11.0–14.2)
5–12 h	1158 (21.7)	171 (13.5)	14.8 (12.8–16.9)
12–24 h	782 (14.7)	170 (13.4)	19.3 (16.7–22.0)
> 24 h	1251 (23.5)	525 (41.5)	42.0 (39.2–44.8)
Don't know	223 (4.2)	75 (5.9)	33.6 (27.5–40.2)
Not relevant	207 (3.9)	110 (8.7)	53.1 (46.1–60.1)
GP-assessed severity			
Potentially severe	1646 (30.9)	113 (8.9)	6.9 (5.7–8.2)
Not severe, but the patient is ill	2777 (52.1)	747 (59.0)	26.9 (25.3–28.5)

Table 1 Characteristics of all OOH-PC telephone contacts and frequency of contacts assessed as medically inappropriate *(Continued)*

Patient is not ill	635 (11.9)	331 (26.1)	52.1 (48.2–56.1)
Don't know	275 (5.2)	75 (5.9)	27.3 (22.1–32.9)
Time of contact (health service perspective)			
Weekday vs. weekend/public holiday			
Weekday	2829 (53.0)	829 (65.5)	29.3 (27.6–31.0)
Weekend/public holiday	2504 (47.0)	437 (34.5)	17.5 (15.0–19.0)
Time in relation to own GP's regular office hours			
< 3 h after office hours	720 (13.5)	269 (21.3)	37.4 (33.8–41.0)
≥ 3 h after/before office hours	4193 (78.6)	852 (67.3)	20.3 (19.1–21.6)
< 3 h before office hours	420 (7.9)	145 (11.5)	34.5 (30.0–39.3)

[a]More than one RFE could be registered
[b]91.8% of contacts had only this RFE; the remaining 8.2% also had other concomitant RFE(s)

(including symptoms of longer duration), or other reason (could be specified in text), and the specific reason(s) for encounter (RFE) were given. The stated RFEs were subsequently coded according to the International Classification of Primary Care (ICPC) [25]. RFEs coded with process code'- 50' (medication - prescription/request/renewal/ injection) were combined across organ systems into one category named 'Request for medication'.

Patient questionnaire

A questionnaire was sent to the patient for each registered contact. The questions covered aspects of the contact to OOH-PC and the patient's general health status. No questionnaire was sent to patients with publicly recorded protection against research participation, unknown postal address, ethically sensitive health problems (e.g., attempted suicide or terminal illness), earlier participation in the study or death registration. Patients received the questionnaire within 1 week after the OOH-PC contact and a reminder with a new questionnaire after 2 weeks if the first questionnaire had not been completed and returned.

From the patient questionnaire we included two items exploring the patient-assessed severity of the health problem and fulfilment of expectations. The patient-assessed severity of the problem at the time of contacting OOH-PC was recoded into two categories: 'Severe' ('Severe and life threatening' and'Severe, but not life threatening') and 'Not severe' ('Not severe, but I found it necessary to talk to a physician' and 'I was not ill, but had some questions'). Fulfilment of patient expectations was recoded into three categories: 'A lot/Completely' and 'A little/Some' and 'Not at all'.

OOH electronic registration system

Information on time and date of contact and patient age and gender was collected from the OOH electronic registration system. Time of contact was recoded into a variable for day ('Weekday' and 'Weekend/public holiday') and a variable for time before/after the office hours of own GP ('<3 h after office hours', '≥ 3 h after or before office hours', and '<3 h before office hours'). Patient age was categorized into five age groups: 18–30, 31–40, 41–60, 61–75, and > 75 years.

Analysis

We included all registered telephone contacts from adults (age ≥ 18 years) (Fig. 1). Three contacts with missing information on appropriateness were excluded; this resulted in a study population of 5,333 OOH-PC patient calls (Study population 1). A total of 1,733 patients responded to the questionnaire, including the questions on problem severity and fulfilment of expectations (Study population 2). We also performed a non-response analysis.

Descriptive statistics were made for Study population 1 on the characteristics of the contacts assessed as medically inappropriate. The rate of contacts assessed as medically inappropriate was defined as the number of such contacts per 100 OOH-PC contacts. This rate was stratified for subgroups and calculated with 95% confidence interval (CI).

The association between contacts being assessed as medically inappropriate and contact characteristics was assessed using logistic regression. Included independent variables were patient characteristics (gender, age group), presented health problem (symptom duration, chronic condition), and time of contact (day, time in relation to regular office hours). Associations were adjusted for all mentioned variables, except for time in relation to office hours as this correlated with time of week.

Descriptive statistics were performed for patient-assessed severity and fulfilment of expectations (Study population 2). The association between medically assessed inappropriateness and both patient-assessed problem severity and fulfilment of expectations was analysed using

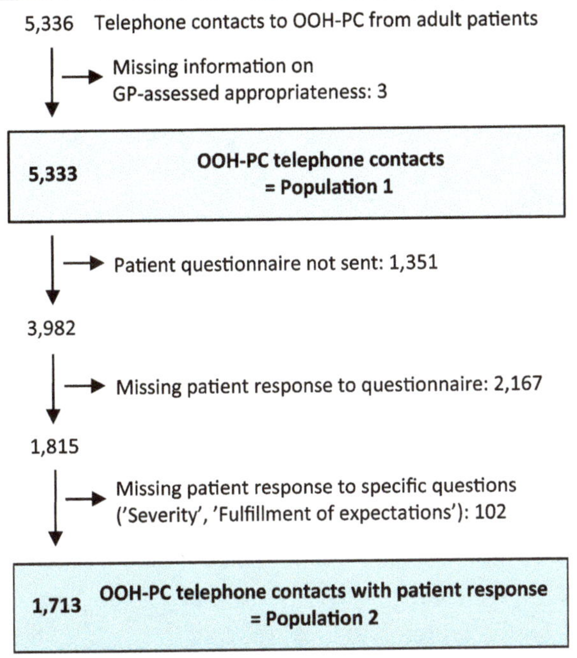

Fig. 1 Flowchart presenting the study population

logistic regression while adjusting for patient age and gender. The analyses of the associations with fulfilment of expectations were additionally adjusted for patient-assessed severity and triage outcome (telephone consultation or subsequent face-to-face contact in OOH-PC or at hospital) as these factors may be associated with patient evaluations of OOH-PC [26]. All associations were calculated as raw and adjusted odds ratios (OR) with 95% CI. P-values ≤ 0.05 were considered statistically significant. Analyses were performed in STATA, version 12.

Results

Contacts assessed by triage GPs as medically inappropriate

According to the triage GPs, 23.7% of contacts should have been directed to daytime primary care (Table 1). In 68.3% of cases, the contact should not have been directed to primary care, and the GP was unsure ('Don't know') in 8% of cases (not shown in table). Of all OOH-PC calls, 45.9% were triaged to a subsequent face-to-face contact in OOH-PC or at hospital, whereas this was the case in only 21.6% of the contacts assessed as medically inappropriate.

Patients aged 18–30 years accounted for 31.3% of the medically inappropriate contacts, and 28.1% (95% CI: 25.8–30.5%) of all contacts from this age group were assessed as inappropriate. For patients aged 75 years or older, only 13.3% (95% CI: 11.0–15.9%) of contacts were assessed as inappropriate. In total, 41.5% of the inappropriate contacts concerned symptoms lasting > 24 h. In 26.1% of the medically inappropriate contacts, the GP assessed that the patient was not ill. In total, 286 different RFEs were registered for contacts assessed as inappropriate. Contacts concerning a medication request were assessed as inappropriate in 54.2% of cases (95% CI: 48.7–59.6%) and accounted for 14.3% of all inappropriate contacts.

Factors related to GP assessed medical inappropriateness

As seen in Table 2, the ORs of assessed medical inappropriateness decreased with increasing patient age (adj. OR = 0.65 (95% CI: 0.51–0.82) for 61–75 years and adj. OR = 0.38 (95% CI: 0.29–0.50) for > 75 years). We found increasing ORs for longer symptom duration (adj. OR = 2.42 (95% CI: 1.92–3.05) for symptom duration of 12–24 h and adj. OR = 6.10 (95% CI: 5.02–7.40) for symptom duration of > 24 h) and for contacts concerning a chronic condition rather than a new episode (adj. OR = 1.29 (95% CI: 1.06–1.56)). Contacts during weekends and holidays were less likely to be assessed as inappropriate than contacts during weekdays (adj. OR = 0.36 (95% CI: 0.31–0.42)). Contacts taken < 3 h before or after own GP's regular office hours were more often assessed as inappropriate than contacts taken ≥ 3 h away from daytime office hours (< 3 h after office hours: adj. OR = 1.63 (95% CI: 1.31–2.02) and < 3 h before office hours: adj. OR = 1.87 (95% CI: 1.44–2.42)).

Patient-assessed severity and fulfilment of expectations

Patients assessed their health problem as severe in 53.4% of the medically inappropriate contacts and in 59.0% of all contacts (Table 3). Patient-assessed severity was not significantly associated with GP-assessed inappropriateness in the adjusted analysis (adj. OR = 0.80, 95% CI: 0.63–1.02). GP-assessed inappropriateness was significantly associated with unfulfilled patient expectations (adj. OR = 1.47 (95% CI: 1.09–2.00) for little/some fulfilment and adj. OR = 3.25 (95% CI: 2.13–4.85) for no fulfilment at all).

The non-response analyses for this population showed a higher proportion of medical inappropriate contacts among patients who did not respond to the questionnaire than among responding patients (25.9% (95% CI: 24.1–27.8) vs. 20.4% (95% CI: 18.5–22.3)). The patient response rate was 45.6% (95% CI: 44.0–47.1) overall, but it was 33.7% (95% CI: 29.4–38.1) for patients assessed by the GP not to be ill.

Discussion

Main findings

About a quarter of OOH-PC telephone contacts should have been directed to daytime primary care according to the triage GPs' medical assessments. Increasing symptom duration was strongly associated with GP-assessed medical inappropriateness, and as many as 40% of the inappropriate contacts were related to symptoms lasting > 24 h. Other

Table 2 Associations between contact characteristics and medical inappropriateness ($N = 4903^{a}$)

	Contacts assessed by triage GP as medically inappropriate			
	OR (95% CI)	P	Adj. OR (95% CI)[b]	$P_{Adj.}$
Patient characteristics				
Sex				
Male	1		1	
Female	1.07 (0.94–1.21)	0.313	1.09 (0.94–1.26)	0.275
Age (years)				
18–30	1		1	
31–40	0.85 (0.70–1.02)	0.076	0.81 (0.65–0.99)	0.046
41–60	0.88 (0.74–1.04)	0.137	0.86 (0.70–1.04)	0.116
61–75	0.70 (0.57–0.86)	0.001	0.65 (0.51–0.82)	< 0.001
> 75	0.39 (0.31–0.50)	< 0.001	0.38 (0.29–0.50)	< 0.001
Symptom characteristics				
Duration of symptoms				
< 5 h	1		1	
5–12 h	1.21 (0.97–1.50)	0.089	1.32 (1.05–1.64)	0.015
12–24 h	1.93 (1.55–2.41)	< 0.001	2.42 (1.92–3.05)	< 0.001
> 24 h	5.04 (4.20–6.04)	< 0.001	6.10 (5.02–7.40)	< 0.001
Reason for contact				
New episode (including symptoms of long duration)	1		1	
Exacerbation of chronic disease	1.50 (1.27–1.77)	< 0.001	1.29 (1.06–1.56)	0.010
Other	3.28 (2.62–4.10)	< 0.001	2.26 (1.60–3.21)	< 0.001
Time of contact				
Weekday vs. weekend/public holiday				
Weekday	1		1	
Weekend/public holiday	0.51 (0.48–0.58)	< 0.001	0.36 (0.31–0.42)	< 0.001
Time in relation to own GP's regular office hours				
< 3 h after office hours	2.33 (1.98–2.77)	< 0.001	1.63 (1.31–2.02)	< 0.001
≥ 3 h after/before office hours	1		1	
< 3 h before office hours	2.07 (1.67–2.56)	< 0.001	1.87 (1.44–2.42)	< 0.001

[a]430 contacts in which the GP responded 'Don't know' or 'Not relevant' to the question on symptom duration were omitted
[b]Adjusted for all presented characteristics of patients and symptoms and whether the contact was taken on weekday or during weekend/public holiday

Table 3 Patient-assessed severity and fulfilment of expectations in relation to assessed medical inappropriateness of contact (Population 2, $N = 1713$)

	All OOH-PC contacts	Contacts assessed by triage GP as medically inappropriate				
	N (%)	n (%)	OR (95% CI)	p	Adj. OR (95% CI)[a]	$P_{Adj.}$
Patient-assessed severity						
Severe	1011 (59.0)	187 (53.4)	0.77 (0.61–0.99)	0.038	0.80 (0.63–1.02)	0.077
Not severe	671 (39.2)	152 (43.4)	1		1	
Not ill, but had some questions	31 (1.8)	11 (3.1)	1.88 (0.88–4.00)	0.103	1.84 (0.86–3.94)	0.119
Fulfilment of expectations						
A lot/completely	1266 (73.9)	217 (62.0)	1		1	
A little/some	325 (19.0)	80 (22.9)	1.58 (1.18–2.11)	0.002	1.47 (1.09–2.00)	0.012
Not at all	122 (7.1)	53 (15.1)	3.71 (2.52–5.47)	< 0.001	3.25 (2.13–4.85)	< 0.001

[a]Analysis of patient-assessed severity adjusted for gender and age group. Analysis of fulfilment of expectations adjusted for gender, age group, patient-assessed severity, and whether the contact was managed by telephone consultation or triaged to face-to-face contact (OOH-PC or hospital)

characteristics associated with inappropriateness were younger patient age, exacerbation of chronic disease, contact during weekdays, and contacts taken < 3 h before/after own GP's opening hours. The RFEs showed wide clinical variation, but medication requests were the most frequent RFE among the medically inappropriate contacts. More than half of the inappropriate contacts concerned symptoms that were considered severe by patients, and contacts assessed by GPs as medically inappropriate were significantly associated with unfulfilled patient expectations.

Comparison with other studies

When comparing studies on inappropriate use of acute health care services it should be held in mind that there is no agreed definition of inappropriateness and that different measures are used [7, 8]. A review found that the prevalence of inappropriate ED use varied from 10 to 90% depending on the criterion used to define inappropriateness [9]. Research on frequency of inappropriate OOH-PC use is very sparse. To our best knowledge, we are the first to examine medical appropriateness of OOH-PC contacts by using triage GPs' medical assessment of whether patients should have contacted their own GP. We found that about one of four OOH-PC contacts was assessed as medically inappropriate. A Norwegian study found that 28% of OOH-PC consultations concerned minor ailments that the patients could easily have handled themselves [4]. In contrast to the Norwegian study medically inappropriate contacts in our study may concern medically relevant requests that should already have been seen by the patients' own GP.

The observed peak in the number of medically assessed inappropriate contacts during the first opening hours of OOH-PC and on weekdays compared with weekends may be explained by limited accessibility and availability of daytime primary care. This is supported by previous studies showing accessibility of daytime care to be associated with consumption of acute care, including OOH-PC services [9–12] Our finding may also reflect that patients are unable or unwilling to attend their own GP during office hours due to daytime commitments [14, 15, 27]. However, in a Dutch study of low-urgency OOH-PC contacts, only 1.5% of patients stated lack of time to go to the GP during the day as a reason for contacting OOH-PC [20]. The observed variation in medical accessed inappropriateness among different age groups may have to do with age-related differences in help-seeking behaviours and type and severity of health problems [28, 29]. Thus, the high rate of medically inappropriate contacts among young adult patients may partly be due to a high overall consumption of OOH-PC services along with a low likelihood of severe illness [30, 31]. The increasing likelihood of inappropriateness with younger age, which was observed in the present study, has also been identified in other studies concerning OOH-PC and ED [9, 20, 32].

As OOH-PC is intended to manage acute health problems, the observed association between long symptom duration and high rate of medically assessed inappropriateness was expected. Long symptom duration has previously been shown to be associated with inappropriateness [9, 20]. With regard to specific RFEs, we found much variation among both medically appropriate and inappropriate contacts. Other studies have also reported considerable variation in RFEs in OOH-PC [33, 34]. As contacts concerning medication request (incl. renewal of prescription) were assessed as inappropriate in more than half of cases and accounted for about 14% of all inappropriate contacts this RFE may be targeted in future effort to optimise OOH-PC utilisation. The gain from targeting specific RFEs other than medication request seems low as each RFE accounted for a low percentage of inappropriate contacts.

The disparity between patient-assessed severity and GP-assessed appropriateness reflects the known gap between patients and healthcare professionals concerning their understanding of urgency and severity of symptoms [3, 8, 17–19]. Also, the association between medically assessed inappropriateness and unfulfilled patient expectations could reflect the mismatch between the perception of appropriateness among the patients and the medical assessments provided by the GPs. The propensity among patients to use OOH care is not only influenced by medical factors but also by feelings (e.g., uncertainty, anxiety), ability to self-manage, practical concerns, and attitudes to and knowledge about health care [8, 13, 14, 16, 35].

Patient worrying and their need for reassurance are important motives for contacting the OOH-PC. Thus, the potential for reducing the number of medically inappropriate contacts to OOH-PC may be limited.

We assume that Danish citizens understand what the intended aim of OOH-PC is: health care for patients with acute health problems that cannot wait until office hours of the own GP. Information on how and when to use Danish OOH-PC including advice on appropriate alternatives is available online Yet, we do not know to what extent Danish citizens are aware of this intended aim. In a Dutch study 46.6% of patients calling OOH-PC for non-urgent health problems thought that the OOH-PC was intended for all health problems and it was suggested that society's experiences with expanded opening hours of other services may have led to increased expectations of healthcare delivery [20].

Strengths and limitations of the study

This study is based on a considerable number of randomly sampled and representative telephone contacts to OOH-PC, which provides our study results with high statistical precision. GP registrations were made immediately after the contact, which reduces the risk of recall bias. Furthermore, the included patients received the questionnaire shortly after their contact to OOH-PC.

The assessment as to whether a health request to OOH-PC is medically appropriate for the setting is not an objective assessment, and there may be some variation among GPs. However, the assessment was performed by fully licensed GPs who were asked to assess appropriateness from a medical perspective (as opposed to a more holistic perspective or a personal opinion). Thus, it can be considered a highly qualified assessment of medical appropriateness. As the triage GPs stated whether the patient should have contacted a GP within office hours, we could not distinguish between OOH contacts that should have been directed to the patient's own GP already and those that could have been postponed. We chose this approach to minimize the triage GPs' workload of responding to the pop-up questionnaire. We obtained a reasonably high response rate (45.6%) for the patient questionnaire, but some selection bias could still be present. The non-response analysis showed a higher proportion of medically inappropriate contacts among non-respondents than among respondents. Additionally, the response rate was lower for contacts in which the patient was assessed not to be ill by the GP. Therefore, the share of inappropriate contacts that were perceived as non-severe by the patients may have been underestimated. Using a more holistic phrasing of the question on appropriateness, including context factors, could possibly have increased the frequency of contacts assessed as appropriate; this may also have strengthened the association between GP-assessed appropriateness and patient-perceived severity. Yet, such phrasing may have reflected the individual GP's personal opinion rather than a medical assessment of appropriateness.

Recommendations and future research

Efforts made to adjust the help-seeking behaviours among patients and reduce the suboptimal use of the OOH-PC should focus on the types of contacts with the highest potential for optimization. It could be relevant to address both the general population and specific patient groups (e.g., young adult patients) to inform them about how and when to use the OOH-PC (e.g., ordering medication on time at their own general practice and contacting own GP during daytime if possible), including the overall aim of OOH-PC. However, more knowledge is needed about potentially avoidable calls to OOH-PC. Future studies should investigate patient perspectives on self-assessed urgency and motives for calling the OOH-PC rather than a GP within office hours in order to plan tailored interventions.

Conclusion

Approximately one out of four calls to OOH-PC was assessed as medically inappropriate by the triage GP, which indicates a potential for optimising OOH-PC utilisation. Strategies should focus on contact types with the highest likelihood of medically assessed inappropriateness such as calls concerning medication requests or long-lasting symptoms and calls from young adult patients. However, the finding that patients frequently assessed the health problem severe and were more likely to report unfulfilled expectations in case of medically assessed inappropriateness emphasizes that 'appropriate' use of OOH-PC is a complex and multifaceted topic. Medical and patient perspectives are not necessarily consistent and strategies to optimise OOH-PC utilisation need to include both perspectives.

Abbreviations

CDR: Central Denmark Region; CI: Confidence interval; ED: Emergency department; GP: General practitioner; ICPC: International Classification of Primary Care; LV-KOS 2011: Survey of reasons for encounter and disease patterns in Danish out-of-hours primary care conducted in 2011; OOH-PC: Out-of-hours primary care; OR: Odds ratio; RFE: Reason for encounter

Acknowledgements

The authors would like to thank all the patients and GPs who took part in this study.

Funding

This project has been supported by the Central Denmark Region, the Danish National Research Foundation for Primary Care, and the Danish foundation TrygFonden.

Authors' contributions

All authors contributed substantially to the design of the study. KBN performed the statistical analyses in consultation with LH and PV. KBN wrote the first draft of the article. LH, GM and PV assisted in writing and revising the manuscript. All authors read and approved the final manuscript.

Competing interests

The authors declare that they have no competing interests.

Consent for publication

Not applicable.

References

1. Smith H, Lattimer V, George S. General practitioners' perceptions of the appropriateness and inappropriateness of out-of-hours calls. Br J Gen Pract. 2001;51(465):270–5.
2. Shipman C, Dale J. Responding to out-of-hours demand: the extent and nature of urgent need. Fam Pract. 1999;16(1):23–7.
3. Hallam L. Primary medical care outside normal working hours: review of published work. BMJ. 1994;308(6923):249–53.
4. Welle-Nilsen LK, Morken T, Hunskaar S, Granas AG. Minor ailments in out-of-hours primary care: an observational study. Scand J Prim Health Care. 2011; 29(1):39–44.
5. Moller TP, Ersboll AK, Tolstrup JS, Ostergaard D, Viereck S, Overton J, Folke F, Lippert F. Why and when citizens call for emergency help: an observational study of 211,193 medical emergency calls. Scand J Trauma Resusc Emerg Med. 2015;23:88.
6. Leutgeb R, Walker N, Remmen R, Klemenc-Ketis Z, Szecsenyi J, Laux G. On a European collaboration to identify organizational models, potential shortcomings and improvement options in out-of-hours primary health care. Eur J Gen Pract. 2014;20(3):233–7.

7. Philips H. Out-of-hours primary care in Belgium, Ph.D thesis. Belgium: Universiteit Antwerpen; 2010.
8. Sanders J. A review of health professional attitudes and patient perceptions on 'inappropriate' accident and emergency attendances. The implications for current minor injury service provision in England and Wales. J Adv Nurs. 2000;31(5):1097–105.
9. Carret ML, Fassa AC, Domingues MR. Inappropriate use of emergency services: a systematic review of prevalence and associated factors. Cad Saude Publica. 2009;25(1):7–28.
10. Rust G, Ye J, Baltrus P, Daniels E, Adesunloye B, Fryer GE. Practical barriers to timely primary care access: impact on adult use of emergency department services. Arch Intern Med. 2008;168(15):1705–10.
11. Smits M, Peters Y, Broers S, Keizer E, Wensing M, Giesen P. Association between general practice characteristics and use of out-of-hours GP cooperatives. BMC Fam Pract. 2015;16:52.
12. Zhou Y, Abel G, Warren F, Roland M, Campbell J, Lyratzopoulos G. Do difficulties in accessing in-hours primary care predict higher use of out-of-hours GP services? Evidence from an English National Patient Survey. Emerg Med J. 2015;32(5):373–8.
13. Campbell SM, Roland MO. Why do people consult the doctor? Fam Pract. 1996;13(1):75–83.
14. Durand AC, Palazzolo S, Tanti-Hardouin N, Gerbeaux P, Sambuc R, Gentile S. Nonurgent patients in emergency departments: rational or irresponsible consumers? Perceptions of professionals and patients. BMC Res Notes. 2012;5:525.
15. Langer S, Chew-Graham C, Hunter C, Guthrie EA, Salmon P. Why do patients with long-term conditions use unscheduled care? A qualitative literature review. Health Soc Care Community. 2013;21(4):339–51.
16. Keizer E, Maassen I, Smits M, Wensing M, Giesen P. Reducing the use of out-of-hours primary care services: a survey among Dutch general practitioners. Eur J Gen Pract. 2016;22(3):189–95.
17. Barry DW, Melhado TV, Chacko KM, Lee RS, Steiner JF, Kutner JS. Patient and physician perceptions of timely access to care. J Gen Intern Med. 2006;21(2): 130–3.
18. Masso M, Bezzina AJ, Siminski P, Middleton R, Eagar K. Why patients attend emergency departments for conditions potentially appropriate for primary care: reasons given by patients and clinicians differ. Emerg Med Australas. 2007;19(4):333–40.
19. Broekhuis SM, van Dijk WD, Giesen P, Pavilanis A. Walk-in clinics in Quebec, Canada: patients and doctors do not agree on appropriateness of visits. Fam Pract. 2014;31(1):92–101.
20. Keizer E, Smits M, Peters Y, Huibers L, Giesen P, Wensing M. Contacts with out-of-hours primary care for nonurgent problems: patients' beliefs or deficiencies in healthcare? BMC Fam Pract. 2015;16(1):157.
21. Flarup L, Moth G, Christensen MB, Vestergaard M, Olesen F, Vedsted P. A feasible method to study the Danish out-of-hours primary care service. Dan Med J. 2014;61(5):A4847.
22. Olesen F, Jolleys JV. Out of hours service: the Danish solution examined. BMJ. 1994;309(6969):1624–6.
23. Pedersen KM, Andersen JS, Sondergaard J. General practice and primary health care in Denmark. J Am Board Fam Med. 2012;25 Suppl 1:S34–8.
24. Christensen MB, Olesen F. Out of hours service in Denmark: evaluation five years after reform. BMJ. 1998;316(7143):1502–5.
25. World Health Organisation: International Classification of Primary Care (ICPC-2). http://www.who.int/classifications/icd/adaptations/icpc2/en/. Accessed June 2016.
26. Shipman C, Payne F, Hooper R, Dale J. Patient satisfaction with out-of-hours services; how do GP co-operatives compare with deputizing and practice-based arrangements? J Public Health Med. 2000;22(2):149–54.
27. Drummond N, McConnachie A, O'Donnell CA, Moffat KJ, Wilson P, Ross S. Social variation in reasons for contacting general practice out-of-hours: implications for daytime service provision? Br J Gen Pract. 2000;50(455):460–4.
28. Glynn LG, Valderas JM, Healy P, Burke E, Newell J, Gillespie P, Murphy AW. The prevalence of multimorbidity in primary care and its effect on health care utilization and cost. Fam Pract. 2011;28(5):516–23.
29. Leventhal EA, Prohaska TR. Age, symptom interpretation, and health behavior. J Am Geriatr Soc. 1986;34(3):185–91.
30. Huibers L, Moth G, Andersen M, van Grunsven P, Giesen P, Christensen MB, Olesen F. Consumption in out-of-hours health care: Danes double Dutch? Scand J Prim Health Care. 2014;32(1):44–50.
31. Huibers LA, Moth G, Bondevik GT, Kersnik J, Huber CA, Christensen MB, Leutgeb R, Casado AM, Remmen R, Wensing M. Diagnostic scope in out-of-
32. McHale P, Wood S, Hughes K, Bellis MA, Demnitz U, Wyke S. Who uses emergency departments inappropriately and when - a national cross-sectional study using a monitoring data system. BMC Med. 2013;11:258.
33. van Charante EP M, van Steenwijk-Opdam PC, Bindels PJ. Out-of-hours demand for GP care and emergency services: patients' choices and referrals by general practitioners and ambulance services. BMC Fam Pract. 2007;8:46.
34. Huber CA, Rosemann T, Zoller M, Eichler K, Senn O. Out-of-hours demand in primary care: frequency, mode of contact and reasons for encounter in Switzerland. J Eval Clin Pract. 2011;17(1):174–9.
35. Gustafsson S, Vikman I, Savenstedt S, Martinsson J. Perceptions of needs related to the practice of self-care for minor illness. J Clin Nurs. 2015.

The 5As team patient study: patient perspectives on the role of primary care in obesity management

Jacqueline Torti[1,2†], Thea Luig[1,3†], Michelle Borowitz[4], Jeffrey A. Johnson[2], Arya M. Sharma[3] and Denise L. Campbell-Scherer[1,5*]

Abstract

Background: Over 60% of people have overweight or obesity, but only a third report receiving counselling from primary care providers. We explored patients' perspectives on the role of primary care in obesity management and their experience with existing resources, with a view to develop an improved understanding of this perspective, and more effective management strategies.

Methods: Qualitative study employing semi-structured interviews and thematic analysis, with a sample of 28 patients from a cohort of 255 patients living with obesity and receiving care to support their weight management in a large Primary Care Network of family practices in Alberta.

Results: Four illustrative themes emerged: (1) the patient-physician relationship plays an important role in the adequacy of obesity management; (2) patients have clear expectations of substantive conversations with their primary care team; (3) complex conditions affect weight and patients require assistance tailored to individual obesity drivers; (4) current services provide support in important ways (accessibility, availability, accountability, affordability, consistency of messaging), but are not yet meeting patient needs for individual plans, advanced education, and follow-up opportunities.

Conclusions: Patients have clear expectations that their primary care physician asks them about weight within a supportive therapeutic relationship. They see obesity as a complex phenomenon with multiple drivers. They want their healthcare providers to assess and address their root causes - not simplistic advice to "eat less, move more". Patients felt that the current services were positive resources, but expressed needs for tailored weight management plans, and longer-term follow-up.

Keywords: Obesity, Primary health care, Qualitative research, Family medicine

Background

Obesity is a prevalent, complex, chronic, relapsing condition associated with medical, genetic, psychological, socio-economic, and cultural root causes and drivers of weight gain as well as multiple comorbidities that require coordinated, long-term, and interdisciplinary care [1–6]. Recognizing this escalating challenge, the Canadian Medical Association declared obesity a chronic disease in 2015 [7]. Both the Canadian and US Task Forces on Preventive Health Care recommend that primary care practitioners screen patients, counsel regarding weight loss, and refer to structured behavioural interventions aimed at weight loss [8–10]. However, only 37% of Canadian patients report that they have received any counselling regarding diet and 24% report receiving any counselling regarding exercise [11, 12]. Many physicians feel ill-equipped to assist patients in weight management, and lack training in the management of obesity [3–5, 13–16]. Obesity counselling and multicomponent interventions in primary

* Correspondence: denise.campbell-scherer@ualberta.ca
†Equal contributors
[1]Department of Family Medicine, University of Alberta, Clinical Research Unit, Edmonton, AB, CanadaT6G 2E1
[5]Department of Medicine, Obesity Research & Management, University of Alberta, Li Ka Shing Building, Rm. 1-116, 87th Avenue and 112th Street, Edmonton, AB T6G 2E1, Canada
Full list of author information is available at the end of the article

care settings, that for example include diet, exercise, and counselling or behavioural therapy, improve obesity prevention and management (referred to herein as weight management) [13, 17, 18]. Patients want their primary care providers to address their weight concerns [5].

The 5As Team program of research aims to address this gap. The program has partnered with a Primary Care Network (PCN) in Alberta, Canada, and worked with frontline interdisciplinary healthcare providers to help them improve their clinical practice [19–22]. As a component program, we wanted to explore patient needs and experience with PCN weight management resources to inform the results of the provider study, and to begin the process of designing an intervention. PCNs in Alberta have the mandate to enhance family practices with access to interdisciplinary teams to improve chronic illness prevention and care using a patient-centred approach [23]. To achieve patient-centeredness it is vital to understand patients' expectations and experiences of healthcare services. We conducted a study answering the questions 1) From the perspective of patients who seek primary care support for weight management, what role do clinicians play in their efforts? 2) How do PCN resources offer meaningful support and satisfy patients' needs? The purpose of this study is to lay the foundation for co-creation with patients of an intervention for a planned randomized control trial.

This paper presents the results of this qualitative study. Unique is our focus on patients' perceptions of the role of primary care providers and PCN programming in overall weight management. This foundational research is needed to develop effective and sustainable interventions.

Methods

The 5As Team intervention study (5AsT) is a longitudinal randomized control trial with convergent mixed-methods evaluation that has been described in detail elsewhere [19]. The qualitative sub-study recruited 28 patients from the 5AsT longitudinal patient cohort. Patients were over 18 years old, had given written informed consent in English, and had a BMI > = 25 kg/m^2. Purposeful sampling targeted individuals who received care of a PCN dietician or participated in a group program to support weight management at least 6 months prior. This ensured that patients were able to comment on the utility of PCN resources for their weight management. Over a 9-week period MB conducted qualitative interviews following a semi-structured interview guide (Appendix 1). The University of Alberta's (U of A) Health Research Ethics Board (HREB) provided institutional ethics approval (Pro00036740).

Interviews were transcribed verbatim, edited for clarity and confidentiality, and formatted for analysis. We used thematic analysis and iteratively coded data revising our list of codes continuously based on emergent patterns that were discussed regularly in analysis discussions with the research team [24, 25]. To ensure validity we used analyst triangulation that included the development of a coding scheme between three investigators (JT, MB, DCS), as well as independent coding of each interview by two investigators (JT, MB). Codes were cross-checked and differences discussed to reach consensus. Emergent themes were critically discussed with the third author (TL) to maintain reflexivity and minimize bias [26]. To maintain confidentiality we used pre-established codes to replace formal names of interviewed patients, primary care providers, and family practice clinics.

Results

A total of 28 individual interviews were conducted with patients from a variety of ages, sexes, socioeconomic status and medical co-morbidities (Table 1). While interviews illustrate the individual character of patients'

Table 1 Participant characteristics and demographics

Age range (years)	*n* (%)
30–45	4 (14)
46–60	12 (43)
61–75	11 (39)
> 75	1 (4)
Median age = 58 (range 30–80 years-old)	
Sex	*n* (%)
Female	19 (68)
Male	9 (32)
Ethnicity	*n* (%)
Caucasian	27 (96)
Aboriginal	1 (4)
Chronic Disease	*n* (%)
Arthritis	12 (43)
Hypertension	12 (43)
Hyperlipidemia	11 (40)
Asthma	7 (25)
Diabetes	7 (25)
COPD[a]	2 (7)
Heart Disease	2 (7)
Kidney Disease	1 (4)
Income	*n* (%)
$15,000–$29,000	5 (23)
$30,000–$49,000	4 (18)
$50,000–$79,000	8 (36)
> $80,000	5 (23)

[a](Chronic Obstructive Pulmonary Disease) COPD

weight management journey, four themes emerged that reflect the commonalities in perspectives, expectations, and needs across all patients:

(1) *Coordinated and person-centred care*: Patients emphasize the need for coordinated, whole-person approaches to address the multiple conditions and drivers that affect weight and weight management;
(2) *The role of family physicians*: Patients have clear expectations of their primary healthcare clinician to initiate a discussion around weight concerns;
(3) *Primary Care Network resources for weight management*: PCN programming and services meet patients' expectations for weight management support by being accessible, providing accountability, and contributing to consistent weight management messaging;
(4) *Patients' weight management needs*: Patients express further needs for weight management supports that are individualized to their medical, socio-economic, and educational needs, better linkages to available resources and programs, and further follow-up.

Coordinated and person-centred care

Patients described their weight management efforts as inseparably tied to other physical, mental, and socio-economic conditions. These conditions pose significant barriers to patients' weight management efforts causing feelings of frustration with their ability to reduce weight (Table 2). Patients emphasized that they needed their providers to adopt a comprehensive perspective addressing their obesity in the context of patients' comorbidities and life circumstances that affect health and their ability to manage weight:

> *"So, I try to work on one aspect of my life. The stressors in my life at the time. But I need something to pull it all together. Yeah. It would seem reasonable that I should be able to find help within the healthcare systems....somebody with a professional background to say, 'Okay, you need help in this area. You need to put all this together now'." (Patients 27)*

Patients explained how painful conditions, such as knee injuries, chronic pain, asthma, osteoarthritis, and plantar fasciitis, impaired their mobility and reduced the amount and level of their physical activity. Some patients reported weight gain from prescription medication, and other mechanical concerns such as sleep apnea. Patients also shared personal stories of their challenges and struggles with obesity and mental health. In these stories, patients link their weight, eating and weight control behaviours to stressful life events, depression, traumatic childhood experiences, fatigue, stress, and addictions. In addition, patients identified Type 2 diabetes, pre-diabetes, hypertension, and gout as associated with their weight. Women described struggling with the effects of menopause. These metabolic conditions often required restricted diets that patients found difficult to realize in their everyday lives. Finally, patients discussed limited

Table 2 Conditions and drivers affecting weight and weight management

Subtheme	Patient Quotes
Mechanical	• I blew my knee out for the first time probably in the late nineties and that's when my weight really started to go up. 'Cause that reduced my physical activity I was doing. (Patient 3)
	• This cough...I just feel that I'm not getting air into my lungs. No ending it. I thought it was a cold, but then after a couple of bottles of cough syrup and no relief, he (family physician) said, 'Throw it away, here's an inhaler.' I've done lung capacity and all kinds of x-rays, and done the sinus and the whole thing and nothing. . .Yeah, snowballs. I think there's a bit of a steroid in this inhaler, because I've noticed the weight has gone up since I started on the inhaler. (Patient 6)
Mental	• I was seeing my physician and we were talking about me being an emotional eater... (Patient 4)
	• I have other issues that relate to the weight because I'm an alcoholic, we're dealing with all of that together. So that's a big part of my weight management is quit (chuckle) drinking. So she's more concerned about that issue than she is about my weight. Because if I stop drinking, the weight is going to come off and I'm noticing that. (Patient 16)
	• . . .because of the weight gain that I'm having. And the stress that's in my life! (chuckle) The two go hand in hand. (Patient 27)
	• My weight issues are connected to mental and emotional issues from childhood so there is a mental component, sort of almost borderline addiction component to my obesity... (Patient 22)
Metabolic	• I can tell you where I got pretty heavy at one point, really heavy, and that's due to the fact I went through prostate cancer. Also, I've taken radiation, and then hormone therapy to knock down your testosterone, which makes you gain weight. . . They just told me it was a common thing to take place when you're taking hormones. So, don't panic! (Patient 10)
Monetary	• When I get paid I go grocery shopping. But I get to a point where I don't have any money. So, I might have to call the Food Bank. Well, last month, I unfortunately had to call the Food Bank. What I got in my basket was bagels, three loaves of bread, cereal, one lettuce, tube things of pasta, two bags of carrots, and a bunch of sweets. Nothing that I could eat except the lettuce! So when you're hungry it's hard because that's all you have. I hardly ever buy canned food, because there's too much garbage in it. If I do I make sure it's things, like tuna, that I know I can eat. I try and keep things like that for my emergencies. But it's really hard when you have no money and you need food. What do you eat? (Patient 16)

finances and time constraints that affect their means to maintain or commit to an obesity management program.

Patients are aware of the connection between their overall health, socio-economic well-being, and comorbidities with their overweight, and they look for support to assess, prioritize, and plan their weight management holistically.

The role of family physicians

Patients had clear and consistent expectations concerning the role of primary care in their weight management. They believed that it is the responsibility of the family physician to initiate the conversation about weight management, and to do so in a non-judgmental, knowledgeable and respectful manner. They felt that the conversation should be guided by a holistic view of weight that acknowledges the patients' overall health and well-being.

Patients discussed how aspects of their encounter with family physicians affect their satisfaction with weight management support (Table 3). These included perceived quality of relationship with the physician, the physician's approach to weight management and knowledge of obesity, and the time spent on the topic.

Some patients reported a positive doctor-patient relationship with their family physician, were at ease discussing their weight, and believed their physician had listened and responded to their needs and concerns. A number of patients perceived their physician as effectively communicating weight management options. In addition, patients appreciated physicians who considered their overall health rather than addressing weight in isolation of other health concerns.

Other patients stated that their family physician never discussed weight. Some patients attributed this to a lack of time during the consultation. Others felt their family physician either ignored or did not recognize their weight concerns and the effect it is has on not only their health and wellbeing, but also their family, social, and work life. Some patients felt that their physician's failure to address weight was due to the patient's general good health. These patients, however, would have preferred their physicians' respond to their concerns and willingness to discuss weight management as a preventative measure. Several patients reported that their physicians expressed weight management was outside their field of expertise and referred them to a dietician or chronic disease management nurse. Some patients experienced their physician's approach to weight management as a variation of '*eat less and move more*', which they found unhelpful and ineffective.

Primary care network resources for weight management

Patients described participation in the PCN educational sessions (Table 4) as useful and beneficial for weight management. Several patients had one-on-one support from dieticians in the PCN. Patients explained that these PCN resources facilitated their weight management through three key elements: *accountability, accessibility, and consistency* (Table 5).

Accountability

Patients expressed that their participation in the programs and the interactions with staff helped to hold them accountable when it came to weight management. They emphasized accountability as a major benefit of using PCN resources. For example, some patients stated regularly scheduled sessions alone increased their commitment. Other key benefits of these programs included explicit goal setting and deliberate follow-up with a PCN clinician to discuss successes and challenges that the

Table 3 The role of family physicians

Subtheme	Patient Quotes
Physicians should initiate weight management conversation	• "I think that having that conversation would be beneficial. I mean even though things are going well now, in the future this could be potentially what being overweight might cause. I think that would be a huge help for a lot of people. It would be a help for me too." (Patient 14)
Physicians should not be judgemental	• "I think a concerned family physician should always talk to you about your weight management, but not denigrate or harass you about it. Because you've achieved this for some reason…You won't change it by medicine, you'll change it by attitude and life." (Patient 15)
Positive experience	• "I love my new doctor because he actually says stuff to you, very nicely. He's very kind and gentle about it but he'll actually say, 'It'll help if you lose weight.' And he encouraged me to come here and encouraged me to take more classes." (Patient 21)
	• "My doctor doesn't deal with the weight management as a completely separate issue. It's affecting my health, my recovery and my ability to exercise. She sees me once a month for a follow-up appointment to check my prescriptions, how I'm feeling, and my weight. So it's part of the bigger picture." (Patient 7)
Negative experience	• "My family physician has never ever talked about my weight." (Patient 5)
	• "My family physician would give me the standard, 'Eat less fat, eat less sugar (chuckle), exercise more,'- and that's not going to cut it" (Patient 2)
	• "They were like, 'Okay, cut your calories and exercise,' and that was their only thing… Eat less and exercise more isn't the end-all-be-all. I'm looking for more concrete strategies." (Patient 11)

Table 4 Examples of some PCN educational programs

Program Title	Duration	Purpose
Weight Management	Full Day or 3 weeks	Information on safe dieting techniques, emotional eating, and setting achievable weight loss goals
Moving for Health	8 weeks	Geared towards people living with chronic disease who want to incorporate exercise into their life to improve health
Grocery Shopping	1 day	Coaching in making better food choices: planning meals, reading nutrition labels, and grocery-shopping tips
Meal Planning	1 day	Coaching in making better food choices: planning meals, reading nutrition labels, choosing healthy take-out options.
Relaxation	4 weeks	Strategies to help patients cope with everyday stress and stress related to various health problems
Managing Emotion	Full Day or 3–4 weeks	Helps patients recognize their strengths and weaknesses to effectively manage stress and choose healthy behaviours
Changeways	6 weeks	Strategies for managing depression and anxiety

patient experienced. Patients expressed that setting goals and working towards achieving them as best as they could, helped them to maintain their motivation.

Accessibility

A major strength of the PCN supports was their accessibility including availability of interdisciplinary clinicians, accommodating schedules, and affordable cost. Patients described benefitting from access to nutritionists, exercise specialists, and behavioural health consultants that focused on underlying psychological issues and behavioural change. In addition, they benefited from access to clinic nurses, which assisted with healthy weight loss and weight maintenance. However, patients also expressed that despite dietician availability, access is insufficient because of lengthy waiting times and lack of capacity to provide individualized support and follow-up.

Weight management sessions were offered after work and on weekends, with PCN clinicians available to patients beyond regular scheduled sessions. In addition, an Alberta Health grant funds the PCNs, as such program fees are either *gratis* or nominal, which considerably lowers the financial barriers to participation. Having affordable access to these weight management resources, patients perceived the PCN as more "caring" and patient-centered as compared with commercial weight loss programs. Patients' experience of the PCN as caring played a significant role in their decision to access the PCN as a weight management resource.

Consistency

Another element of PCN resources and supports that emerged as significant for patient satisfaction was consistent weight management messaging. Patients remarked that a core point in this messaging was that weight loss is not a 'quick fix' and they should consider their weight management as a journey that will take commitment and time.

Table 5 PCN programming meets patients' expectations in important ways

Subtheme	Patient quotes
Accountability	• Well, I think it (regular attendance of PCN programs) sort of keeps you accountable a little bit when it's a regular thing, you know. (Patient 8) • Like certain things like how many laps you could do in a circle… And they would compare it when you're done the workshop at the end of the eight weeks, I think…. And I noticed I did increase because I think it held me accountable. (Patient 1)
Accessibility	• I'm glad that they did evening sessions because then I could go. (Patient 16) • They seemed to really let you know what they had available, that they wanted to be able to help you out, which is nice. (Patient 14) • Well I'm just totally happy with PCN. I just think it's like a gold mine! Like, you know. And it's really nice to have…like services are, you know, not real expensive or free here. (Patient 2) • Maybe I'm just more appreciative that it doesn't cost me any money, so psychologically I have been more acceptable to the (PCN) program. I feel it's a caring kind of a thing, not a business kind of a thing. (Patient 11)
Consistency	• I felt that they were all pulling together. They weren't necessarily communicating deeply with one another, but I never felt like I was getting conflicting messages. The message was always the same. What one person was saying was building…I could take what the doctor said, what the dietician said, what the PCN people said, and what the exercise people said and put it all together and build on it. There was no confusion. (Patient 27)

Patients' weight management needs

Four additional areas of weight management support were identified: (1) more individualized weight management resources; (2) addition of more advanced educational sessions; (3) enhanced advertisement; and, (4) further follow-up (see Table 6).

Strategies for individual sets of comorbidities

Patients had a good understanding of the multifactorial issues at play in their weight management and expressed the need for resources tailored to their particular situation. While patients appreciated that group programs provided a venue to share experiences with other patients, they found that the content remained too broad, thus not providing strategies that are applicable to their particular situation. They suggested that increasing the opportunity for one-on-one interaction would help them to address their individual weight management challenges.

Advanced weight management knowledge

Although patients understood the broad nature of the educational sessions and appreciated that they start at a very basic level, they felt that they would also benefit from more advanced educational resources.

Linking and advertising resources

Patients indicated the need for better promotion and advertisement of weight management resources and programs. Improved descriptions of programs would allow patients to make informed decisions about which resources would benefit their weight management best.

Follow-up

Patients expressed that extended follow-up with primary healthcare providers would improve their overall weight management experience, increase patient and provider accountability to meet their weight management goals, and help address any challenges patients may be experiencing. In addition, sometimes patients felt overwhelmed with the volume of information given in one consultation and would prefer long-term weight management resources. They felt ongoing access to resources and programming would be supportive in establishing new and improved eating behaviours, and encourage commitment to sustainable behaviour change.

Discussion

Family physicians should play a vital role in weight management, which is consistent with current literature [3, 13, 15, 17, 27, 28]. Physicians should play a dual role in initiating weight management consultations with a

Table 6 Further patient needs for weight management

Subtheme	Patient quotes
Individualized weight management resources	• ...when you do a group session, there are people with so many different dietary needs. There were a lot of people in that class that had...were looking at needing bariatric surgery and all kinds of other things. So the needs of all people were so different that it's hard to get the answers to what you want because everybody is different. (Patient 16)
Advanced educational sessions	• I would like there to be more of the *Moving for Health*. It would be nice if there was different levels, because they've got a lot of equipment there. It would be great to learn how to use. There's just that first one to get you moving and then it's up to you to carry on. It would be great if they would do classes. I think a lot of people would come here to do it because one if it's free, and two when everybody else is overweight, you're more comfortable. You're not as comfortable when you're having to go to a gym and everybody is all healthy and skinny and running on that track, so if you could come here and do Jazzercise or that kind of thing in the gym. (Patient 19)
Enhanced advertisement	• I think the one thing that I would say was if this were more readily advertised...The PCN programs were advertised that they were available, I think I would have jumped on them a lot faster 'cause it is something that is interesting and motivating for me. (Patient 14)
Follow-up sessions	• The other thing that would be really helpful in these programs is the commitments from patients. Again, it comes down to accountability. So the patient says, 'I'm going to do this, this, and this.' When you check back, whoever it is that you're checking in with is asking, 'Have you done this?' 'Why?' 'Why not?' 'How did it work?' 'What can you do further?' 'If that's not work, what can we do instead?' (Patient 23)
	• The other part would be accountability. That there is an opportunity either at the PCN or at the doctor, whoever wants to take the lead that can be an ongoing follow-up. I think the programs are great, but when the program ends, what happens next to that patient? . . . And, the thing is this is a lifestyle thing. So all of those things are great building blocks on your lifestyle, but what is going to keep you working on that lifestyle, to improve in general. So, it would be an ongoing connection, I think, with a PCN or with the doctor. I think PCN would be a great place to continue because they have some resources that the doctor's offices don't always have. (Patient 23)
	• I'd love something that could be ongoing! Almost like a course where it was a whole year long and you make a commitment to it...Yeah I'd love something like that where you're more accountable, there's more follow up, and you can ask questions and express your concerns. (Patient 2)

comprehensive assessment and coordinating care of conditions and comorbidities that affect weight. In addition, we found that PCN services support weight management in important ways that meet patient needs for accessibility, accountability, and consistency. Finally, the results point to where patients' needs are not met and future efforts are warranted.

Patients clearly articulated that they would like their family physician to initiate weight counselling, which is consistent with existing literature [3, 5, 16, 29]. However, our findings emphasize the need to assess root causes and drivers of weight gain, comorbidities, and psychosocial barriers of individual patients in order to develop a care plan that offers realistic and sustainable strategies according to patients' particular constraints and strengths. Patients felt that their weight is a complex phenomenon impacted by a multitude of factors. Consistent with literature that categorizes common conditions associated with obesity into the "4Ms of obesity management" [6], patients discussed mechanical, mental, metabolic, monetary issues as inseparable from their weight trajectory and has having decisive impact on their weight management efforts. This resonates with the mounting evidence showing that obesity is a complex condition that is impacted by multiple factors beyond diet and exercise [3, 5, 16, 30, 31]. Consequently, weight management in primary care must build on an individual assessment of a person's history with weight, attempts at weight control, comorbidities, mental health, and socio-economic situation. Findings underscore that patients want personalized information about physiology of obesity, its chronicity and resistance to treatment in order to formulate personal strategies with realistic expectations, and a focus on prevention and patient-important health outcomes rather than numbers on a scale. In addition, treatment plans must be guided by the recognition that behaviour and behaviour change arises at the intersection of cultural and social environments with individual factors such as automatic responses, conscious choice, values, and physiology [3, 5, 32, 33]. Family physicians are ideally positioned to develop such personalized care plans based on their long-term relationship with patients and the lifecycle approach of primary care.

Our findings show that while patients expect physicians to initiate and coordinate weight management; extended interdisciplinary health teams contribute valuable care and resources beyond the constraints of physicians' time and expertise. This echoes previous research calling for multidisciplinary teams to address obesity [3, 5, 15, 16].

Patients appreciated the sense of accountability to their weight management goals through PCN programming. The importance of accountability for behaviour change has been found previously and points to the relational quality of human behaviour [2, 32]. Goal setting and follow-up, in concert with social support, facilitates the establishment of healthy habits [34, 35]. Patients value consistent messaging around prioritizing health improvement instead of focusing on weight alone, realistic expectations for weight loss, and the holistic understanding of obesity. Such consistency in conceptualizing and framing weight management for patients supports their sense-making of their condition and their ability to manage it [21]. These findings support the potential of the Patient Medical Home model, that the PCN structure is based on for improving weight management and obesity care [23, 36].

Beyond these benefits of current weight management resources, patients emphasized the lack of personalized care plans including information that applies to patients' particular combination of challenges and offers knowledge that is appropriate for diverse levels of education. They also emphasized the need for long-term, sustainable approaches and for better coordination of existing resources in the community. Challenges to address these needs include a lack of physician education in obesity physiology and training in weight management skills resource constraints for patient-centeredness of the current health care model and the lack of an evidence-based, yet flexible and adaptable, intervention [3, 13, 17, 29, 30].

Practice implications of our findings include a clear need for personalized weight management interventions that are practical and sustainable for interdisciplinary primary care clinicians. The "5As for obesity management™" (Ask-Assess-Advise-Agree-Assist) offer a promising framework that can guide practitioners in addressing patients' individual weight management needs in a way that is patient-centred, comprehensive, and coordinated [13, 15, 21, 22, 27, 37]. The 5As are gaining traction in the US and Canada [13, 15, 19, 27, 37–40], have been shown to improve provider self-efficacy, increase weight management visits [13], and result in clinically significant patient weight loss at 12 months post-intervention with a physician trained in the 5As [24]. However, considering the chronicity and complexity of obesity as well as research questioning the utility of weight loss as measure for successful management [41], there is a pressing need for further research identifying appropriate patient outcome measures.

Furthermore, research is needed to understand how a comprehensive, personalized assessment and weight management plan can be implemented in diverse health care settings, in particular where extended interdisciplinary teams are not available and budget is limited, and how to build capacity in other interdisciplinary team members to support patient weight management.

There are some limitations of this study. All patients in this cohort had a family physician and received PCN weight management care. While 85% of Canadians have a family physician, and over 80% of Albertans belong to a PCN, the services and structures vary across different geographic regions. Although we achieved diversity of patients for gender, age, and stages of obesity, the majority of the group identified as Euro-Canadian and as urban/suburban residing in a major city in Alberta. The themes that emerged from the data reflect the perspectives of patients who are concerned about their weight and willing to work with clinicians to improve their health. While our conclusions are not generalizable to all patients living with obesity, they are foundational to developing an intervention that is effective for patients who seek support for their weight management within primary care.

Conclusion

These results further our understanding of patients' perception of if, when, and how primary care clinicians and resources can support weight management. The study is part of the larger 5AsT research program to improve weight management in primary care. Moving beyond patient experiences of living with and managing excess weight, this research examined how patients perceive the weight management support provided by extended interdisciplinary teams embedded in family medicine practices, such as the PCN model in Alberta, Canada.

Overall, patients expressed the need for weight management that is tailored to their individual set of comorbidities and provides strategies that are realistic and sustainable under their personal circumstances.

Appendix 1: Interview guide

To provide some *background*, I would like to hear about *your weight management experience*. So, can we begin with...

1) Where do you go or where have you gone to get help with weight management?
   a. What professionals, programs or resources have you used for weight management?
   b. What types of healthcare providers, if any, have you talked to for weight management?
      i. Prompt - If not mentioned: Have you talked to your family physician or their clinic team about weight management?
      ii. Prompt - If not mentioned: Have you talked to PCN staff (nurse, dietician, mental health worker, behavioural health consultant, exercise specialist) about weight management?

Family practice office

2) Tell me about your experience with your family physician including with members of their clinic team when you've talked about weight management.
   a. What types of programs or resources were you provided with OR referred to for weight management?
   b. What healthcare providers have you seen at your family physician's office for weight management?
   c. What types of programs or resources would you like from your family physician and/or clinic-based team to support your weight management? If no programs or resources, why not?
   d. Were/Are you comfortable talking about your weight and weight management with your family physician and/or their clinic team?
   e. Do you think your family physician and/or clinic team should talk with you about weight management? If yes, when should this occur? If not, why?

PCN healthcare providers, weight management programs and resources

3) I would like to hear about your experiences with the PCN healthcare providers and their programs and resources for weight management.
   a) How did you come to use PCN programs and/or resources for weight management?
   b) What type of PCN programs have you used to support your weight management?
   c) Are you using other PCN programs and/or resources for your health?
      i) If yes, are these a part of your weight management?
   d) Are there PCN programs and/or resources that you would like to use to support your weight management but do not?
   e) Are/were you comfortable talking about your weight with PCN healthcare providers?
   f) What PCN healthcare providers have you talked to about your weight management?
      i) How are they providing the help you want in your weight management?
   g) Are there PCN healthcare providers who you have not had access to but would like to talk to about your weight management?
      i) How would you want them to help you in your weight management?

Additional questions

4) Thinking to a time before you talked about weight management with your family physician and their clinic team and/or PCN healthcare providers would you have considered primary healthcare providers as a resource to help you with weight management?

5) Do your family physician and PCN staff work together for your weight management?
6) How similar was the information you were told by your family physician and PCN staff about managing weight and setting goals?
7) Do you receive information about weight management from specialists? If yes, is it similar information that you received from your family physician and/or PCN healthcare providers?
8) Ideally, thinking about your weight management in the context of your health, how would you like to see your family physician and/or PCN healthcare providers helping you with your weight management?
9) Is there anything you would like to tell me about your weight management experience that we have not discussed?

Abbreviations

4M's: Mechanical, Mental, Metabolic, Monetary issues; 5A's: 5A's for Obesity Management (Ask – Assess – Advise – Agree – Assist); 5AsT: 5As team; BMI: Body mass index; HREB: Health research ethics board; PCN: Primary care network; UofA: University of Alberta

Acknowledgements

The grant generation and oversight of the overall 5AsT Project, of which this project was a sub-study, was supported by Sheri Fielding, nurse practitioner and clinical director of the Primary Care Network partner, Christian Rueda-Clausen, MD, PhD (post-doctoral fellow, Dept. of Medicine), Andrew Cave, MD (professor, Dept. of Family Medicine), Donna Manca, MD (associate professor, Dept. of Family Medicine). Jodie Asselin PhD (post-doctoral fellow) supported the protocol and initial semi-structured interview guide creation. Melanie Heatherington MEd (study coordinator) supported the ethics submission, and study logistics.

Funding

The 5AsT study is funded by Alberta Innovates-Health Solutions CRIO grant, with significant in kind support from the Primary Care Network. The researchers are independent of the study funder. The funder had no access to study data, no involvement in the design or execution of the study, no involvement in analysis, and no role in the decision to publish.

Author's contributions

DCS and AMS, supported by JAJ, conceived of the study, wrote the grant, and supervised the project. DCS supported by the 5AsT study team wrote the ethics and protocol, and oversaw the 5AsT patient cohort project. MB conducted the patient interviews. MB and JT supported by DCS did the coding. MB and JT supported by TL did the analysis. TL supported by DCS, MB and JT synthesized the findings and integrated them with the literature, formulating the argument. JT and TL supported by MB and DCS wrote the manuscript. All authors had access to data and analyses, reviewed the manuscript and provided comments, and can take responsibility for data integrity and accuracy. All authors read and approved the final manuscript.

Competing interests

JT, TL, MB, and JAJ have nothing to disclose. AMS is a member of an Advisory Board with a commercial organization (Novo Nordisk: Advisory Board for anti-obesity drug); AMS was a member of the Data Safety Monitoring Board for an anti-obesity trial (Takeda).
DLCS is an unpaid board chair for the Primary Care Network that partnered in this study.

Consent for publication

Not applicable.

Author details

[1]Department of Family Medicine, University of Alberta, Clinical Research Unit, Edmonton, AB, CanadaT6G 2E1. [2]School of Public Health, University of Alberta, Edmonton, AB, CanadaT6G 2E3. [3]Department of Medicine, Division of Endocrinology, University of Alberta, Edmonton, AB, CanadaT6G 2E1. [4]Department of Anthropology, University of Alberta, Edmonton, AB, CanadaT6G 2H4. [5]Department of Medicine, Obesity Research & Management, University of Alberta, Li Ka Shing Building, Rm. 1-116, 87th Avenue and 112th Street, Edmonton, AB T6G 2E1, Canada.

References

1. Government of Canada SC. Body mass index, overweight or obese, self-reported, adult, by age group and sex (Number of persons). 2016. http://www.statcan.gc.ca/tables-tableaux/sum-som/l01/cst01/health81a-eng.htm. Accessed 4 Feb 2016.
2. Metzgar CJ, Preston AG, Miller DL, Nickols-Richardson SM. Facilitators and barriers to weight loss and weight loss maintenance: a qualitative exploration. J Hum Nutr Diet. 2015;28(6):593–603.
3. Janke EA, Ramirez ML, Haltzman B, Fritz M, Kozak AT. Patient's experience with comorbidity management in primary care: a qualitative study of comorbid pain and obesity. Prim Health Care Res Dev. 2016;17(01):33–41.
4. Greener J, Douglas F, van Teijlingen E. More of the same? Conflicting perspectives of obesity causation and intervention amongst overweight people, health professionals and policy makers. Soc Sci Med. 2010;70(7):1042–9.
5. Kirk SF, Price SL, Penney TL, Rehman L, Lyons RF, Piccinini-Vallis H, et al. Blame, shame, and lack of support a multilevel study on obesity management. Qual Health Res. 2014;24(6):790–800.
6. Sharma AM. M, M, M & M: a mnemonic for assessing obesity A. M. Sharma Obesity mnemonic. Obes Rev. 2010;11(11):808–9.
7. Canadian Medical Association. CMA recognizes obesity as a disease. 2015. https://www.cma.ca/En/Pages/cma-recognizes-obesity-as-a-disease.aspx. Accessed 14 Mar 2016.
8. Brauer P, Connor Gorber S, Shaw E, Singh H, Bell N, Shane AR, et al. Recommendations for prevention of weight gain and use of behavioural and pharmacologic interventions to manage overweight and obesity in adults in primary care. CMAJ. 2015;187(3):184–95.
9. Moyer VA. Screening for and management of obesity in adults: U.S. preventive services task force recommendation statement. Ann Intern Med. 2012;157(5):373–8.
10. Wee CC, McCarthy EP, Davis RB, Phillips RS. Physician counseling about exercise. JAMA J Am Med Assoc. 1999;282(16):1583–8.
11. Sinclair J, Lawson B, Burge F. Which patients receive advice on diet and exercise? Do certain characteristics affect whether they receive such advice? Can Fam Physician Médecin Fam Can. 2008;54(3):404–12.
12. Brauer PM, Sergeant LA, Davidson B, Goy R, Dietrich L. Patient reports of lifestyle advice in primary care. Can J Diet Pract Res Publ Dietit Can Rev Can Prat Rech En Diététique Une Publ Diététistes Can. 2012;73(3):122–7.
13. Rueda-Clausen CF, Benterud E, Bond T, Olszowka R, Vallis MT, Sharma AM. Effect of implementing the 5As of Obesity Management framework on provider-patient interactions in primary care: 5As of obesity management in primary care. Clin Obes. 2014;4(1):39–44.
14. Jay M, Kalet A, Ark T, McMacken M, Messito M, Richter R, et al. Physicians' attitudes about obesity and their associations with competency and specialty: a cross-sectional study. BMC Health Serv Res. 2009;9(1):106.
15. Fitzpatrick SL, Wischenka D, Appelhans BM, Pbert L, Wang M, Wilson DK, et al. An evidence-based guide for obesity treatment in primary care. Am J Med. 2016;129(1):115. e1–115.e7.
16. Thomas SL, Hyde J, Karunaratne A, Herbert D, Komesaroff PA. Being "fat" in today's world: a qualitative study of the lived experiences of people with obesity in Australia. Health Expect. 2008;11(4):321–30.
17. Kirk SFL, Penney TL, McHugh T-L, Sharma AM. Effective weight management practice: a review of the lifestyle intervention evidence. Int J Obes. 2012;36(2):178–85.

18. Loureiro ML, Nayga Jr RM. Obesity, weight loss, and physician's advice. Soc Sci Med. 2006;62(10):2458–68.
19. Campbell-Scherer DL, Asselin J, Osunlana AM, Fielding S, Anderson R, Rueda-Clausen CF, et al. Implementation and evaluation of the 5As framework of obesity management in primary care: design of the 5As Team (5AsT) randomized control trial. Implement Sci. 2014;9(1):78.
20. Ogunleye A, Osunlana A, Asselin J, Cave A, Sharma AM, Campbell-Scherer DL. The 5As team intervention: bridging the knowledge gap in obesity management among primary care practitioners. BMC Res Notes. 2015;8(1): 1–12. http://www.biomedcentral.com/1756-0500/8/810. Accessed 21 Jan 2016.
21. Asselin J, Osunlana AM, Ogunleye AA, Sharma AM, Campbell-Scherer D. Challenges in interdisciplinary weight management in primary care: lessons learned from the 5As team study: challenges in interdisciplinary weight management. Clin Obes. 2016;6(2):124–32.
22. Osunlana AM, Asselin J, Anderson R, Ogunleye AA, Cave A, Sharma AM, et al. 5As Team obesity intervention in primary care: development and evaluation of shared decision-making weight management tools. Clin Obes. 2015;4:219.
23. Nielsen M, Olayiwola J, Grundy P, Grumbach K, for the Patient-centred Primary Care Collaborative. The patient centred-centred medical home's impact on cost and quality: an annual update of the evidence 2012–2013. Millbank Memorial Fund. 2014. http://www.milbank.org/uploads/documents/reports/Patient-Centered_Medical_Homes_Impact_on_Cost_and_Quality.pdf. Accessed on 25 Nov 2015.
24. Fereday J, Muir-Cochrane E. Demonstrating rigor using thematic analysis: a hybrid approach of inductive and deductive coding and theme development. Int J Qual Methods. 2008;5(1):80–92.
25. Vaismoradi M, Turunen H, Bondas T. Content analysis and thematic analysis: implications for conducting a qualitative descriptive study. Nurs Health Sci. 2013;15(3):398–405.
26. Johnson B. Examining the validity structure of qualitative research. Education. 1997;118(3):282–92.
27. Jay M, Gillespie C, Schlair S, Sherman S, Kalet A. Physicians' use of the 5As in counseling obese patients: is the quality of counseling associated with patients' motivation and intention to lose weight? BMC Health Serv Res. 2010;10(1):1–10.
28. Rose S, Poynter P, Anderson J, Noar S, Conigliaro J. Physician weight loss advice and patient weight loss behavior change: a literature review and meta-analysis of survey data. Int J Obes. 2013;37:118–28.
29. Kirk SF, Tytus R, Tsuyuki RT, Sharma AM, et al. Weight management experiences of overweight and obese Canadian adults: findings from a national survey. Chronic Inj Can. 2012;32(2):63–9.
30. Dietz WH, Baur LA, Hall K, Puhl RM, Taveras EM, Uauy R, et al. Management of obesity: improvement of health-care training and systems for prevention and care. Lancet Lond Engl. 2015;385(9986):2521–33.
31. Sharma AM, Padwal R. Obesity is a sign - over-eating is a symptom: an aetiological framework for the assessment and management of obesity. Obes Rev. 2010;11(5):362–70.
32. Kelly MP, Barker M. Why is changing health-related behaviour so difficult? Public Health. 2016;136:109–116. doi:10.1016/j.puhe.2016.03.030.
33. Michie S, West R, Campbell R, Brown J, Gainforth H. ABC of behaviour change theories: an essential resource for researchers, policy makers and practitioners. London: Silberback; 2014.
34. The Primary Care Alliance. Evolving primary care networks in Alberta. A companion document to the PCN evolution vision and framework of the primary care alliance. 2013. www.health.alberta.ca/documents/PHC-PCN-Evolution-Evolving-2013.pdf. Accessed on 23 Nov 2015.
35. Mann T, de Ridder D, Fujita K. Self-regulation of health behavior: social psychological approaches to goal setting and goal striving. Health Psychol. 2013;32(5):487–98.
36. The College of Family Physicians of Canada. A vision for Canada: family practice the patient's medical home. [Internet]. 2011 [cited 2015 Nov 23]. Available from: www.cfpc.ca/uploadedFiles/Resources/Resource_items/PMH_A_Vision_for_Canada.pdf
37. Vallis M, Piccinini–Vallis H, Sharma AM, Freedhoff Y. Modified 5 As minimal intervention for obesity counseling in primary care. Can Fam Physician. 2013;59(1):27–31.
38. Plourde G, Prud'homme D. Managing obesity in adults in primary care. Can Med Assoc J. 2012;184(9):1039–44.
39. Sharma AM. The 5A model for the management of obesity. CMAJ Can Med Assoc J. 2012;184(14):1603.
40. Jay MR, Gillespie CC, Schlair SL, Savarimuthu SM, Sherman SE, Zabar SR, et al. The impact of primary care resident physician training on patient weight loss at 12 months. Obes Silver Spring Md. 2013;21(1):45–50.
41. Padwal RS, Pajewski NM, Allison DB, Sharma AM. Using the Edmonton obesity staging system to predict mortality in a population-representative cohort of people with overweight and obesity. CMAJ. 2011;183(14):e1059–66.

21

Effective team-based primary care: observations from innovative practices

Edward H. Wagner[1*], Margaret Flinter[2], Clarissa Hsu[3], DeAnn Cromp[3], Brian T. Austin[1], Rebecca Etz[4], Benjamin F. Crabtree[5] and MaryJoan D. Ladden[6]

Abstract

Background: Team-based care is now recognized as an essential feature of high quality primary care, but there is limited empiric evidence to guide practice transformation. The purpose of this paper is to describe advances in the configuration and deployment of practice teams based on in-depth study of 30 primary care practices viewed as innovators in team-based care.

Methods: As part of LEAP, a national program of the Robert Wood Johnson Foundation, primary care experts nominated 227 innovative primary care practices. We selected 30 practices for intensive study through review of practice descriptive and performance data. Each practice hosted a 3-day site visit between August, 2012 and September, 2013, where specific advances in team configuration and roles were noted. Advances were identified by site visitors and confirmed at a meeting involving representatives from each of the 30 practices.

Results: LEAP practices have expanded the roles of existing staff and added new personnel to provide the person power and skills needed to perform the tasks and functions expected of a patient-centered medical home (PCMH). LEAP practice teams generally include a rich array of staff, especially registered nurses (RNs), behavioral health specialists, and lay health workers. Most LEAP practices organize their staff into core teams, which are built around partnerships between providers and specific Medical Assistants (MAs), and often include registered nurses (RNs) and others such as health coaches or receptionists. MAs, RNs, and other staff are heavily involved in the planning and delivery of preventive and chronic illness care. The care of more complex patients is supported by behavioral health specialists, RN care managers, and pharmacists. Standing orders and protocols enable staff to act independently.

Conclusions: The 30 LEAP practices engage health professional and lay staff in patient care to the maximum extent, which enables the practices to meet the expectations of a PCMH and helps free up providers to focus on tasks that only they can perform.

Keywords: Primary care, Practice team, Patient-centered medical home

Background

The coordinated involvement of teams in patient care has emerged as an essential feature of patient-centered medical homes (PCMHs) capable of achieving the quadruple aim—improving patient health, enhancing patient experience, reducing health care costs, and improving the work life of providers and staff [1, 2]. Clinical trials show that the involvement of medical assistants, nurses and other staff in delivering clinical services to diabetic, hypertensive, and depressed patients leads to substantial improvements in disease control [3–7]. Qualitative studies of exemplary primary care practices conclude that practices without effective teams have difficulty performing functions such as population management, care coordination and care management that are critical to the success of a PCMH [2, 8, 9]. If patients experience care by well-organized teams, both satisfaction with overall care and with their provider increase [10, 11]. Lastly, recent studies indicate that more effective teams are

* Correspondence: wagner.e@ghc.org
[1]MacColl Center for Health Care Innovation, Group Health Research Institute, 1730 Minor Ave., Suite 1600, Seattle, WA 98101, USA
Full list of author information is available at the end of the article

associated with less job exhaustion and burnout for physicians and other staff [12, 13].

Despite the growing recognition of the importance of teams, there is relatively little empiric evidence to guide practices wanting to create high-performing primary care teams. In response, the Robert Wood Johnson Foundation created The Primary Care Team: Learning from Effective Ambulatory Practices (PCT-LEAP), a national program devoted to helping primary care practices develop more effective primary care teams using insights and examples gleaned from the study of innovative, high-performing practices [14]. In an earlier paper, we described preliminary findings on the changing roles of key staff across LEAP practices [14]. Since the publication of that paper, we have completed the site visits to all 30 practices, distilled key themes from the data, developed a web-based technical assistance program (www.improvingprimarycare.org), and used the program to help practices implement team-based primary care. In this paper, we describe major themes in team configuration and team-based care observed in LEAP practices, and highlight specific changes in staff composition or deployment that appear to be promising departures from traditional practice.

Methods

Setting

LEAP is co-directed by EW and MF, and is based at the MacColl Center for Health Care Innovation. A National Advisory Committee (NAC) has played important roles in the selection of practices, conduct of site visits, and development of the technical assistance program.

Site selection

Practice selection involved a multi-stage process comprised of: first, nomination by national primary care experts of primary care practices that creatively use their workforce to improve care quality and efficiency; second, data collection from nominated practices; and finally, data review and grading. From a literature review of primary care workforce innovations [15], we identified 50 thought leaders and asked them to recommend potentially relevant practices and additional nominators. Ultimately, we elicited names of 435 practices from 387 individuals. Roughly ½ of the nominated organizations were eliminated, most commonly because they were not primary care. One of the authors (RE) completed 45 min telephone interviews with a leader in the remaining 227 practices. Information collected included: practice organization and size, patient characteristics, payment mix, workforce innovations, practice team composition and roles; and practice performance and quality improvement. The descriptive and interview data from each practice were summarized in a two-page structured report for 154 practices deemed to have workforce innovations.

Four NAC members and staff independently reviewed each two-page report and rated the practice team innovations. We then requested available data on quality of care and patient experience from the 70 highest rated practices. Based on the practice team innovativeness ratings and the review of performance data, the NAC selected 30 practices that reflect a range of geographic locations/settings, practice organizational types, and populations served. Within each multi-site organization, data collection focused on a single practice site where we could best observe high functioning practice teams. Table 1 describes the 30 LEAP practice sites, which comprise 15 Federally Qualified Health Centers (FQHCs) including a nurse-managed center, and 15 private practices, nine of which were part of multi-specialty groups or integrated systems. Four sites are major medical residency training sites, and one serves as a Nurse Practitioner residency site. Most (77%) LEAP sites are part of multi-site practice organizations. Panel sizes per primary care provider range from 800 to 2750. Panel sizes tend to be larger in private practices with smaller Medicare populations. Twenty-one of the 30 sites were NCQA level 3 PCMH's and 3 more had state-based PCMH certification. Most LEAP private practices primarily depend on fee-for-service reimbursement from commercial plans, Medicare, and Medicaid. FQHCs largely rely on Medicaid and their federal grant. Only one LEAP site reported that the majority of their revenue was from capitation.

We sought to compare the staffing of LEAP practices with less highly selected American primary care practices. A recent paper described the staffing of 496 practices in seven regions of the U.S. that participated in the Centers for Medicare and Medicaid Services Comprehensive Primary Care Initiative (CPC) [16]. Federally Qualified Health Centers and Rural Health Clinics were excluded from CPC.

Site visits

Each of the 30 LEAP practice sites hosted a 3-day site visit by a team of 3–5 individuals that included a clinician investigator, a qualitative researcher, and a research assistant. All site visitors received training in qualitative data collection. Site visit activities were generally limited to the single practice location described above. The site visits included: tours of clinic space and the EMR; formal semi-structured (recorded and transcribed) and informal interviews with practice leaders, providers, and staff; staff and patient shadowing; observations of huddles and other team meetings; a staff survey; and collection of photographs, practice materials and tools. Site visits took place between August 2012 and September 2013. Guides for interviews conducted and observations made during site visits are listed in the Additional files 1, 2 and 3.

Table 1 Characteristics of LEAP Practice Sites

Organizational Type	
Federally Qualified Health Center	15 (50%)
Private Practice	
Multi-specialty Group	9 (30%)
Primary Care	6 (20%)
Residency Training Program	
Medical	4 (13%)
Nurse Practitioner	1 (3%)
No residency	25 (83%)
Region	
New England (MA, ME,NH)	5 (17%)
Middle Atlantic (NY, PA,WV,DC)	7 (23%)
Southeast (SC,LA)	2 (7%)
Midwest (OH,IN,IA,WI,MN)	5 (17%)
Southwest (TX,NM,CO)	5 (17%)
Pacific Coast (CA,OR,WA)	6 (20%)
Location	
Urban	9 (30%)
Suburban	8 (27%)
Rural	11 (37%)
Multiple	2 (7%)
Number of Sites in the Practice Organization	
One	7 (23%)
2–5	6 (20%)
6–10	8 (27%)
11–20	4 (13%)
21+	5 (17%)
Panel Size per full-time PCP	
< 1500	10 (33%)
1500–1999	9 (30%)
2000–2500	10 (33%)
> 2500	1 (3%)
PCMH Certification	
NCQA level 3	20 (67%)
JCAHO	1 (3%)
State Certification	3 (10%)
No PCMH Certification	6 (20%)

Data analysis

We used a modified Delphi process with all site visitors to identify advances in team configuration and roles observed during site visits [17]. We verified these advances and related themes with LEAP sites through an in-person convening of representatives from all sites. We used Atlas.ti to help organize and store the qualitative data from site visits and the in-person meeting of practice representatives. We developed codes to capture the key domains of interest, which were influenced by the findings from the Delphi process and the in-person meeting. We coded site visit interview transcripts, site visitor notes and summaries, field notes from shadowing staff and patients, staff survey comments, and notes from the in-person meeting. Coded segments were then reviewed and themes identified and confirmed.

Technical assistance

We summarized major themes and related findings from the study of LEAP practices in a web-based technical assistance program to help other primary care practices build and deploy effective teams. The website–"Primary Care Team Guide" (www.improvingprimarycare.org) –became publicly available in October 2014. Since its release, the Primary Care Team Guide has supported technical assistance for developing effective teams in three different learning collaboratives involving over 60 primary care practices and a national webinar series.

Results

Table 2 describes the major advances in team-based care identified by site visitors and confirmed by LEAP practice leaders and qualitative data analysis. It includes both major trends across sites and less common innovations with the potential to substantially change traditional practice.

Team structure

The primary care staff in LEAP sites is generally divided into: smaller core teams that work with specific providers and their panels; and an extended team that serves all providers and patients at the site. LEAP core teams are generally built around a single or small group, sometimes called a pod of stable Provider—Medical Assistant partnerships. Table 3 shows the composition of core teams, as defined by practice leaders at each site. Core teams in a large majority of LEAP sites include multiple provider/MA dyads, and often include registered nurses (RNs) and other staff. Licensed practical nurses (LPNs) on core teams are most commonly used in MA roles and included with MAs in Table 3. In one-third of practices, front desk staff works with specific core teams, are encouraged to develop personal relationships with patients, and help collect and collate patient information prior to visits. In 5 practices with high psychosocial morbidity, Behavioral Health Specialists are members of core teams.

The ratio of MAs to providers is 1:1 in most practices, but 6 LEAP practices link multiple MAs (1.5–3 MAs) with each provider. One LEAP practice assigns 2 MAs to each provider, which allows one MA to remain with each patient throughout their clinic visit. The MA enters

Table 2 Primary Care Staff Organization, Roles and Activities in LEAP Practices

Innovation Area	Major Trends	Promising Innovations
Primary care team structure	• Providers and their panels are supported by a core team built around strong provider-MA partnerships. • Multi-provider core teams often include, RNs, and front desk staff. • Core team members including PCPs share offices and work spaces. • Extended practice teams often include RN care managers, behavioral health specialists, and pharmacists.	• Each PCP works with 2 MAs, who remain with each patient throughout their visit—doing intake, scribing for the PCP, and handling post-visit questions and issues.
Enhanced role of medical assistants	• MAs review charts of scheduled patients and lead core team huddles to plan care. • MAs arrange or deliver most preventive care procedures. • MAs often involved in outreach to patients with care gaps or needing follow-up. • MAs are actively involved in Quality Improvement and play leadership roles.	• MAs with additional training in self-management support and diabetes care conduct individual and small group visits with diabetic patients.
Roles of Registered Nurses	• Core team RNs provide follow-up care, skills training, and self-management support to chronically ill patients in nurse encounters or conjoint visits. • Team RNs use nurse visits and standing orders to manage common acute illnesses. • RN care managers work with small panels of high risk patients.	• RNs use delegated order sets to titrate medications for patients with common chronic conditions—e.g., warfarin, anti-hypertensive drugs.
Layperson Patient Care Roles	• Laypersons help patients address needs for information, community resources, and coordination of their care.	• Laypersons trained in self-management counseling serve as health coaches. • Layperson EMR experts make changes to the EMR supportive of quality improvement.
Managing Complex Illness	• RN Care Managers work with small panels of sicker patients, including those discharged from hospital. • Behavioral Health Specialists, other social workers, and lay care coordinators/community health workers address psychosocial needs. • Pharmacists provide Medication Therapy Management services to multi-problem patients.	• Weekly or bi-weekly case conferences convene multi-disciplinary clinic staff to discuss challenging patients and develop a comprehensive care plan, and review progress of previously discussed patients.
Behavioral Health Integration	• Core team (MAs and RNs) involved in depression screening and follow-up. • On-site Behavioral Health Specialists facilitate warm handoffs and provide short-term therapy and crisis management. • Advice on psychotropic drugs is obtained from on-site or consulting Psychiatrists or Psychiatric NPs.	• Patients on chronic opioid therapy are tracked, asked to sign contracts, and offered in-clinic buprenorphine therapy if warranted.
Clinic-Community Connections	• Practices hire staff from populations served by the clinic. • Designated practice team members help patients identify and access community services. • Practice actively cultivates partnerships with community organizations to address social and environmental issues.	• The practice works with other agencies in the community to address social determinants of health.

the provider's description of the findings and plan into the EHR (often called scribing) [18], while the other MA is checking in the next patient. The innovation is being disseminated throughout the practice, as a pilot test demonstrated that PCPs were more satisfied AND could see more patients.

LEAP extended teams often include RN care managers, BHSs, and Pharmacists who support all core teams, either working with a subpanel of patients or by referral from the core team. Table 4 compares the availability of various staff roles in LEAP sites (on both core and extended teams) with 496 private practices (FQHCs

Table 3 Core Team Composition in LEAP Practices: Number and Percentage of Practices

	1 Primary Care Provider* n = 6	2-3 Primary Care Providers* n = 15	4+ Primary Care Providers* n = 9	All Practices n = 30
Medical Assistants**	6 (100%)	15 (100%)	9 (100%)	30 (100%)
Registered Nurses	1 (17%)	6 (40%)	7 (78%)	14 (47%)
Licensed Practical Nurses (LPNs)	0	4 (27%)	0	4 (13%)
Front Desk Staff	1 (17%)	8 (53%)	1 (11%)	10 (33%)
Behavioral Health	0	3 (20%)	2 (22%)	5 (17%)
Health Coach	1 (17%)	1 (7%)	2 (22%)	4 (13%)
Lay Care Coordinator	0	1 (7%)	1 (11%)	2 (7%)
Social Worker	0	0	1 (11%)	1 (3%)

*Number of Paneled Providers (MD, DO, ND, NP, PA) on each core team
**Includes LPNs if used as Medical Assistants

were excluded) selected for the Centers for Medicare and Medicaid Services Comprehensive Primary Care Initiative (CPC) [16]. We classified RNs in LEAP practices either as team RNs or care managers depending on their primary functions. RN care managers were more prevalent in LEAP practices than in CPC practices. Pharmacists and social workers were much more available in LEAP practices (37 and 63%, respectively) than in CPC practices (7 and 5%, respectively). Most social workers in LEAP practices are licensed therapists and function as BHSs. Table 4 also shows some differences in staffing between LEAP private practices and FQHCs of similar size with the latter less likely to employ RN care managers and more likely to employ BHSs.

The enhanced role of medical assistants

LEAP practices encourage MAs to develop personal relationships with patients and be more involved in patient care [2, 19]. Role expansion generally includes the previsit review of the charts of scheduled patients (chart-scrubbing) to identify needed preventive and chronic care services. These "care gaps" are discussed in presession huddles with their provider partner(s) and the visit planned. MAs deliver or arrange many preventive services by standing orders before the provider enters the examination room. Between visits, they make phone calls to check on recently seen patients. In some LEAP practices, MAs receive additional training in chronic disease management and self-management counseling and act as health coaches [20, 21]. In one practice, diabetes control improved when MAs trained in self-management support and diabetes care started meeting individually or in small groups with diabetic patients.

The changing roles of Registered Nurses (RN)

There was considerable variation among LEAP practices in RN roles. One-half of LEAP sites had designated RN care managers who work with sicker, more complex patients outside of clinic visits (See Complex Care Management below). RN role variability was predominantly seen among those working on or with core teams in the care of patients visiting the clinic. While team RNs in some LEAP sites are mostly responding to patient phone calls, doing procedures, and teaching patients, RNs in a number of LEAP practices are providing direct patient care via independent nurse visits, conjoint visits with a provider, or electronic communications. These nurses play major roles in the routine management of patients with chronic illness including teaching and follow-up [22]. RNs in 13 practices use delegated order sets to

Table 4 Percentage of CPC and LEAP Practices with Different Types of Staff

	<5 Primary Care Providers*		5+ Primary Care Providers*		
	CPC N = 364	LEAP Private Practices N = 3	CPC N = 132	LEAP Private practices N = 12	LEAP FQHCs N = 15
Administrative staff	98	100	100	100	100
Medical assistants	86	100	95	100	100
Team Registered Nurses	29	33	54	50	53
Registered Nurse Care managers	20	33	36	75	33
Pharmacists	4	0	17	42	40
Social Workers	2	33	13	58	73
Nutritionists	3	50	8	20	14

*Number of providers in the practice site

manage patients on warfarin, and in a few practices RNs titrate anti-hypertensive and hypoglycemic medications. Some practices also use independent nurse visits and standing orders to provide care for a variety of common acute illnesses.

The growing involvement of lay roles in patient care

One-half of LEAP practices employ staff without formal health training or certification (lay roles) in patient-facing roles such as health coach, care navigator/coordinator, or community health worker. In 20% of LEAP practices, lay staff are important members of core teams. These layperson roles tend to fall into two categories: health coaching or self-management support [20, 21, 23, 24] and/or assisting in patient follow-up or care coordination [25, 26]. Other lay roles help patients obtain specialist consultations or community resources.

One-half of LEAP practices employed health coaches. While the majority of health coaches were MAs or nurses, some were laypersons trained in self-management counseling. A couple of LEAP sites have hired computer-savvy laypersons who receive intensive training in the functionality and adaptability of the practice's EMR. Their primary role is to work closely with quality improvement teams and care teams to ensure that the EMR reflects and supports new care processes.

Closing the loop

During site visits, we frequently heard staff talk about "closing the loop" on gaps or failures in care—e.g., poorly controlled chronically ill patients without appointments, or preventive services that are overdue. To close these loops, LEAP practices have exploited or developed data systems that enable them to track critical patient information. In most LEAP sites, multiple members of the practice team routinely review data on different patient populations and reach out to those needing further care. For example, patients recently hospitalized are tracked by RN care managers while MAs or panel managers look for patients overdue for preventive care or chronic disease follow-up.

A few LEAP practices have created a referral manager/coordinator position to help patients access specialty and other community services, and ensure that all parties receive the information they need [27].

Managing complex illness

Essentially all LEAP practices have made the care of patients with multiple health problems including recent hospital discharges a priority, and altered the composition and functioning of their practice teams accordingly. One-half of practices have RN care managers. These nurse care managers sometimes collaborate with other staff knowledgeable about community resources to better address the psycho-social needs of patients. 40% of LEAP practice teams have pharmacists, most of whom work with patients on complex drug regimens.

A few practices regularly review complex patients in multi-disciplinary case conferences. In one FQHC, the entire clinic staff meets weekly to discuss how they might better care for 1 or 2 of their most challenging patients.

Behavioral health integration

Nineteen LEAP practices (63%) employ one or more BHSs who consult with the team about mental health, substance abuse, and other behavioral health issues, and provide short-term crisis management and therapy. Most commonly in LEAP practices, the BHS is a Licensed Clinical Social Worker. A few practices have added psychiatrists or psychiatric nurse practitioners to consult on psychoactive drugs. Multiple team members participate in providing mental health care– e.g., MAs perform depression screening before the provider enters the room, and RNs or BHSs make follow-up phone calls to depressed patients started on treatment.

Most LEAP practices are addressing the opioid epidemic in various ways. Patient contracts, urine drug testing, and medication monitoring to control drug-seeking behavior are common. A handful of practices with interested providers have successfully instituted buprenorphine treatment programs.

Clinic-community connections

A long-term relationship with and commitment to their community draws many health professionals and staff to primary care. Among LEAP practices, this community focus manifests in different ways. Many try to hire staff representative of their patient populations to help them communicate with their patients and understand the cultural and environmental issues that may be influencing their health and treatment. Some, including a few private practices, provide or collaborate with other agencies to provide programs that reach beyond their patients to support the health of the broader community such as healthy eating and active living activities, community gardens, etc. For example, a LEAP site in a low-income rural community was the driving force behind the community's efforts to reduce childhood obesity.

Discussion

The Affordable Care Act makes clear that American primary care must be strengthened and improved through transformation of existing practice organizations to PCMHs [28]. By most definitions of a PCMH, practices are expected to provide comprehensive, high quality care in the office, use data to identify and eliminate gaps in care, track and support patients between office visits, and address comprehensive patient needs including behavioral health issues [1, 2, 29]. The innovative, high performing LEAP practices have expanded the roles of existing staff and added new personnel to provide the person power and skills needed to achieve the quadruple aim and perform the tasks and functions expected of a PCMH [1, 2, 30–32].

Recent policy-maker enthusiasm for strengthening the primary care sector stems in part from the expectation that high cost patients, generally those with multiple chronic conditions, can be effectively managed in the community. In response, many LEAP practices either employ or have access to RN care managers, BHSs, and Pharmacists to augment services to high risk patients. While LEAP practice teams include a somewhat broader array of disciplines than teams in more traditional practices, the expanded roles of traditional staff such as MAs or RNs and their involvement in care delivery probably has the largest impact on care quality. To sustain role expansion, staff are being continuously trained, mentored, and assessed. Workflows are documented and incorporated into staff training. Several LEAP practices have modified their EMR to support new and improved workflows. In addition, widespread use of protocols and standing orders increases efficiency by allowing staff to work independently.

In addition to the general trends in staffing described above, we saw promising advances in staffing and care delivery with the potential to fundamentally change primary care practice [33]. For example, with additional training and support: MAs or laypersons can take on much of the responsibility for documenting encounters or providing self-management support; RNs can titrate medications for common illnesses; and laypersons can substantially improve care coordination or the utility of the EMR.

Practice leaders reported that the largest barrier to the development of effective practice teams was dependence of the practice on fee-for-service reimbursement because of the premium placed on provider involvement in care. Bundled or capitated payments facilitate shifting clinical tasks from providers to other staff. While LEAP practice leaders generally feel that they are aligning their organizations with future payment reforms, most are currently relying on grant funds or negotiated arrangements with local health insurers to support workforce innovation.

The major limitations of LEAP and this paper are the reliance on cross-sectional data collected from a limited number of highly selected practices 3–4 years ago. Site selection involved a rigorous process that looked for practices that demonstrated workforce innovation, quality improvement infrastructure, and quality of care. Although we reviewed clinical performance data collected by each practice, the variability in the content and quality of measurement from site to site limited our confidence in attesting to the quality of care provided. However, direct observations of care delivery in the 30 practices confirmed that these were high performing practices. In selecting practices for LEAP, we sought diversity in geography, business models, and patient populations served. While the practice diversity potentially made data interpretation more difficult, the trends in the configuration and deployment of practice teams described above were shared across the range of practices and bridged key distinctions such as between FQHC's and private practices. We have engaged leaders from LEAP sites in our technical assistance activities over the years since the site visits, which gives us some assurance that the observations presented above reflect current practice. Our recent involvement in practice transformation efforts focused on building more effective primary care teams suggests that the advances in team-based care described above are not widespread.

Primary care teams are complex adaptive systems [34], consisting of interdependent and constantly changing parts. As a consequence, it will be very difficult to empirically test each of the many moving parts. Nonetheless, we urgently need comparative trials to help clarify the optimal structure and functioning of cost-effective teams capable of providing the comprehensive, high quality services expected of PCMHs. In the absence of data from rigorous trials, innovative, high quality practices are perhaps the best source of information and ideas on which to base efforts to transform primary care practices.

Conclusion

To build more effective practice teams, the 30 LEAP practices have expanded the roles of existing staff and added new staff and new competencies. In particular, MAs play important patient care roles such as delivering preventive care or health coaching, and RNs are more involved in face-to-face care delivery. Most practices have developed in-house training activities since external training programs for key roles such as MAs or RNs generally aren't preparing trainees for these expanded roles. Key new competencies include behavioral health, RN care management, and pharmacy. These richer, more effective teams enable practices to achieve high levels of performance and helps free up providers to focus on tasks that only they can perform.

Additional files

Additional file 1: LEAP Interview Guide – Clinic Staff. Guide for conducting recorded interviews with various staff members in each visited clinic.

Additional file 2: LEAP Interview Guide – Leadership. Guide for conducting recorded group interviews with administrative and clinical leaders in each visited clinic

Additional file 3: PCT LEAP Site Visit Observation Guide – Clinical Expert. The guide includes instructions as to what clinical site visitors should observe and document during site visits

Abbreviations
BHS: Behavioral health specialist; CPC: Comprehensive primary care initiative; EMR: Electronic medical record; FQHC: Federally qualified health center; LPN: Licensed practical nurse; MA: Medical assistant; NAC: National Advisory Committee; NCQA: National Committee on quality assurance; PCMH: Patient-centered Medical Home; PCP: Primary care provider; PCT-LEAP: Primary care team-learning from effective ambulatory practices; RN: Registered nurse

Acknowledgements
We would like to thank Sylvia Hoffmeyer, Sarah McDonald, Leah Tuzzio, Nitzali Rivera, Elaine Skoch and Drs. Tom Bodenheimer, Lisa Letourneau, Michael Parchman, James Ralston, and Carolyn Shepherd for their involvement in the site visits and development of major themes. This work gracious hospitality, and candor of the leaders and staff of the 30 LEAP would not have been possible without the generous commitment of time, practices. The names and information about the LEAP sites can be accessed at http://www.improvingprimarycare.org/start/about-sites.

Funding
Study design, data collection, analysis and manuscript preparation were supported by a grant from the Robert Wood Johnson Foundation.

Authors' contributions
EW participated in securing funding, study design, data collection, data analysis and drafting the manuscript. MF participated in securing funding, study design, data collection, and manuscript review. CH participated in study design, data collection and analysis, and manuscript preparation. DC participated in study design, data collection and analysis, and manuscript preparation. BA participated in securing funding, study design, data collection, and manuscript review. RE participated in study design, recruiting practices, data analysis, and manuscript review. BC participated in study design, recruiting practices, data analysis, and manuscript review. ML participated in study design, recruiting practices, data collection, and manuscript review. All authors have read and approved the final version of the manuscript.

Competing interests
The authors declare that they have no competing interests.

Consent for publication
Not applicable.

Author details
[1]MacColl Center for Health Care Innovation, Group Health Research Institute, 1730 Minor Ave., Suite 1600, Seattle, WA 98101, USA. [2]Community Health Center, Inc., Middletown, CT, USA. [3]Center for Community Health and Evaluation, Group Health Research Institute, Seattle, WA, USA. [4]Department of Family Medicine, Virginia Commonwealth University, Richmond, VA, USA. [5]Department of Family Medicine and Community Health, Rutgers-Robert Wood Johnson Medical School, Piscataway Township, NJ, USA. [6]Robert Wood Johnson Foundation, Princeton, NJ, USA.

References
1. Wagner EH, Coleman K, Reid RJ, Phillips K, Abrams MK, Sugarman JR. The changes involved in patient-centered medical home transformation. Prim Care. 2012;39(2):241_59.
2. Bodenheimer T, Ghorob A, Willard-Grace R, Grumbach K. The 10 building blocks of high-performing primary care. Ann Fam Med. 2014;12(2):166–71.
3. Shojania KG, Ranji SR, McDonald KM, Grimshaw JM, Sundaram V, Rushakoff RJ, Owens DK. Effects of quality improvement strategies for type 2 diabetes on glycemic control: a meta-regression analysis. JAMA. 2006;296(4):427–40.
4. Walsh JM, McDonald KM, Shojania KG, Sundaram V, Nayak S, Lewis R, Owens DK, Goldstein MK. Quality improvement strategies for hypertension management: a systematic review. Med Care. 2006;44(7):646–57.
5. Thota AB, Sipe TA, Byard GJ, Zometa CS, Hahn RA, McKnight-Eily LR, Chapman DP, Abraido-Lanza AF, Pearson JL, Anderson CW, et al. Collaborative care to improve the management of depressive disorders: a community guide systematic review and meta-analysis. Am J Prev Med. 2012;42(5):525–38.
6. Proia KK, Thota AB, Njie GJ, Finnie RK, Hopkins DP, Mukhtar Q, Pronk NP, Zeigler D, Kottke TE, Rask KJ, et al. Team-based care and improved blood pressure control: a community guide systematic review. Am J Prev Med. 2014;47(1):86–99.
7. Tricco AC, Ivers NM, Grimshaw JM, Moher D, Turner L, Galipeau J, Halperin I, Vachon B, Ramsay T, Manns B, et al. Effectiveness of quality improvement strategies on the management of diabetes: a systematic review and meta-analysis. Lancet. 2012;379(9833):2252–61.
8. Wagner EH, Gupta R, Coleman K. Practice transformation in the safety net medical home initiative: a qualitative look. Med Care. 2014;52(11 Suppl 4): S18–22.
9. Friedberg MW, Rosenthal MB, Werner RM, Volpp KG, Schneider EC. Effects of a Medical Home and Shared Savings Intervention on Quality and Utilization of Care. JAMA Intern Med. 2015;175(8):1362–8.
10. Gilfillan RJ, Tomcavage J, Rosenthal MB, Davis DE, Graham J, Roy JA, Pierdon SB, Bloom Jr FJ, Graf TR, Goldman R, et al. Value and the medical home: effects of transformed primary care. Am J Manag Care. 2010;16(8):607–14.
11. Day J, Scammon DL, Kim J, Sheets-Mervis A, Day R, Tomoaia-Cotisel A, Waitzman NJ, Magill MK. Quality, satisfaction, and financial efficiency associated with elements of primary care practice transformation: preliminary findings. Ann Fam Med. 2013;11 Suppl 1:S50–59.
12. Willard-Grace R, Hessler D, Rogers E, Dube K, Bodenheimer T, Grumbach K. Team structure and culture are associated with lower burnout in primary care. J Am Board Fam Med. 2014;27(2):229–38.
13. Helfrich CD, Dolan ED, Simonetti J, Reid RJ, Joos S, Wakefield BJ, Schectman G, Stark R, Fihn SD, Harvey HB, et al. Elements of team-based care in a patient-centered medical home are associated with lower burnout among VA primary care employees. J Gen Intern Med. 2014;29 Suppl 2:S659–666.
14. Ladden MD, Bodenheimer T, Fishman NW, Flinter M, Hsu C, Parchman M, Wagner EH. The Emerging Primary Care Workforce: Preliminary Observations From the Primary Care Team: Learning From Effective Ambulatory Practices Project. Acad Med. 2013;88(12):1830–4.
15. Friedman A, Hahn KA, Etz R, Rehwinkel-Morfe AM, Miller WL, Nutting PA, Jaen CR, Shaw EK, Crabtree BF. A typology of primary care workforce innovations in the United States since 2000. Med Care. 2014;52(2):101–11.
16. Peikes DN, Reid RJ, Day TJ, Cornwell DD, Dale SB, Baron RJ, Brown RS, Shapiro RJ. Staffing patterns of primary care practices in the comprehensive primary care initiative. Ann Fam Med. 2014;12(2):142–9.
17. Jones J, Hunter D. Consensus methods for medical and health services research. BMJ. 1995;311:376–80.
18. Sinsky CA, Willard-Grace R, Schutzbank AM, Sinsky TA, Margolius D, Bodenheimer T. In search of joy in practice: a report of 23 high-functioning primary care practices. Ann Fam Med. 2013;11(3):272–8.
19. Naughton D, Adelman AM, Bricker P, Miller-Day M, Gabbay R. Envisioning new roles for medical assistants: strategies from patient-centered medical homes. Fam Pract Manag. 2013;20(2):7–12.
20. Bodenheimer T. A 63-year-old man with multiple cardiovascular risk factors and poor adherence to treatment plans. JAMA. 2007;298(17):2048–55.
21. Willard-Grace R, Chen EH, Hessler D, DeVore D, Prado C, Bodenheimer T, Thom DH. Health coaching by medical assistants to improve control of diabetes, hypertension, and hyperlipidemia in low-income patients: a randomized controlled trial. Ann Fam Med. 2015;13(2):130–8.
22. Bodenheimer T, Bauer L. Rethinking the primary care workforce - an expanded role for nurses. N Engl J Med. 2016;375(11):1015–7.
23. Margolius D, Bodenheimer T, Bennett H, Wong J, Ngo V, Padilla G, Thom DH. Health coaching to improve hypertension treatment in a Low-income, minority population. Ann Fam Med. 2012;10(3):199–205.
24. Thom DH, Ghorob A, Hessler D, De Vore D, Chen E, Bodenheimer TA. Impact of peer health coaching on glycemic control in low-income patients with diabetes: a randomized controlled trial. Ann Fam Med. 2013;11(2):137–44.

25. Adair R, Wholey DR, Christianson J, White KM, Britt H, Lee S. Improving chronic disease care by adding laypersons to the primary care team: a parallel randomized trial. Ann Intern Med. 2013;159(3):176–84.
26. Garson Jr A, Green DM, Rodriguez L, Beech R, Nye C. A new corps of trained Grand-Aides has the potential to extend reach of primary care workforce and save money. Health Aff (Millwood). 2012;31(5):1016–21.
27. Wagner EH, Sandhu N, Coleman K, Phillips KE, Sugarman JR. Improving care coordination in primary care. Med Care. 2014;52(11 Suppl 4):S33–38.
28. Abrams M, Nuzum R, Mika S, Lawlor G. Realizing health reform's potential: how the Affordable Care Act will strengthen primary care and benefit patients, providers, and payers. Issue Brief (Commonw Fund). 2011;1:1–28.
29. Stange KC, Nutting PA, Miller WL, Jaen CR, Crabtree BF, Flocke SA, Gill JM. Defining and measuring the patient-centered medical home. J Gen Intern Med. 2010;25(6):601–12.
30. Parchman M, Kaissi AA. Are elements of the chronic care model associated with cardiovascular risk factor control in type 2 diabetes? Jt Comm J Qual Patient Saf. 2009;35(3):133–8.
31. Stellefson M, Dipnarine K, Stopka C. The chronic care model and diabetes management in US primary care settings: a systematic review. Prev Chronic Dis. 2013;10:E26.
32. Friedberg MW, Schneider EC, Rosenthal MB, Volpp KG, Werner RM. Association between participation in a multipayer medical home intervention and changes in quality, utilization, and costs of care. JAMA. 2014;311(8):815–25.
33. Christensen CM. Disruptive innovation: can health care learn from other industries? A conversation with Clayton M. Christensen. Interview by Mark D. Smith. Health Aff (Millwood). 2007;26(3):w288–295.
34. Plsek PE, Greenhalgh T. Complexity science: the challenge of complexity in health care. BMJ. 2001;323(7313):625–8.

Permissions

All chapters in this book were first published in FP, by BioMed Central; hereby published with permission under the Creative Commons Attribution License or equivalent. Every chapter published in this book has been scrutinized by our experts. Their significance has been extensively debated. The topics covered herein carry significant findings which will fuel the growth of the discipline. They may even be implemented as practical applications or may be referred to as a beginning point for another development.

The contributors of this book come from diverse backgrounds, making this book a truly international effort. This book will bring forth new frontiers with its revolutionizing research information and detailed analysis of the nascent developments around the world.

We would like to thank all the contributing authors for lending their expertise to make the book truly unique. They have played a crucial role in the development of this book. Without their invaluable contributions this book wouldn't have been possible. They have made vital efforts to compile up to date information on the varied aspects of this subject to make this book a valuable addition to the collection of many professionals and students.

This book was conceptualized with the vision of imparting up-to-date information and advanced data in this field. To ensure the same, a matchless editorial board was set up. Every individual on the board went through rigorous rounds of assessment to prove their worth. After which they invested a large part of their time researching and compiling the most relevant data for our readers.

The editorial board has been involved in producing this book since its inception. They have spent rigorous hours researching and exploring the diverse topics which have resulted in the successful publishing of this book. They have passed on their knowledge of decades through this book. To expedite this challenging task, the publisher supported the team at every step. A small team of assistant editors was also appointed to further simplify the editing procedure and attain best results for the readers.

Apart from the editorial board, the designing team has also invested a significant amount of their time in understanding the subject and creating the most relevant covers. They scrutinized every image to scout for the most suitable representation of the subject and create an appropriate cover for the book.

The publishing team has been an ardent support to the editorial, designing and production team. Their endless efforts to recruit the best for this project, has resulted in the accomplishment of this book. They are a veteran in the field of academics and their pool of knowledge is as vast as their experience in printing. Their expertise and guidance has proved useful at every step. Their uncompromising quality standards have made this book an exceptional effort. Their encouragement from time to time has been an inspiration for everyone.

The publisher and the editorial board hope that this book will prove to be a valuable piece of knowledge for researchers, students, practitioners and scholars across the globe.

List of Contributors

Reimar W. Thomsen and Mette Søgaard
Department of Clinical Epidemiology, Aarhus University, Olof Palmes Alle 43-45, 8200 Aarhus N, Denmark

Steffen Haldrup
Department of Clinical Epidemiology, Aarhus University, Olof Palmes Alle 43-45, 8200 Aarhus N, Denmark
Department of General Practice, Institute of Public Health, Aarhus University, Aarhus, Denmark

Flemming Bro
Department of General Practice, Institute of Public Health, Aarhus University, Aarhus, Denmark

Robert Skov
Antimicrobial Resistance Reference Laboratory and Surveillance Unit, Department of Microbiology and Infection Control, Statens Serum Institut, Copenhagen, Denmark

Lars Bjerrum
Section and Research Unit of General Practice, Department of Public Health, Copenhagen University, Copenhagen, Denmark

Rahul Alam, Sudeh Cheraghi-Sohi, Maria Panagioti and Aneez Esmail
NIHR Greater Manchester Primary Care Patient Safety Translational Research Centre (Greater Manchester PSTRC), The University of Manchester, Williamson Building, Oxford Road, Manchester M13 9PL, UK

Stephen Campbell
NIHR Greater Manchester Primary Care Patient Safety Translational Research Centre (Greater Manchester PSTRC), The University of Manchester, Williamson Building, Oxford Road, Manchester M13 9PL, UK
Centre for Research and Action in Public Health, University of Canberra, ACT 2601, Australia

Efharis Panagopoulou
Medical School, Department Social Medicine, Aristotle University, Thessaloniki, Greece

Makoto Kaneko
Musashikoganei Clinic, Japanese Health and Welfare Co-operative Federation, 1-15-9, Honcho, Koganei-shi, Tokyo 184-0004, Japan
Division of Clinical Epidemiology, Jikei University School of Medicine, 3-25-8, Nishishimbashi, Minato-ku, Tokyo 105-8461, Japan

Masato Matsushima
Division of Clinical Epidemiology, Jikei University School of Medicine, 3-25-8, Nishishimbashi, Minato-ku, Tokyo 105-8461, Japan

Ryuichi Ohta
Unnan City Hospital, Faculty of Community Care, 96-1, Iida, Daito-cho, Unnan city, Shimane 699-1221, Japan

Naoki Nago and Motoharu Fukushi
Musashi Kokubunji Park clinic, 2-16-34-127, Nishimoto-machi, Kokubunji-shi, Tokyo 185-0023, Japan

Allison J. Ober, Katherine E. Watkins, Sarah B. Hunter, Brett Ewing, Kirsten Becker Karen C. Osilla and Claude M. Setodji
RAND Corporation, 1776 Main Street, Santa Monica, CA 90407, USA

Allison L. Diamant
RAND Corporation, 1776 Main Street, Santa Monica, CA 90407, USA
UCLA Department of Internal Medicine, Division of General Internal Medicine, 911 Broxton Avenue, Los Angeles, CA 90024, USA

Karen Lamp and Mimi Lind
Venice Family Clinic, 2509 Pico Boulevard, Santa Monica, CA 90405, USA

Keith Heinzerling
UCLA Department of Family Medicine, UCLA Family Health Center, 1920 Colorado Avenue, Santa Monica, CA 90404, USA

Agneta Pettersson
Medical Management Centre, Department of Learning, Informatics, Management and Ethics, Karolinska Institutet, Tomtebodavägen 18 A, SE-171 77 Stockholm, Sweden
Swedish Agency for Health Technology Assessment and Social Assessment, SE-102 33 Stockholm, Sweden

Sonja Modin
Division of Family Medicine, Department of Neurobiology, Care Sciences and Society, Karolinska Institutet, Alfred Nobels allé 23 D2, SE-141 83 Huddinge, Sweden

Rolf Wahlström
Department of Public Health Sciences, Karolinska Institutet, Tomtebodavägen 18 A, SE-171 77 Stockholm, Sweden

Sandra af Winklerfelt Hammarberg
Department for Neurobiology, Care Sciences and Society, Karolinska Institutet, Alfred Nobels allé 23 D2, SE 141 83 Huddinge, Sweden

Ingvar Krakau
Department of Medicine, Clinical Epidemiology Unit T2, 14, Karolinska Institutet, SE-171 77 Stockholm, Sweden

Jolien Janssen, Paula S. Koekkoek and Guy E. H. M. Rutten
Julius Centre for Health Sciences and Primary Care, University Medical Centre Utrecht, Utrecht, The Netherlands

L. Jaap Kappelle and Geert Jan Biessels
Department of Neurology, Brain Centre Rudolf Magnus, University Medical Centre Utrecht, Utrecht, The Netherlands

Eric P. Moll van Charante
Department of General Practice, Academic Medical Centre, Amsterdam, The Netherlands

Mette Tranberg
Department of Public Health Programmes, Randers Regional Hospital, Østervangsvej 68, 8930 Randers NØ, Denmark

Peter Vedsted, Morten Bondo Christensen and Grete Moth
Research Unit for General Practice, Department of Public Health, Aarhus University, Bartholins Allé 2, 8000 Aarhus C, Denmark

Bodil Hammer Bech
Section for Epidemiology, Department of Public Health, Aarhus University, Bartholins Allé 2, 8000 Aarhus C, Denmark

Søren Birkeland
Department of Psychology, Faculty of Health Sciences, University of Southern Denmark, Campusvej 55, 5230 Odense M, Denmark

Kathy Ellis, Henrietta Mulnier and Angus Forbes
Florence Nightingale Faculty of Nursing, Midwifery and Palliative Care, King's College London, 57 Waterloo Road, London SE1 8WA, UK

Stephanie Brooks Holliday, Layla Parast, Elizabeth J. D'Amico and Brett A. Ewing
RAND Corporation, 1776 Main Street, Santa Monica, CA 90407-2138, USA

Lisa S. Meredith
RAND Corporation, 1776 Main Street, Santa Monica, CA 90407-2138, USA
VA HSR&D Center for the Study of Healthcare Innovation, Implementation and Policy, California, Los Angeles, USA

Bradley D. Stein and William G. Shadel
RAND Corporation, Pittsburgh, PA, USA

Evi Matthys, Roy Remmen and Peter Van Bogaert
University of Antwerp, Campus Drie Eiken DR334, Universiteitsplein 1, 2610 Wilrijk, Belgium

Elizabeth H. Evans, Kirby Sainsbury, Alex Bolster, Vera Araujo-Soares and Falko F. Sniehotta
Institute of Health & Society, Newcastle University, Newcastle upon Tyne NE2 4AX, UK

Dominika Kwasnicka
School of Psychology and Speech Pathology, Curtin University, GPO Perth, WA 6845, Australia

Mairead Murphy, Sandra Hollinghurst and Chris Salisbury
Population Health Sciences, Bristol Medical School, University of Bristol, Canynge Hall, 39 Whatley Road, Bristol BS8 2PS, UK

Tessa C. C. Quanjel and Dirk Ruwaard
Department of Health Services Research, Care and Public Health Research Institute, Faculty of Health Medicine and Life Sciences, Maastricht University, Maastricht, The Netherlands

Jeroen N. Struijs
Department for Quality of Care and Health Economics, Centre for Nutrition, Prevention and Health Services, National Institute for Public Health and the Environment, Bilthoven, The Netherlands

Marieke D. Spreeuwenberg
Research Centre for Technology in Care, Zuyd University of Applied Sciences, Heerlen, The Netherlands

Caroline A. Baan
Scientific Centre for Transformation in Care and Welfare (Tranzo), University of Tilburg, Tilburg, The Netherlands

Carolina S. Monsalve-Reyes
Departamento de Ciencias Sociales, Universidad Católica de La Santísima Concepción, Concepción, Chile
Doctorado en Psicología de la Salud, Facultad de Psicología, Universidad Nacional de Educación a Distancia (UNED), Madrid, Spain

Concepción San Luis-Costas
Spanish University of Distance Education, Madrid, Spain

Jose L. Gómez-Urquiza
Nursing Department, University of Granada, Granada, Spain
Faculty of Health Sciences, University of Granada, Cortadura del Valle Street S/N, 51001 Ceuta, Spain

Luis Albendín-García
Andalusian Health Service and University of Granada, Granada, Spain

Raimundo Aguayo
Psychology Department, University of Granada, Granada, Spain

Guillermo A. Cañadas-De la Fuente
Nursing Department, University of Granada, Granada, Spain

Ranita Hisham, Chirk Jenn Ng, Su May Liew, Pauline Siew Mei Lai, Ee Ming Khoo, Nik Sherina Hanafi and Sajaratulnisah Othman
Department of Primary Care Medicine, Faculty of Medicine, University of Malaya, Kuala Lumpur, Malaysia

Yook Chin Chia
Department of Primary Care Medicine, Faculty of Medicine, University of Malaya, Kuala Lumpur, Malaysia
Department of Medical Sciences School of Healthcare and Medical Sciences Sunway University, Selangor, Malaysia

Ping Yein Lee
Department of Family Medicine, Faculty of Medicine and Health Sciences, Universiti Putra Malaysia, UPM Serdang, Selangor, Malaysia

Khatijah Lim Abdullah
Department of Nursing Sciences, Faculty of Medicine, University of Malaya, Kuala Lumpur, Malaysia

Karuthan Chinna
Department of Social and Preventive Medicine, Julius Centre University of Malaya, University of Malaya, Kuala Lumpur, Malaysia

Jacobi Elliott, Paul Stolee, Lora Giangregorio and George Heckman
University of Waterloo, 200 University Avenue West, Waterloo, ON N2L 3G1, Canada

Veronique Boscart
Conestoga College, 299 Doon Valley Dr, Kitchener, ON N2G 4M4, Canada

Rune Aakvik Pedersen, Halfdan Petursson and Irene Hetlevik
General Practice Research Unit, Department of Public Health and Nursing, NTNU, Norwegian University of Science and Technology, N-7491 Trondheim, Norway

Stefan Markun, Vera Aemissegger and Thomas Rosemann
Institute of Primary Care, University Hospital of Zurich, University of Zurich, Pestalozzistrasse 24, 8091 Zurich, Switzerland

Nathalie Scherz
Institute of Primary Care, University Hospital of Zurich, University of Zurich, Pestalozzistrasse 24, 8091 Zurich, Switzerland
Arud Centres for Addiction Medicine, Zurich, Switzerland

Ryan Tandjung
Institute of Primary Care, University Hospital of Zurich, University of Zurich, Pestalozzistrasse 24, 8091 Zurich, Switzerland
Federal Office of Public Health, Bern, Switzerland

Karen Busk Nørøxe, Linda Huibers, Grete Moth and Peter Vedsted
Department of Public Health, Research Unit for General Practice, Aarhus University, Bartholins Alle 2, 8000 Aarhus C, Denmark

Jacqueline Torti
Department of Family Medicine, University of Alberta, Clinical Research Unit, Edmonton, AB, CanadaT6G 2E1
School of Public Health, University of Alberta, Edmonton, AB, CanadaT6G 2E3

Thea Luig
Department of Family Medicine, University of Alberta, Clinical Research Unit, Edmonton, AB, CanadaT6G 2E1
Department of Medicine, Division of Endocrinology, University of Alberta, Edmonton, AB, CanadaT6G 2E1

Jeffrey A. Johnson
School of Public Health, University of Alberta, Edmonton, AB, CanadaT6G 2E3

Arya M. Sharma
Department of Medicine, Division of Endocrinology, University of Alberta, Edmonton, AB, CanadaT6G 2E1

Michelle Borowitz
Department of Anthropology, University of Alberta, Edmonton, AB, CanadaT6G 2H4

Denise L. Campbell-Scherer
Department of Family Medicine, University of Alberta, Clinical Research Unit, Edmonton, AB, CanadaT6G 2E1
Department of Medicine, Obesity Research & Management, University of Alberta, Li Ka Shing Building, Rm. 1-116, 87th Avenue and 112th Street, Edmonton, AB T6G 2E1, Canada

Edward H. Wagner and Brian T. Austin
MacColl Center for Health Care Innovation, Group Health Research Institute, 1730 Minor Ave., Suite 1600, Seattle, WA 98101, USA

Margaret Flinter
Community Health Center, Inc., Middletown, CT, USA

Clarissa Hsu and DeAnn Cromp
Center for Community Health and Evaluation, Group Health Research Institute, Seattle, WA, USA

Rebecca Etz
Department of Family Medicine, Virginia Commonwealth University, Richmond, VA, USA

Benjamin F. Crabtree
Department of Family Medicine and Community Health, Rutgers-Robert Wood Johnson Medical School, Piscataway Township, NJ, USA

MaryJoan D. Ladden
Robert Wood Johnson Foundation, Princeton, NJ, USA

Index

www.ingramcontent.com/pod-product-compliance
Lightning Source LLC
LaVergne TN
LVHW080720210926
848485LV00003B/495